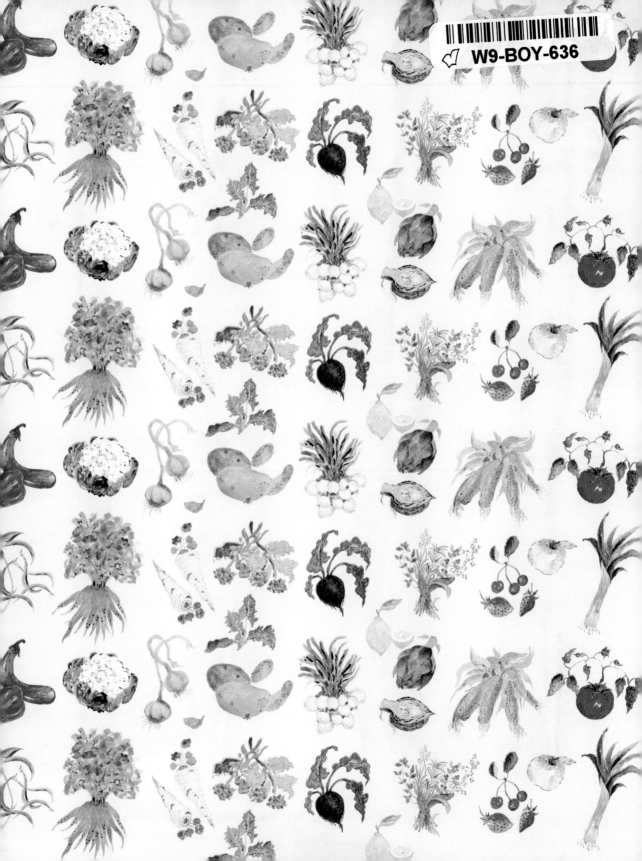

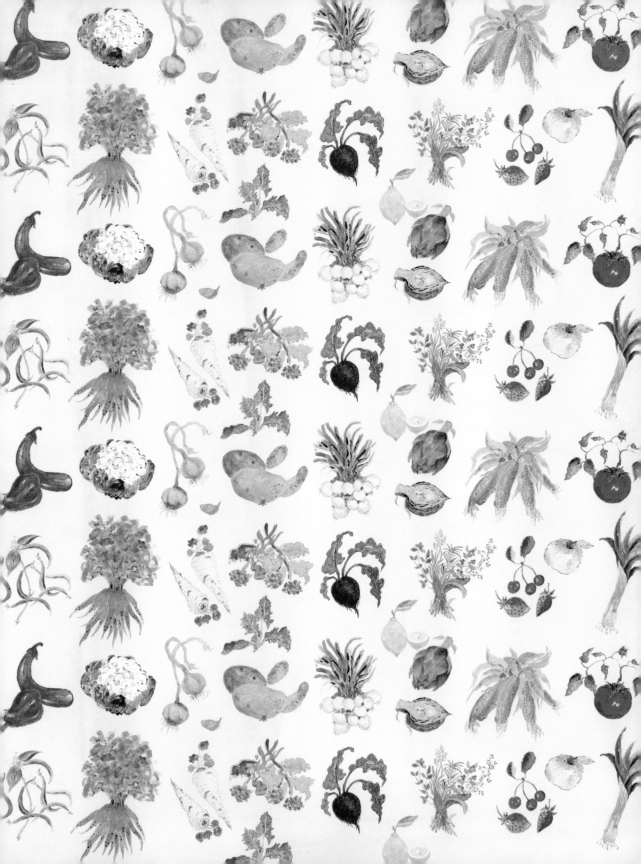

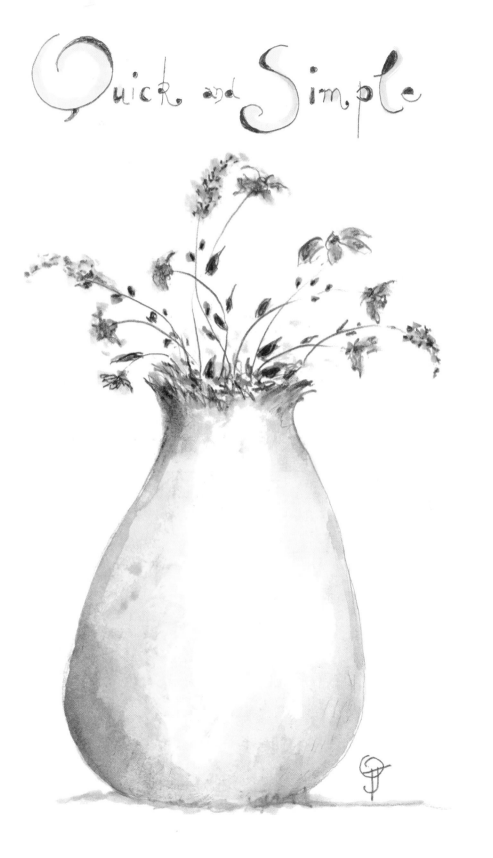

Quick and Simple

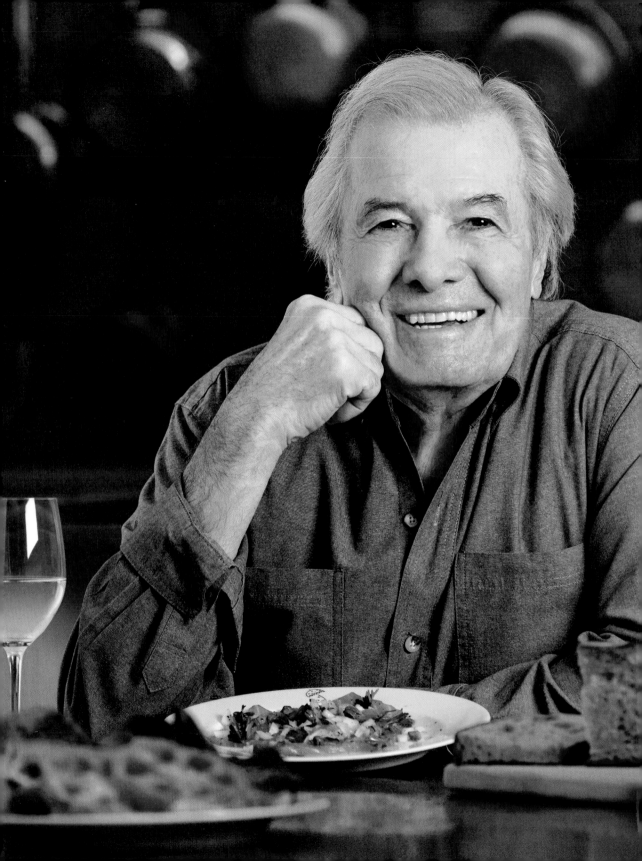

JACQUES PEPIN

Quick + Simple

SIMPLY WONDERFUL MEALS
with SURPRISINGLY LITTLE EFFORT

ILLUSTRATIONS BY JACQUES PEPIN
PHOTOGRAPHS BY TOM HOPKINS

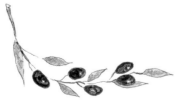

Houghton Mifflin Harcourt
Boston New York 2020

Library of Congress Cataloging-in-Publication Data
Names: Pépin, Jacques, author. | Hopkins, Tom, photographer.
Title: Jacques Pépin quick + simple : simply wonderful meals with
    surprisingly little effort / Jacques Pépin ; photographs by Tom
    Hopkins.
Other titles: Quick and simple : simply wonderful meals with surprisingly
    little effort
Description: Boston : Houghton Mifflin Harcourt, 2020. | Includes index. |
    Summary: "250 of master chef Jacques Pépin's classic and timeless
    recipes for unexpectedly polished and satisfying meals with minimal prep
    and cleanup"-- Provided by publisher.
Identifiers: LCCN 2020016359 (print) | LCCN 2020016360 (ebook) |
    ISBN 9780358352556 (hardback) | ISBN 9780358352563 (ebook)
Subjects: LCSH: Quick and easy cooking.
Classification: LCC TX833.5 .P465 2020 (print) | LCC TX833.5 (ebook) |
    DDC 641.5/12--dc23
LC record available at https://lccn.loc.gov/2020016359
LC ebook record available at https://lccn.loc.gov/2020016360

Book design by Toni Tajima

Printed in the United States of America

DOC 10 9 8 7 6 5 4 3 2

4500812225

To Claudine.

May these recipes make your life easier and your love for cooking even greater.

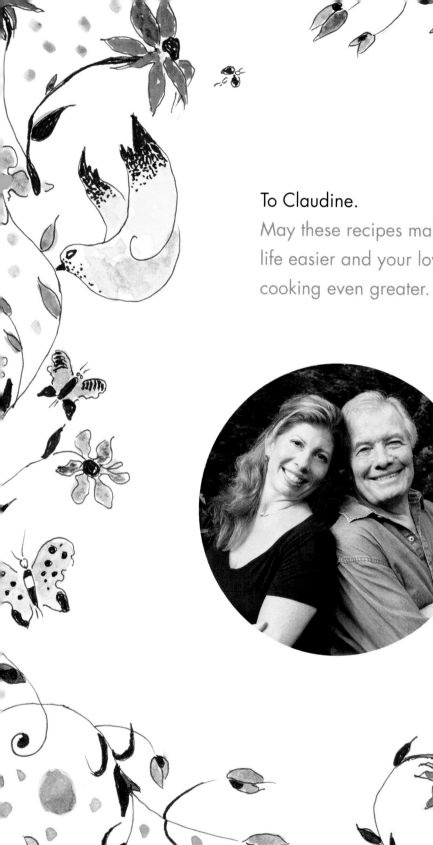

Acknowledgments

This book was not a solitary endeavor, and I have many people to thank for it: My wife, Gloria, the best in the world. My daughter, Claudine, and son-in-law, Rollie. And, among my many friends, Tom, Christine, Jared, Charlie, Priscilla, Reza, and Paula, who dutifully and happily consume my creations.

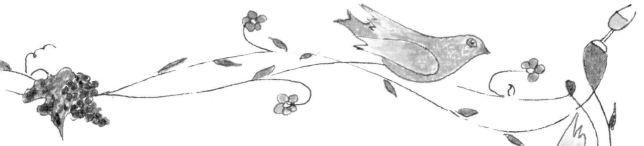

Contents

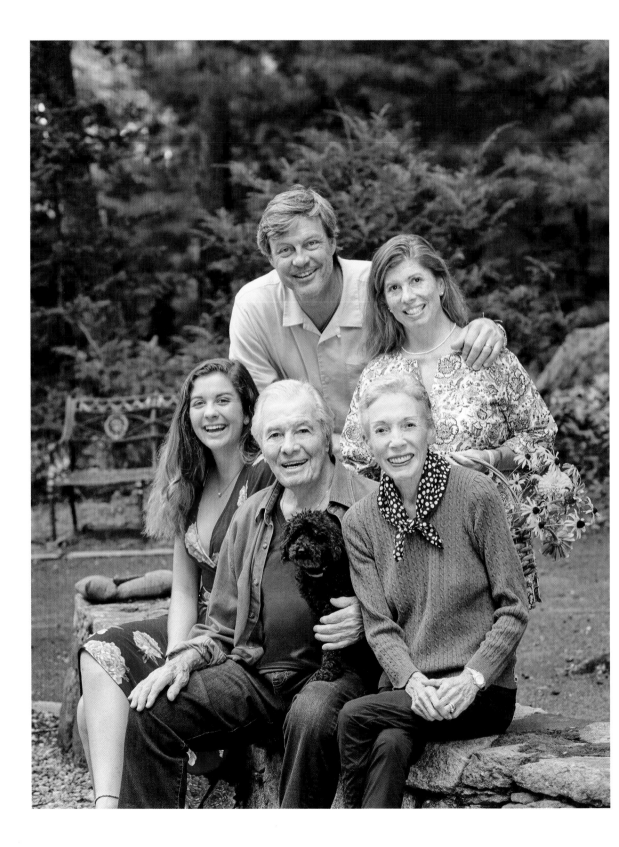

Introduction

This book is intended to make your life easier. In it I share streamlined cooking techniques, teach you how to make use of good-quality convenience foods, suggest supplies for a well-stocked freezer and pantry, and specify the most useful cooking equipment and utensils. The cuisine that emerges in the two hundred–plus recipes here is one born of the necessity to accommodate today's fast-paced lifestyles, a cuisine that is rewarding without being demanding. The book celebrates simple, satisfying fare that can be prepared easily and cooked quickly at the end of a busy day.

Many styles of cooking are represented on these pages, with dishes created to satisfy a variety of needs and fit a host of occasions. Just as it's not "right" or "wrong" to eat in the kitchen rather than the dining room, simple food is not "better" than elaborate food: The food and the setting should be compatible with the occasion, and if something tastes good, it doesn't matter whether it is "authentic" or prepared "correctly"—what works, works.

With very little time to cook today, people often eat in fast-food restaurants or buy expensive and often inferior precooked food. My way of cooking—based on years of professional experience—makes use of fresh foods from farmers' markets and the supermarket, preferably organic, to which I apply a personal touch to make them my own.

All supermarkets today offer precut meats and poultry, grated cheeses, presliced mushrooms, and washed spinach. Although these convenience foods are a bit more expensive, the savings in time and effort are worth the additional cost—and the quality of your cooking is not diminished because someone else has done some of the preparation for you. Store-bought mayonnaise and already-peeled squash are just a few examples of useful basic products that can be given your personal signature with a little ingenuity.

Small restaurants—pressed for time and short of skilled hands—often proceed along similar lines. They buy small quantities of peeled and diced fresh vegetables, cleaned salad greens, trimmed lamb racks, and filleted fish. Although these products are more expensive than when bought in bulk, the savings in time and labor offset the higher cost and often provide the only possible course of action.

The term "homemade" has taken on a righteous tone: In today's terminology, it means better, more virtuous, truer to nature—in short, the "proper" way to do things. But homemade food is good only when it is superior in taste to its store-bought counterpart. In reality, many homemade breads, cakes, croissants, jams, and condiments are inferior to similar items available at the local supermarket.

In France it is quite common for even great home cooks to buy certain prepared foods—those renowned for their exceptional quality—at the market. Items like breads, pâtés, dumplings, basic doughs, jams, and relishes are rarely made at home. To quote Montaigne, the sixteenth-century French writer, "The bees go from flower to flower to gather the pollen, but with it they create their own honey." I am proposing the same course of action here: Select superior items at the market and use them in ways that make them your own.

Selectively mixing fresh with canned, bottled, or frozen foods can result in great dishes. For example, quickly sauté fresh scallops and toss them in a delicious sauce made of commercial mayonnaise that you've flavored with lemon juice, scallions, Worcestershire sauce, and Tabasco sauce (see Scallops in a Skillet, page 224). Or, for an elegant dessert, mold rectangles of store-bought puff pastry around fresh Bartlett pear halves and bake (see Bartlett Pears in Puff Pastry, page 352). Your delighted guests will not know or care that such dishes weren't made exclusively with "fresh" food.

Cooking is not the only part of food preparation that can be simplified. Food shopping is a time-consuming activity that benefits from thoughtful advance planning. Even the use and cleaning of cooking utensils can be streamlined. And having a well-stocked larder (see page 8) means you are able to create meals on short notice. An impromptu visit from friends can often be the occasion for a "cuisine of opportunity," with dishes prepared from what is at hand.

Understanding the basic mechanics of cooking is also helpful. If you decide to cook a stew, for example, know that although it would take a couple of hours to cook it conventionally on top of the stove, a pressure cooker can reduce the cooking time by half. If you double or triple the recipe, you can freeze the leftovers for use later on or refrigerate them to make a soup or a puree for a meal later that week.

Techniques are important too. Peel vegetables directly into a sink equipped with a garbage disposal, or place an oversize garbage can (mine is on wheels) in a convenient position and let the peelings drop directly into it. If neither of these options is feasible, spread newspapers on your work surface to catch the peelings and so simplify the cleanup.

Whenever possible, line baking pans with nonstick aluminum foil to eliminate time-consuming cleaning afterward. Fill a dirty pot or roasting pan with water as soon as you have finished using it to loosen solidified bits of food and make washing up easier. Roll dough out between sheets of plastic wrap to keep the work surface and rolling pin clean. Cook in gratin dishes attractive enough to go directly from the oven to the table. And freeze food in dishes that can go right from the freezer to the oven to the table. When sautéing meat—whether it be pork chops or veal scaloppini—sauté a vegetable to serve with it in the unwashed skillet once you've cooked the meal; a cleanup step is eliminated, and the juices from the meat will enhance the flavor of the vegetable.

Give some thought beforehand to your use of a food processor. If a menu calls for pureed vegetables and fresh bread crumbs, for example, process the bread first so the processor won't need washing between the two uses. Merely rinse your pots between uses and whenever possible, progress from cooking "clean" foods to sticky ones. A mistake many people make when preparing a pasta dish is to wait until the sauce is finished before they put the pasta cooking water on to boil. Put the pot on the heat when you begin cooking so the water will be boiling when you need it. And when selecting a menu consisting of three dishes, make sure that one or two of them can be made ahead, or you will be too involved in cooking to create a hospitable atmosphere when your guests arrive.

Follow my time-and-labor-saving techniques and then come up with some of your own, equip your kitchen with the best-possible cooking equipment and utensils to make the work easier, and seek out good-quality convenience foods that you can combine appetizingly with fresh foods to create sumptuous meals. Simple, speedy, sensible, and smart, this is quick and simple cooking—ideal for people on the run who demand good food.

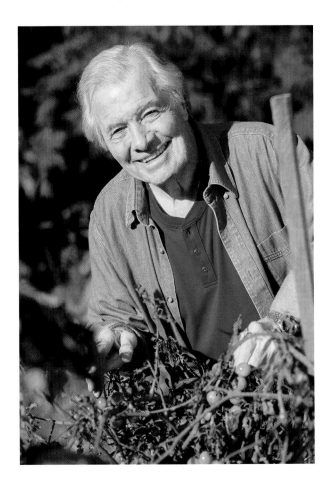

EQUIPMENT

To be a good cook, you need high-quality equipment. Anyone who has attempted to chop vegetables or cut meat with a dull knife, or has had to run to the store to buy sugar in the midst of baking a cake, knows how frustrating a poorly organized kitchen can be, even if you're not rushed. And when you don't have much time, inadequate equipment can turn you against cooking altogether. Here's a list of kitchen equipment I find especially useful, followed by pantry items I like to have on hand.

A microwave oven is wonderful, but be discriminating in your use of it. It is especially good for cooking individual portions of vegetables, fish, and fruit, and it is the best choice for reheating food. And it doesn't require much cleaning.

A toaster oven is a wise purchase. It heats very quickly, is big enough for two servings—or sometimes even three or four—and is much more economical to operate than a conventional oven. It's particularly good for toasting nuts, cooking hot sandwiches, and browning the tops of grains and other dishes.

The pressure cooker is another labor-saving device that is a favorite in my kitchen. A stew can be prepared in a pressure cooker in less than half the time it would take to cook in a conventional pot, and the quality is not sacrificed. In addition to helping preserve the nutritional value of foods, a pressure cooker retains their moisture as well. And the modern version of this old invention is completely safe.

A food processor is invaluable. Chopping, pureeing, and grating can be completed in seconds thanks to this miraculous machine.

A mini-chop is also handy. This small version of a food processor has a blade that spins much faster than that of its larger relative and is good for grinding dry ingredients like peppercorns, dried mushrooms, and dried tomatoes and for chopping spices, herbs, and garlic, which in small quantities get lost in a conventional food processor. The mini-chop is easy to clean too.

An **immersion blender** is also very good to have. The shaft of this handheld appliance goes directly into a soup or vegetable mixture to puree it in seconds, and there is nothing to wash except the shaft and blade, which rinse clean when held under hot water.

Nonstick pans are essential for most sautéing, since they are easy to clean. For other cooking needs, select pans made of good solid stainless steel or thick aluminum lined with stainless steel; they give an excellent result and clean up easily. Good **stainless steel strainers** are a must, as are **rubber spatulas, high-quality carbon steel knives,** and a **good knife sharpener,** all of which will make your job easier.

A **salad spinner** is indispensable. Use the base of the spinner as a container to wash the salad greens, then lift the greens from the water and place them in the strainer insert before spinning them dry. Packed in plastic bags and refrigerated, washed greens will keep in the refrigerator for a few days.

I buy large boxes of **plastic wrap and nonstick aluminum foil,** as I use a great deal of both. I find the large rolls are easier to work with and their boxes have a better cutting edge than smaller ones. Line cookie sheets and pans with nonstick aluminum foil to avoid time-consuming cleanup. Plastic wrap seals foods well, preventing spillage from refrigerated leftovers or defrosting foods.

A **good-size freezer** is also vital to shortcut cooking. It enables you to keep soup and sauce bases, ice cream, and frozen fruits and vegetables on hand.

It's fun to cook in a well-equipped modern kitchen.

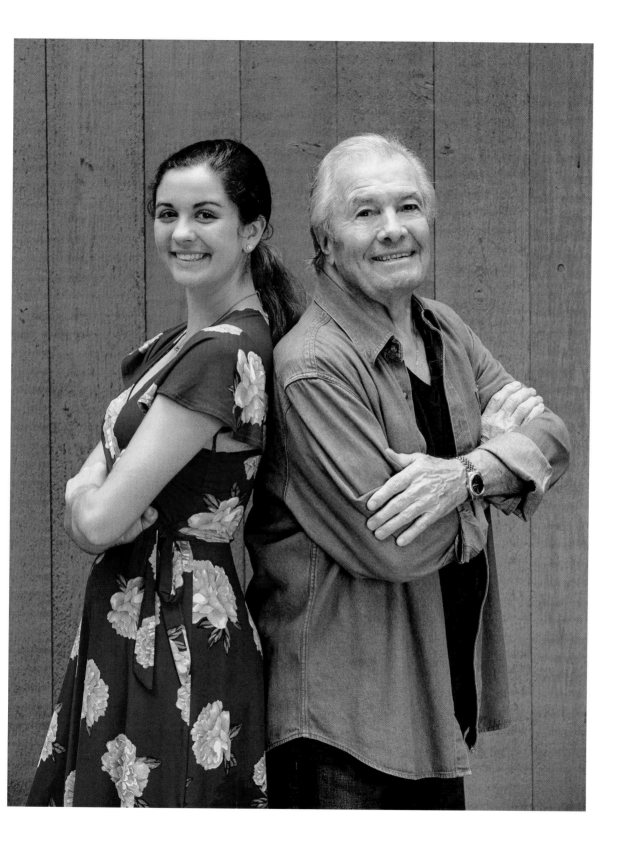

PANTRY

A well-stocked larder is a most important aspect of shortcut cooking. If you keep an abundance of dry products, canned goods, frozen foods, and fresh ingredients on hand, with a little imagination and help from this book, you can easily create terrific meals in no time at all.

Dry products keep for many months. These include dried beans—red, white, and black, as well as chickpeas—pasta, rice, dried tomatoes and mushrooms, and chicken bouillon cubes. I always have a supply of thickeners on hand for soups and stews: Flour, potato starch, oatmeal, farina, couscous, bulgur wheat, and potato flakes are all very useful for this purpose. In the pastry area, keep a stock of cookies, chocolates, and nuts.

Among the canned products you should have on your pantry shelves are chicken broth, Italian tomatoes, tomato paste, smoked mussels, smoked oysters, shrimp, crabmeat, sardines, herring, salmon, chili, pumpkin puree, and different types of vegetables, including button mushrooms.

Jarred products include mayonnaise, chutneys, Worcestershire sauce, soy sauce, steak sauce, hoisin sauce, Chinese chili-garlic sauce, teriyaki sauce, duck sauce, sparerib sauce, fish sauce, and plum sauce. I also keep on hand hot chili oil, toasted sesame oil, olive oil, vegetable oil, various vinegars, hot salsa, and artichoke hearts, as well as pepperoncini, cherry peppers, sweet peppers, mixed pickles, and marinated mushrooms, along with an assortment of mustards, cocktail sauces, and horseradish.

If you have enough freezer space, you can stock frozen foods such as shrimp, squid, stuffed pasta (manicotti, ravioli, tortellini, lasagna), fruit juice concentrates (orange, pineapple, grapefruit), and different desserts or ingredients like cakes, brownies, ice creams and sherbets, and doughs—from puff pastry to bread, pie, and cookie dough. Frozen strawberries and raspberries, as well as peaches and cherries, are very good to have on hand. Very useful, too, are mixed and individually quick-frozen vegetables from petite peas to corn, tiny pearl onions, French green beans, spinach leaves, cauliflower, and mustard greens. Homemade chicken stock, several types of sausages—from kielbasa to Italian sausage—and chicken breasts are among my freezer staples.

When buying **fresh products,** remember that some items will keep longer than others. Garlic, carrots, and eggs can be stored in the refrigerator for a long time; potatoes and onions should be stored in a cool pantry. Take advantage of all the peeled and cleaned packaged vegetables in the supermarket, not forgetting to occasionally make use of the salad bar to pick up ready-to-eat seasonal vegetables. Take advantage, too, of precut meat and poultry, fish in pre-portioned packages, and the bounty of supermarket deli departments with their different types of olives, salads—from chicken to pasta to potato to smoked fish—pickles, cold cuts, and sausages.

If you have at least some of the equipment listed here and know at all times what food items you have in your pantry, refrigerator, and freezer, you can happily and easily accommodate your family and any surprise visitors.

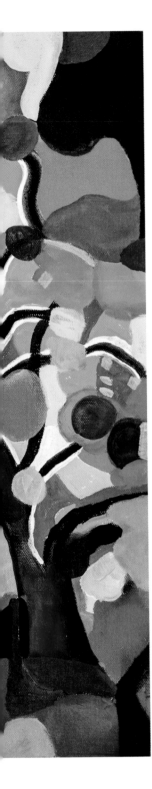

BASICS

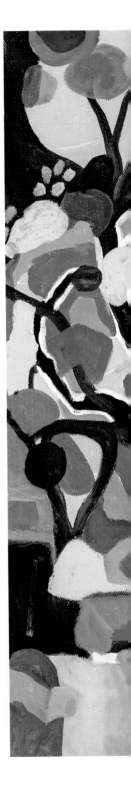

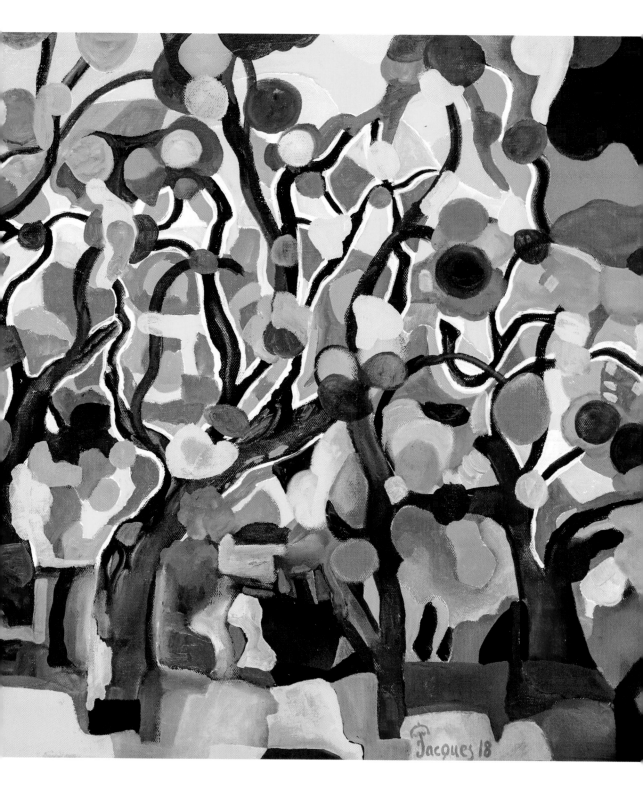

MUSTARD VINAIGRETTE

∘ MAKES ABOUT 1¼ CUPS
(20 SERVINGS)

1 cup oil, preferably half extra-
virgin olive oil and half peanut,
canola, or corn oil

2 tablespoons tarragon red wine
vinegar

1½ tablespoons Dijon-style
mustard, preferably "hot"

½ teaspoon salt

½ teaspoon freshly ground
black pepper

At our house, we eat salad with almost every meal, and nine out of ten times the dressing is a standard vinaigrette. I make the vinaigrette in a jar with a tight-fitting lid and store it in the refrigerator so it is available whenever I need it—it will keep for up to 2 weeks.

Occasionally, if I want to vary the taste, I add some crushed garlic to the dressing in the salad (but not to the dressing in the jar, because the garlic will lose its freshness after a few days and adversely affect the dressing's flavor). I like a tarragon-flavored vinegar, but you might want to try another type for a different taste.

This dressing is not emulsified, because the oil is added along with the other ingredients, not whisked in at the end. So no matter how long or how hard you shake the jar, the vinaigrette won't become creamy. It will blend somewhat, which is what you want, but then it will separate again. This means that the salad greens will be glossy and flavorful without being heavily coated. Just shake the jar briefly before each use to partially blend the ingredients again.

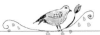

Place all the ingredients in a 12-ounce glass jar, cover tightly, and shake well to mix. Refrigerate until ready to use.

When you are ready to use the dressing, shake the jar briefly to recombine the ingredients.

> This dressing is made and stored in the
> same jar, ready for immediate use.

Although salsa is readily available at most supermarkets, you might enjoy this homemade version. Use as a dip for chips or add to salads and stews. It will keep for up to 2 weeks in the refrigerator.

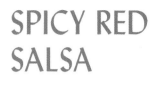

Place the jalapeño, garlic, and cilantro in a food processor and process for 5 to 10 seconds, until coarsely chopped. Add the tomato pieces, water, ketchup, and salt and process until the mixture is chunky, with no pieces larger than ½ inch. Transfer to a jar and refrigerate until ready to use.

SPICY RED SALSA

◦ MAKES ¾ CUP

1 jalapeño pepper, coarsely chopped (2½ teaspoons)

1 large clove garlic, peeled and crushed

2 tablespoons cilantro leaves

2 small plum tomatoes (4 ounces total), quartered

1 tablespoon water

1 tablespoon ketchup

⅛ teaspoon salt

This sauce is excellent with clams or oysters on the half shell, and it gives added zip to salad dressings, barbecue sauces, and tomato sauces. It will keep in the refrigerator for a couple of weeks.

Combine all the ingredients in a jar with a tight-fitting lid and mix thoroughly. Store, refrigerated, in the covered jar until ready to use.

HORSERADISH SAUCE

◦ MAKES 1 CUP (6 SERVINGS)

½ cup ketchup

¼ cup grated fresh horseradish, or 6 tablespoons bottled

2 teaspoons rice vinegar

½ teaspoon Tabasco sauce

TAPENADE

1¼ cups oil-cured black olives, pitted

¼ cup extra-virgin olive oil

4 dried figs (4 ounces total), cut into ¼- to ½-inch pieces

3 tablespoons capers, drained

One 2-ounce can anchovy fillets in oil

½ teaspoon freshly ground black pepper

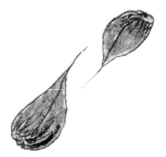

This olive spread is a staple in Provence, where it is usually served with aperitifs or as an appetizer. Try it on pita toasts (page 106), bagel chips, or *fougasse*, the famous bread of Provence (see page 93. Serve with chilled white wine or rosé. The tapenade can also be added to sauces or to ratatouille, or used as a garnish with smoked salmon and other smoked fish or pâtés.

The traditional recipe for tapenade doesn't contain dried figs, but I think they are a great addition. Be careful not to overprocess the mixture; it should be chunky, not creamy. Tightly covered, it will keep for up to 2 weeks in the refrigerator.

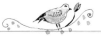

Place all the ingredients in a food processor and process for 4 to 5 seconds. Scrape down the sides of the bowl and process for 7 to 8 seconds longer, until the mixture holds together but is still somewhat chunky. Transfer to a small bowl and serve, or store in an airtight container in the refrigerator.

When I see packages of chicken necks, backs, and gizzards at the supermarket, I buy them and store them in the freezer. Then, when I find myself spending a day in the kitchen preparing other recipes, I take them out and use them to make a stock. When the stock has finished cooking, I strain it, cool it, defat it completely, pour it into plastic containers with tight-fitting lids, and store it in the freezer. That way I always have it on hand for use in soups.

Place the chicken parts and water in a large stockpot and bring to a boil over high heat. Reduce the heat and boil gently for 30 minutes. Most of the fat and impurities will rise to the surface during this time; skim off and discard as much of them as you can.

Add the remaining ingredients, return the liquid to a boil, and boil gently for 2 hours. Strain the stock through a fine-mesh sieve or a colander lined with a dampened kitchen towel or dampened paper towels. Allow the stock to cool, then remove the surface fat and discard. Freeze the stock in plastic containers with tight-fitting lids to use as needed.

NOTE: If you do not have herbes de Provence, make your own. Mix together dried oregano and rosemary, and equal amounts of any of the following: dried marjoram, thyme, summer savory, or sage.

BASIC CHICKEN STOCK

∘ MAKES 3¼ QUARTS (13 CUPS)

3 pounds chicken necks, backs, and gizzards, skinless or with as little skin as possible

6 quarts lukewarm water

1 large onion (about 8 ounces), peeled and cut into 4 pieces

6 whole cloves

1 tablespoon herbes de Provence (see Note)

1 tablespoon dark soy sauce

1 teaspoon celery seeds

▷ **If your finished stock doesn't have enough flavor, add 1 tablespoon chicken base, preferably organic.**

 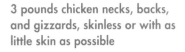

QUICK TOMATO SAUCE

◦ MAKES 4 CUPS (6 SERVINGS)

2½ pounds very ripe tomatoes

3 tablespoons olive oil

1 onion (4 to 5 ounces), peeled
and chopped fine (1 cup)

1 teaspoon herbes de Provence
(see Note, page 15) or Italian
seasoning

3 cloves garlic, peeled, crushed,
and chopped very fine (about
1½ teaspoons)

1 teaspoon salt

½ teaspoon freshly ground
black pepper

½ teaspoon sugar

1 tablespoon tomato paste

Because the tomatoes are not cooked much here—
the other ingredients are cooked first and then the
tomatoes are added and just heated briefly—the sauce
has a very fresh taste.

Tomato paste adds color, texture, and flavor to
the tomatoes—especially valuable out of season, when
fresh tomatoes tend to be watery and bland. I suggest
you use the paste that comes in a tube. You can
squeeze out only as much as you need and then recap
it so the remainder doesn't dry out, and it keeps for a
long time in the refrigerator.

In addition to making a delicious topping for
pasta, the sauce can be used as a garnish for fish or
broiled meats. You can even mix it into tomato soup
(see Cold Raw Tomato Soup, page 80, and Tomato
Soup with Chives, page 78).

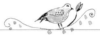

Plunge the tomatoes into a pot of boiling water for
10 to 15 seconds. Drain in a colander. Peel off the
skin and cut the tomatoes crosswise in half. Squeeze
them gently, pressing out the seeds and juices
(reserve the juices to add later if you like). Cut the
tomato flesh into ½-inch pieces (you should have
4 cups).

Heat the olive oil in a large skillet or saucepan
(preferably stainless steel to prevent discoloration).
When the oil is hot, add the onion and herbes de
Provence and sauté for about 1½ minutes. Add the
garlic and stir it into the onion. Add the tomatoes,
salt, pepper, sugar, and tomato paste. Bring the
mixture to a strong boil, reduce the heat, and boil
gently for 1 to 2 minutes. You can strain the tomato
juice into the sauce, discarding the seeds, if you like.

This is a staple at our house; we like its spiciness and crunch. Put it in sandwiches, mix it into salads, or serve it as a condiment with meats. Chopped, the relish makes an excellent sauce (see Salmon Croquettes with Cucumber Salsa, page 237). Stored in a jar or bowl in your refrigerator, it will keep for several weeks.

After you have eaten all the cucumbers, you can reuse the marinade a couple of times, adding more fresh cucumbers.

Peel the cucumber and cut it into very thin slices by hand or using a food processor fitted with the 1-millimeter slicing blade. Transfer the slices to a bowl and add the remaining ingredients. Mix well, cover, and refrigerate for at least 2 hours before serving.

NOTE: Add about ¼ cup coarsely chopped cilantro for a different flavor.

SPICY CUCUMBER RELISH

◦ MAKES 4 CUPS (6 SERVINGS)

1 large English ("seedless") cucumber (about 1 pound)

1 cup boiling water

½ cup white or cider vinegar

2 tablespoons sugar

2 teaspoons Sriracha or other hot sauce

1 teaspoon salt

CRANBERRY RELISH WITH LIME

◦ MAKES 2½ CUPS (8 SERVINGS)

1 small lime (about 3 ounces)

One 12-ounce package fresh cranberries

1 cup light maple syrup

¼ teaspoon cayenne pepper

¼ teaspoon ground ginger

¼ teaspoon ground mace

▷ **Packaged cranberries come cleaned, so they don't need to be washed.**

This relish is delicious with roast turkey (page 287) as well as with game, roast chicken, and roast pork. It has a spicy but sweet citrus flavor that goes well with rich foods such as pâtés. It takes only a few minutes to make and will keep for weeks in the refrigerator.

Cut the lime lengthwise into quarters, then cut each quarter into thin triangular slices. Place them in a medium stainless steel saucepan and add the remaining ingredients. Stir well, cover, and bring to a boil over high heat. Mix thoroughly, cover again, reduce the heat to medium, and boil gently for about 5 minutes. All the cranberries should be broken and the mixture well combined.

Transfer the relish to a bowl and allow it to cool, then refrigerate until ready to serve.

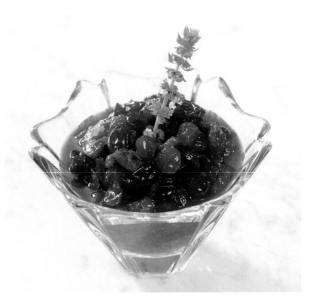

This is a very versatile mixture, delicious in salads, sauces, stews, and sandwiches. I use it in several recipes in this book; it helps to season everything from pasta to cheese to salad.

Place the mushrooms and tomatoes in a bowl and add boiling water to cover. Soak for 5 minutes. Drain (reserve the liquid for use in stock or soup). Chop the mushrooms and tomatoes into ½-inch pieces.

Place the mushrooms and tomatoes in a jar and add all the remaining ingredients. Allow the mixture to steep for at least a few hours before serving. It will keep, tightly covered, for up to 4 weeks in the refrigerator.

MUSHROOM, TOMATO, AND NUT MIX

∘ MAKES ABOUT 3½ CUPS

1 cup dried porcini mushrooms

4 cups sun-dried tomatoes (not packed in oil)

1 cup olive oil

3 large cloves garlic, peeled and sliced thin (about 1½ tablespoons)

1 tablespoon thinly sliced jalapeño pepper

¼ cup sunflower seeds

¼ teaspoon hot pepper flakes

¼ teaspoon dried tarragon

½ teaspoon salt (optional, if the sun-dried tomatoes are not salted)

RED PEPPER DIP

○ MAKES ABOUT 2 CUPS

2 cloves garlic, peeled and crushed

½ large jalapeño pepper, seeded and chopped coarsely (1 tablespoon)

1 cup drained roasted sweet peppers or pimento peppers

⅓ cup pecan pieces

⅓ cup extra-virgin olive oil

¼ teaspoon salt

This dip has a fresh, clean taste and is easy to make with jarred or canned roasted sweet peppers or pimentos. I add pecans for a somewhat unusual combination. The dip is a big hit at parties, served with bagel chips, Melba toast, freshly toasted bread, or Pita Cheese Toasts (page 106). It also makes a great pasta sauce (see Rigatoni with Red Pepper Sauce, page 129).

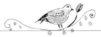

Place the garlic and jalapeño in a food processor and process for 10 to 15 seconds, until pureed. Add the remaining ingredients and process until the mixture is smooth. Transfer to a bowl and serve.

▷ Roasted red peppers from a jar or can are the main ingredient in this delicious, piquant, easy-to-make dip.

This spread can be served as an appetizer or as an hors d'oeuvre with aperitifs. Easy to make, it is particularly good on Pita Cheese Toasts (see page 106) or black pumpernickel bread, and it will keep for up to a week in the refrigerator. You can also use it as a pasta sauce. Or serve it hot as a side dish with meat or fish.

Preheat the oven to 400 degrees. Place the eggplants (whole and untrimmed) on a cookie sheet lined with nonstick aluminum foil. Bake for 45 minutes, or until soft. Remove from the oven and let cool slightly.

While the eggplant is cooking, heat the canola oil in a large skillet over medium heat, then add the onions and sauté for 3 to 4 minutes. Stir in the garlic, then transfer the mixture to a bowl. Add the remaining ingredients. Stir to combine.

When the eggplant has cooled enough to handle, peel off and discard the skin and mince the flesh by hand or in a food processor (you should have 1¾ to 2 cups). Add the eggplant to the ingredients in the bowl and mix well.

EGGPLANT "CAVIAR"

○ MAKES 3 CUPS

1 or 2 Chinese or Japanese eggplants (the long, narrow type; 1 pound total)

1 tablespoon canola oil

2 onions (about 6 ounces total), peeled and chopped (1½ cups)

3 large cloves garlic, peeled, crushed, and chopped (2 teaspoons)

2 ripe tomatoes (about 12 ounces total), halved, seeded, and cut into ¼-inch dice (1½ cups)

2 tablespoons olive oil

1½ tablespoons chopped cilantro

1 tablespoon cider vinegar

1 teaspoon salt

½ teaspoon freshly ground black pepper

½ teaspoon sugar

½ teaspoon Tabasco sauce

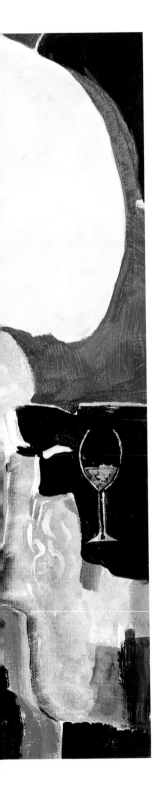

APPETIZERS & SALADS

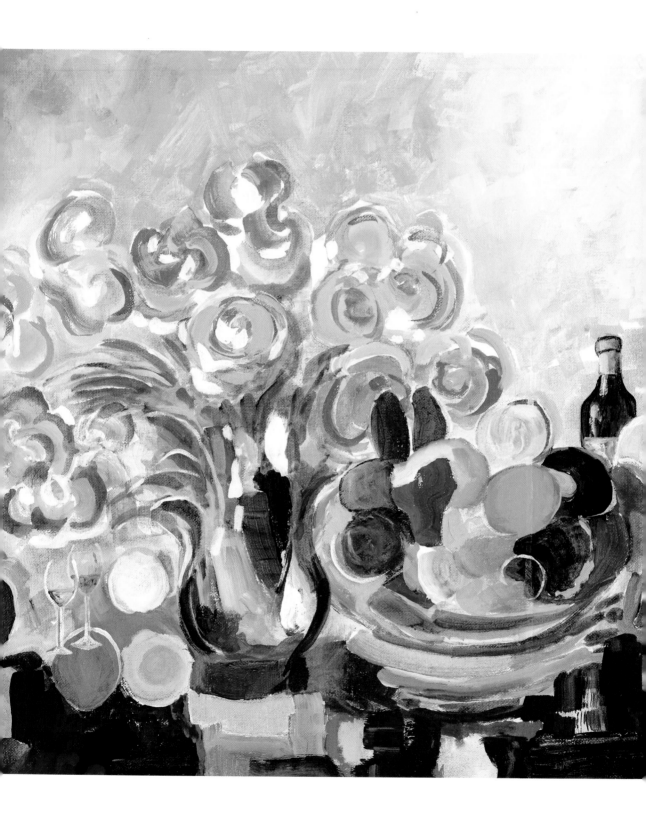

SALMON–CREAM CHEESE ROLL-UPS

◦ MAKES ABOUT
25 HORS D'OEUVRES

One 8-ounce package cream cheese, cold

5 or 6 slices smoked salmon (about 5 ounces)

½ teaspoon freshly ground black pepper

About 25 small round slices (about 2-inch diameter) pumpernickel or other dark bread or rice crackers or Ritz crackers

▷ **Rolling the cream cheese out between sheets of plastic wrap eliminates a messy cleanup chore.**

Preparing the roll-ups ahead of time and placing them in the freezer for a couple of hours makes slicing them much easier.

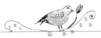

Place the cream cheese on a 12-inch square of plastic wrap. Cover it with another 12-inch square and, with your hands, spread the cream cheese out to form a square approximately 8 by 8 inches. Peel off and discard the top piece of plastic wrap and arrange the salmon on the cheese. Sprinkle the pepper evenly over the salmon. Lifting up the plastic wrap, roll the cream cheese up tightly, enclosing the salmon (don't let the plastic get rolled up inside). Use the plastic wrap to help tighten the roll; it should measure about 9 inches long by 1½ inches. Seal it well in the plastic wrap and place in the freezer for 1½ to 2 hours.

Remove the partially frozen roll from the plastic wrap and, using a sharp thin-bladed knife, cut it into ½-inch-wide slices. Place the slices on the bread rounds. Work quickly while the cream cheese is still cold, so it doesn't stick too much to your fingers or to the knife. If it gets sticky, return it to the freezer for a few minutes to harden.

Arrange the hors d'oeuvres on a large serving plate and serve cold.

VEGETABLE-CREAM CHEESE ROLL-UPS

In place of the salmon, use 1 large carrot, peeled and sliced lengthwise into thin strips with a vegetable peeler, 8 sun-dried tomatoes from the Mushroom, Tomato, and Nut Mix (page 19), and 12 mint leaves. Arrange the vegetables and mint over the cheese (omit the pepper) and roll up as described.

NOTES: If you don't have the tomato mix on hand, you can use sun-dried tomatoes packed in oil or reconstituted dehydrated tomatoes. Try other vegetables as well, for variations in flavor and color.

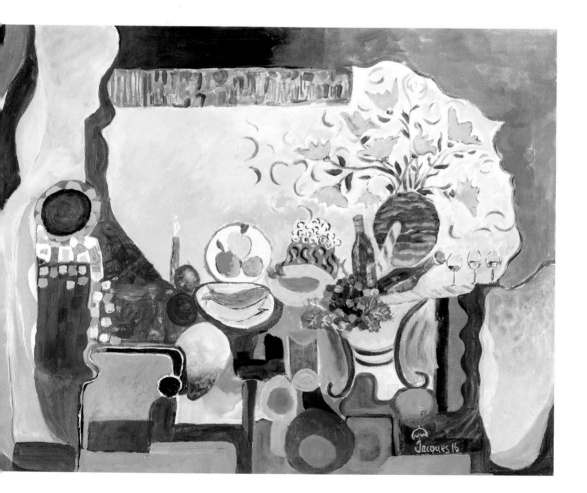

ANCHOVY, PARSLEY, AND CARROT SALAD IN TOMATO BOATS

∘ MAKES ABOUT
40 HORS D'OEUVRES

One 2-ounce can anchovy fillets in oil (about 12)

4 cups flat-leaf parsley leaves

8 to 10 cloves garlic, peeled and chopped fine (3 tablespoons)

About 5 carrots (1½ pounds), trimmed, peeled, and shredded (about 4 cups)

¼ teaspoon salt (optional)

1 teaspoon freshly ground black pepper

⅓ cup olive oil or vegetable oil

1 tablespoon red wine vinegar

2 pounds small plum tomatoes (about 20)

We often serve this salad with toast as a first course, and it is a great recipe for a large party. When serving it as an hors d'oeuvre, I either mound it in hollowed-out plum tomato halves, as here, or present it as a dip with toast, bagel chips, or pita toasts (see page 106). It also makes a delicious sauce for hot pasta.

The salad will keep in the refrigerator for as long as 2 weeks.

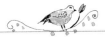

Cut the anchovy fillets into ¼-inch pieces. Place them in a bowl and mix in the parsley, garlic, carrots, salt, if using, pepper, olive oil, and vinegar. Cover tightly (or transfer to a jar) and refrigerate until ready to use.

Cut the tomatoes lengthwise in half and carefully hollow them out with a spoon that has a sharp edge (reserve the insides for soup, if desired). When you are ready to serve, arrange the tomato shells on a serving platter and fill with the salad.

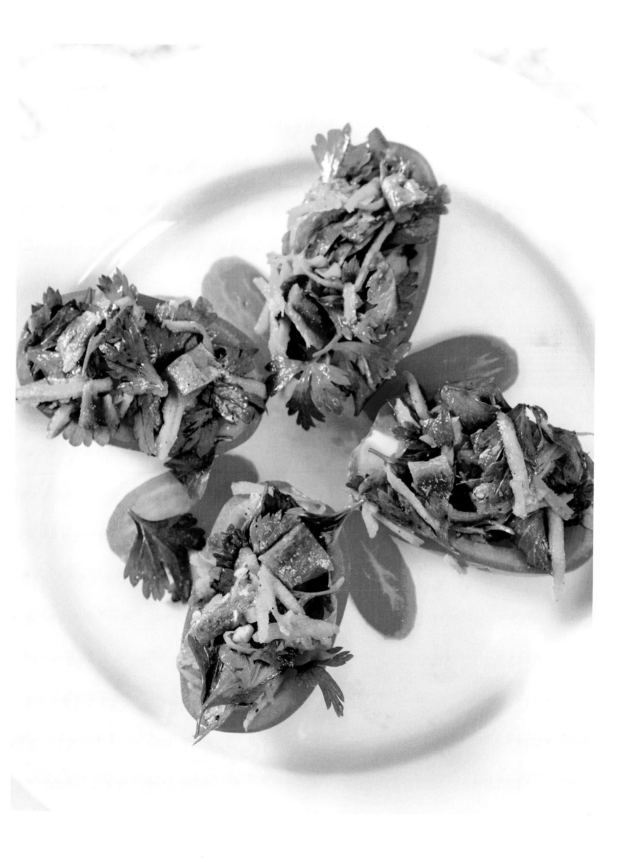

TUNA TARTARE ON DAIKON RADISH

○ SERVES 6 AS A FIRST COURSE

1 pound very fresh tuna steak (preferably belly), any skin and tough sinews removed

½ cup chopped red onion

3 tablespoons minced scallions (about 2)

½ teaspoon chopped garlic (1 clove)

3 tablespoons virgin olive oil

1 teaspoon salt

½ teaspoon freshly ground black pepper

2 teaspoons red wine vinegar

1 teaspoon chirashi sauce

1 teaspoon chopped tarragon

1 small white or red daikon radish (about 8 ounces and 1½ inches in diameter)

White toast or black bread, for serving (optional)

Use very fresh sashimi-grade tuna (or salmon or black sea bass) for this recipe. The spiciness of the daikon radish complements the raw tuna. If you like, you could also make tiny sandwiches by placing spoonfuls of the tartare between slices of radish, or serve it on a bed of shredded daikon.

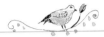

Coarsely chop the tuna by hand—it should not be chopped too fine.

If the chopped red onion has a strong odor, rinse it in a sieve under cool water (this removes the sulfuric acid compound that tends to sting your eyes). Drain well and pat dry.

Combine the tuna, onion, scallions, garlic, olive oil, salt, pepper, vinegar, chirashi, and tarragon in a small bowl and mix well.

Peel the daikon and slice it into thin rounds. Place about 1 tablespoon of the tuna mixture on each radish slice. Arrange them on a platter and serve with toast or black bread, if desired.

NOTE: For another way to serve the dish, cut the daikon into julienne strips instead of rounds. Mound some tartare in the center of each individual plate, sprinkle with a little olive oil, and garnish with the radish strips. Serve with toast or black bread, if you like.

I like my guacamole fairly well seasoned. The important factor is the ripeness of the avocados, of course. They should yield to the touch but not have turned brown. Serve the guacamole with packaged natural fried corn chips, or with store-bought corn or flour tortillas that you fry yourself.

Rinse the red onion in a sieve under cold water, drain, and pat dry.

Cut the avocados in half, remove the pits and set aside, and spoon the flesh into a bowl. Mash it coarsely with a fork or potato masher. Add the red onion, garlic, tomato, scallions, lime juice, olive oil, salt, Tabasco, and jalapeño, if using. Stir well, then embed the avocado pits in the mixture (see Note). Cover tightly with plastic wrap, pressing it directly against the surface of the guacamole, and set aside until ready to serve.

At serving time, remove the avocado pits and stir some of the cilantro into the guacamole. Transfer to a serving dish, sprinkle the remaining cilantro on top, and serve with chips.

NOTE: You can make the guacamole ahead of time. It won't turn brown if you submerge the avocado pits in the mixture and cover it tightly as described above.
    Another way to prevent the avocado from turning brown is to rinse the avocado flesh under cold water.

GUACAMOLE PIQUANTE

∘ MAKES 4 CUPS

¾ cup diced (¼-inch pieces) red onion

4 avocados (about 2 pounds) preferably organic

2 cloves garlic, peeled and chopped (1 teaspoon)

1 very ripe tomato (about 4 ounces), halved, seeded, and cut into ¼-inch dice (1 cup)

2 scallions, minced (⅓ cup)

3 tablespoons lime juice

2 tablespoons olive oil

1½ teaspoons salt

1 teaspoon Tabasco sauce

1 small jalapeño pepper, seeded and chopped (optional)

¼ cup coarsely chopped cilantro

Corn chips or fresh or frozen tortillas, prepared according to the package instructions, for serving

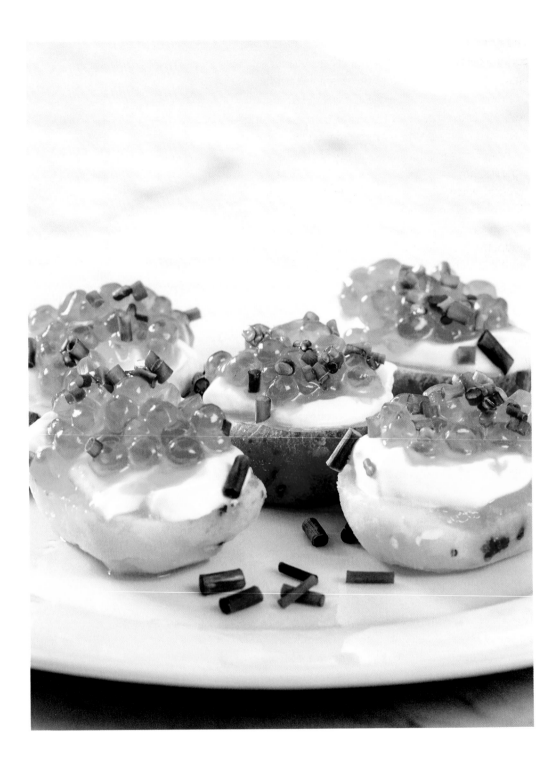

This is delightful as an hors d'oeuvre for a special cocktail party or as a first course for a sit-down dinner. It is best while the potatoes are still warm.

There are two types of red caviar: "natural" and "red," which has a deeper color than the natural. Good natural caviar has an eye (a darker spot inside each egg). The eggs in either variety should be separate, not part of a mushy mass. Each one should "crunch" when bitten, yet still be delicate enough to almost melt in your mouth. The caviar should have a lightly salty, nutty flavor, with no bitter aftertaste. To ensure that the caviar is of good quality, buy it at a reputable store that has a high turnover.

Wash the potatoes in cool water and place them in a saucepan. Cover with water, bring to a boil over high heat, and boil gently until just tender, 20 to 22 minutes for small potatoes, longer for larger ones. Drain and set aside to cool slightly. (The heat in the potatoes will absorb any remaining moisture, producing a better-tasting potato than if they were cooled under cold water.)

When they are cool enough to handle, peel the potatoes, trim slightly on two opposite sides (to enable the halves to stand upright), and cut in half. (If using larger potatoes, cut into slices ¾ to 1 inch thick.)

Mix the oil with the caviar to make it looser and easier to serve. Place 2 teaspoons of the sour cream on each potato (or slice) and top each with a generous teaspoon of the caviar. Arrange on a tray and serve immediately, sprinkled with the chives.

POTATOES WITH RED CAVIAR

∘ MAKES 40 HORS D'OEUVRES

3 pounds small red potatoes (about 20)

1½ cups sour cream

12 ounces good natural or red salmon caviar (or trout caviar)

2 teaspoons peanut oil

3 tablespoons minced chives

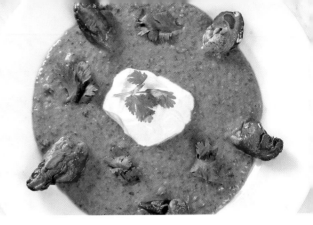

BLACK BEAN HUMMUS WITH SMOKED OYSTERS AND SOUR CREAM

○ MAKES 2 CUPS (6 SERVINGS)

One 16-ounce can black beans

3 cloves garlic, peeled and crushed

⅓ cup oil, preferably half olive oil and half walnut or peanut oil

1 tablespoon toasted sesame oil

1 tablespoon red wine vinegar

1 teaspoon Tabasco sauce

½ teaspoon salt

2 tablespoons coarsely chopped cilantro, plus whole leaves for garnish

1 cup sour cream

Two 3¾-ounce cans smoked oysters (about 30)

Toast triangles or Melba toast, for serving

This interesting variation on traditional Middle Eastern chickpea hummus was inspired by the black bean purees found in Mexico. Served with sour cream and smoked oysters, it makes an exciting dish.

I use canned black beans, but of course you can cook your own, which will tend to be darker than the canned variety. This is also good made with red kidney or other types of beans. I suggest serving it as a first course, but it can also be served as a dip with corn chips or Melba or other toasts.

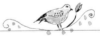

Drain the black beans in a sieve and place them in a food processor, along with the garlic. Process until the garlic is finely chopped and the mixture is smooth. Add the oils, vinegar, Tabasco, and salt and process for another 5 to 10 seconds to blend. Transfer to a serving bowl and stir in the chopped cilantro. Cover and refrigerate until ready to serve.

At serving time, spoon about ⅓ cup of the hummus onto each of six plates and spread it out in the middle of the plate. Place a generous spoonful of sour cream in the center and top with cilantro leaves. Arrange the oysters around the hummus, dividing them evenly. Serve the toasts alongside.

This is a summertime special, to be made when tomatoes are at their juiciest and basil is tender and fresh. The contrast with the crisp toasts is delightful. You can also use this tomato mixture as a sandwich filling, a cold pasta sauce, or a topping for poached or grilled fish.

Plunge the tomatoes into boiling water for 15 to 30 seconds, then drain. When they are cool enough to handle, peel off the skins. Cut the tomatoes crosswise in half and squeeze out the juice and seeds. Cut the tomato flesh into ¼-inch dice (you should have about 4½ cups).

Rinse the red onion in a sieve under cold water, drain, and pat dry.

Combine the tomatoes, onion, scallions, basil, olive oil, salt, pepper, and Tabasco in a serving bowl and mix well. Place a serving spoon in the bowl, set the bowl on a tray, and serve surrounded by the toasts.

NOTE: You can use crackers, bagel chips, Melba toasts, or grilled slices of bread or pita.

TOMATO-BASIL TOASTS

○ MAKES ABOUT
40 HORS D'OEUVRES

2 pounds ripe beefsteak or plum tomatoes

1 cup diced (⅛-inch pieces) red onion

6 scallions, cleaned and sliced thin (about 1 cup)

½ cup shredded basil leaves

⅓ cup virgin olive oil

1¼ teaspoons salt

1 teaspoon freshly ground black pepper

¼ teaspoon Tabasco sauce

40 crackers or toasts, for serving (see Note)

> **The easiest way to shred basil is to gather the leaves into a pile, roll them, and then cut them crosswise into fine strips (this is called chiffonade).**

CHEESE, APPLE, AND NUT BALLS

∘ MAKES 40 TO
45 HORS D'OEUVRES

12 ounces cheese: a combination
of Camembert, Brie, and blue

2 apples, such as Golden Delicious
(12 ounces total), unpeeled

1 teaspoon freshly ground
black pepper

1 cup coarsely chopped
or crushed hazelnuts

1 large carrot (1 to 1½ inches
in diameter)

2 tablespoons chopped chives,
for garnish (optional)

> Make this tasty hors
> d'oeuvre with your choice
> of cheeses and nuts—or
> offer a selection of different
> combinations for variety
> and serve on toast, crackers,
> or even salad leaves or
> cucumber slices.

I use Camembert, Brie, and blue cheeses for this flavorful hors d'oeuvre, but try other combinations with cheeses you have on hand—and if you don't have hazelnuts, other nuts can be substituted. The little balls can also be served on small toasts instead of carrot rounds.

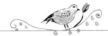

Preheat the oven to 400 degrees. Cut the cheese into pieces and transfer to a food processor. Pulse for 10 to 15 seconds to combine the textures and tastes (or crush and mix the pieces of cheese in a bowl with a fork). Place the cheese in a bowl.

Halve and core the apples, then cut them into thin sticks about ½ inch long. Stir them into the cheese mixture. Sprinkle with the pepper.

Arrange the nuts in a single layer on a cookie sheet and toast in the oven until lightly browned, 6 to 8 minutes. Add the nuts to the cheese mixture and stir together thoroughly. Refrigerate for at least 1 hour to firm the cheese.

Meanwhile, peel the carrot and cut it crosswise into slices about ⅛ inch thick (you should have 40 to 45 rounds).

Form the cold cheese mixture into small balls and place one ball on each carrot slice. Sprinkle with the chives, if desired, and serve.

　Jacques Pépin ⓔ Quick+Simple

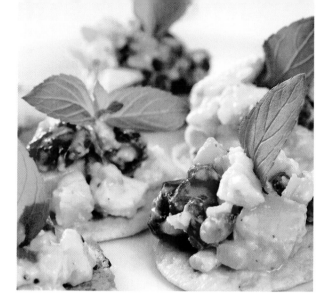

CHEESE MISHMASH

○ MAKES ABOUT
36 HORS D'OEUVRES

About 12 ounces assorted leftover cheeses (such as feta, blue, Gouda, mozzarella, Muenster, Port Salut, Swiss, Fontina, and/or goat)

⅓ cup sunflower or pumpkin seeds

⅓ cup dried cranberries

⅓ cup honey

2 tablespoons lemon juice

1 teaspoon freshly ground black pepper

About 3 dozen savory wafers or rice crackers

Small mint leaves, for garnish

Cheese is expensive, and I hate to discard any of it when it gets old. I use it in many ways, most often in *fromage fort,* a recipe inspired by my father. I clean away any surface damage from the cheese and process it in a food processor with white wine, garlic, and pepper to make a smooth puree to enjoy on crackers or toast. I also use this mixture in *gougères,* in soups, in gratins, and even on pizza. It freezes well.

The recipe below is a sweet version that tastes great on thin wafers or toast. Depending on what's in your refrigerator, the recipe will always vary. *Vive la difference!*

Trim or scape off any dry or damaged areas from the surface of the cheese. Cut or crumble the cheese into ½-inch pieces.

Combine the cheese, sunflower seeds, cranberries, honey, lemon juice, and pepper in a medium bowl and stir with a spoon briefly to combine. Mound a heaping teaspoon of the cheese mixture on top of each wafer, garnish each with a mint leaf, and serve.

MOM'S CHEESE AND SPINACH SOUFFLÉ

∘ SERVES 4

3 tablespoons plus 1 teaspoon unsalted butter

3 tablespoons all-purpose flour

1¼ cups cold milk

¼ teaspoon salt

⅛ teaspoon freshly ground black pepper

⅛ teaspoon ground nutmeg

3 cups baby spinach leaves

1½ cups grated Gruyère or Beaufort cheese (about 4 ounces)

4 large eggs, lightly beaten

3 tablespoons coarsely chopped flat-leaf parsley or basil

> This is the ideal soufflé to assemble ahead and cook at the last moment.

I have a very personal attachment to this soufflé. The recipe comes from my mother, who told me that when she was a young bride, she wanted to make a soufflé for my father, who loved them, but she didn't know how. A friend told her that a cheese soufflé was composed of a béchamel (white sauce), which she knew how to make, grated cheese, and eggs. So she proceeded to make one with these ingredients, not knowing that in a classic soufflé the eggs are separated—the yolks mixed into the white sauce first and the beaten whites folded in later. So she beat the whole eggs into the béchamel and was so happy with the result that she made her soufflés in this manner ever afterward!

This kind of soufflé has many advantages, the most important being that you can prepare the base mixture up to a day ahead, so there is no hectic last-minute preparation involved. Although it takes a little longer to cook than a standard soufflé and has a slightly less airy texture, it rises beautifully, browns well, and is delicious. The soufflé is made in a gratin dish rather than a soufflé mold so that it cooks faster, is crustier, and is easier to divide into portions.

Melt 3 tablespoons of the butter in a medium saucepan over high heat. Add the flour and stir with a whisk until well combined and sizzling, then whisk in the cold milk and bring to a boil, stirring and mixing with the whisk so the mixture doesn't stick as it thickens. Boil for about 20 seconds, mixing continuously with the whisk. Add the salt, pepper, and nutmeg and remove the pan from the heat.

»—>

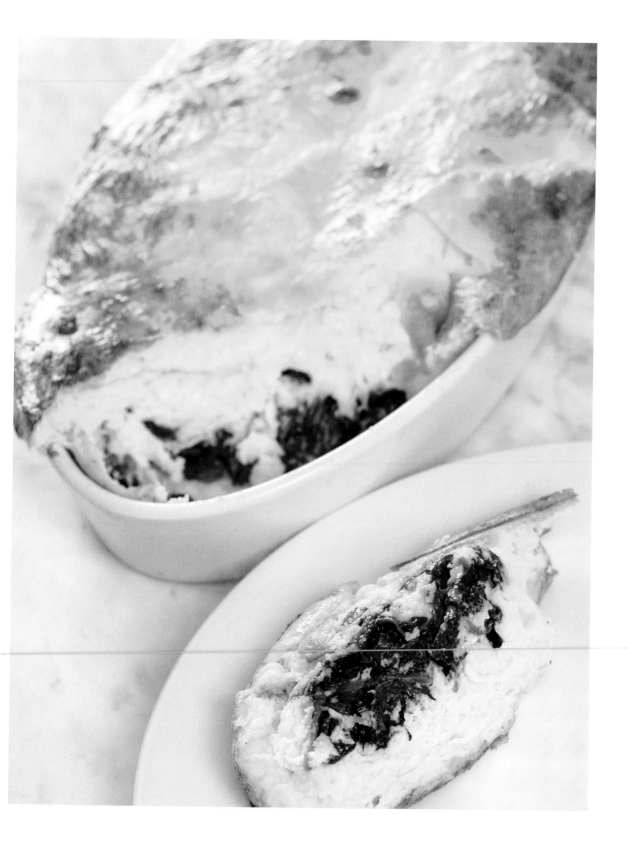

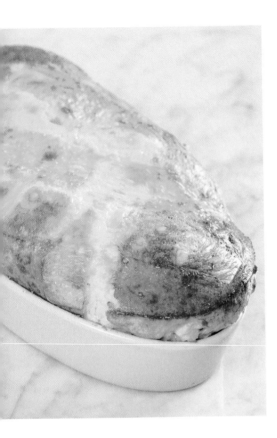

Use the 1 remaining teaspoon butter to grease the bottom of a 3- to 4-cup oval gratin dish. Place the spinach in a bowl and microwave for 2 minutes, or until wilted.

By now, the white sauce should have cooled a little. Add the spinach and cheese to it and mix with the whisk. Add the eggs and parsley and mix well. Pour the mixture into the prepared gratin dish. This step can be done a couple of hours ahead and the dish kept in the refrigerator until cooking time.

When you are ready to cook the soufflé, preheat the oven to 400 degrees. Place the gratin dish on a cookie sheet lined with nonstick aluminum foil for easy cleanup and bake for approximately 40 minutes, until well puffed and brown. Serve immediately.

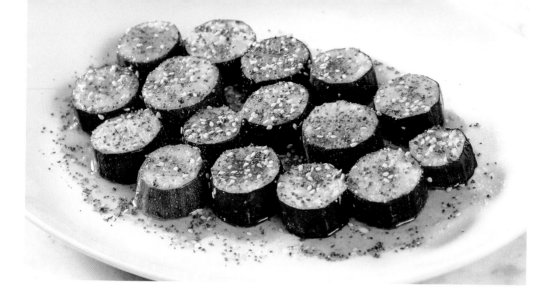

I use slices of young, thin, firm zucchini for these crisps that I serve as an hors d'oeuvre. The slices are cooked briefly in a microwave oven, then topped with *piment d'Espelette* (or, if unavailable, smoked paprika), grated Parmesan cheese, poppy seeds, sesame seeds, and olive oil and served at room temperature. The recipe takes only a few minutes to make.

ZUCCHINI CANAPÉS

○ MAKES ABOUT
20 HORS D'OEUVRES

Cut the zucchini crosswise into ½-inch-thick slices (to get about 20) and place in a bowl. Sprinkle with the salt and microwave for 2 minutes.

Arrange the zucchini slices in one layer on a serving plate (discard any liquid left in the bowl) and sprinkle with the cheese and then the piment d'Espelette, poppy seeds, and olive oil. Serve.

▷ **Piment d'Espelette is a mildly spicy pepper from Espelette, a town in the French Basque area.**

2 to 3 small zucchini
(1¼ inches in diameter)

½ teaspoon salt

2 tablespoons grated Parmesan cheese

½ teaspoon piment d'Espelette or smoked paprika

½ teaspoon poppy seeds

½ teaspoon toasted sesame seeds

2 tablespoons extra-virgin olive oil

CAESAR SALAD

○ SERVES 6

1 head romaine lettuce, as pale as possible

Croutons
___

2 cups ½-inch diced firm country bread

¼ cup peanut oil

Dressing
___

⅓ cup extra-virgin olive oil

2 cloves garlic, peeled, crushed, and chopped coarsely (about 1 tablespoon)

2 tablespoons lemon juice

1 tablespoon Worcestershire sauce

½ teaspoon salt

¼ teaspoon freshly ground black pepper

1 large egg

4 canned anchovy fillets in oil

½ cup grated Parmesan cheese

¼ cup crumbled Roquefort, Stilton, or other blue cheese

I had never had Caesar salad until I came to the United States. My wife, Gloria, made it for me when we first met, and we've used her recipe at home ever since. You can prepare the salad, dressing, and croutons ahead and combine them at the last minute.

Trim the lettuce and break it into 2-inch pieces (you should have about 8 cups). Rinse and dry thoroughly in a salad spinner. Set aside.

Prepare the croutons: Preheat the oven to 375 degrees. Toss the bread with the oil and spread on a cookie sheet. Bake until nicely browned, 12 to 14 minutes. Set aside.

Prepare the dressing: Place the olive oil, garlic, lemon juice, Worcestershire sauce, salt, pepper, and egg in a bowl and beat with a fork until well combined. Cut the anchovy fillets into ¼-inch pieces and add them to the dressing.

At serving time, toss the greens with the dressing in a large serving bowl. Add the cheeses and toss again. Scatter the croutons on top of the salad and serve immediately.

I love Greek salads, with their distinctively flavored kalamata olives, feta cheese, and tomatoes. Happily, a reasonable facsimile can be made at home in a few minutes, since the ingredients are readily available at your local market. The main difference between the salads you would find in Greece and this recipe is that I use much less oil in mine.

I make this salad a few hours ahead so the flavors have time to blend and develop. Refrigerate it if you make it ahead, but serve it at room temperature, taking the chill off by heating it momentarily in a microwave oven just before serving. Serve with crunchy bread.

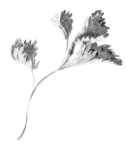

Mix all the ingredients together in a salad bowl and set aside until serving time. (You can make the salad a few hours ahead and refrigerate it, but bring it back to room temperature before serving.)

GREEK SALAD

◦ SERVES 4

16 cherry tomatoes, cut in half

4 ounces kalamata olives (about 20)

6 ounces feta cheese in brine, drained and broken into ½- to 1-inch pieces

1 red onion (about 5 ounces), peeled and sliced thin

1½ teaspoons dried oregano

½ teaspoon salt

½ teaspoon freshly ground black pepper

6 tablespoons virgin olive oil

4 teaspoons red wine vinegar

¼ cup flat leaf parsley leaves

About 4 cloves garlic, peeled and sliced thin (1½ tablespoons)

SALADE NIÇOISE

○ SERVES 6

8 cups salad greens (such as Boston, red-leaf, or romaine lettuce)

½ cup Mustard Vinaigrette (page 12)

4 large cloves garlic, peeled and sliced thin (1½ tablespoons)

6 scallions, cleaned and minced (1 cup)

¼ teaspoon salt

One 2-ounce can anchovy fillets in oil (about 12), drained

One 6½-ounce can tuna in olive oil, drained and crumbled

About 3 ripe tomatoes (1 pound total), cut into 6 wedges each

¾ pound haricot vert

3 hard-cooked eggs (see Notes), peeled and quartered

About 12 basil leaves, coarsely shredded

About 6 ounces olives (see Notes)

A traditional dish from the South of France, specifically Provence, salade Niçoise is served everywhere there, from large bistros to fancy restaurants, and the variations are practically infinite. My rendition includes canned tuna, anchovy fillets, olives, tomatoes, and basil. Make the salad according to your own taste—some versions include onions (red or yellow), cooked fava beans, artichokes, peppers, tiny string beans (haricots verts), and/or cucumbers—but always include tomatoes, garlic, olives, and greens.

This salad makes an ideal lunch. It is excellent served with pita toasts (see page 106) broken into pieces on top, or with bagel chips, but I especially like it with fougasse (page 93), the classic bread from the South of France.

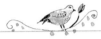

Wash the salad greens thoroughly and dry well in a salad spinner.

Place the dressing in a large bowl and stir in the garlic and scallions. Add the salad greens and salt and toss to mix well.

Arrange the salad on six plates. Decoratively arrange 2 anchovy fillets, about 2 tablespoons of the crumbled tuna, 2 or 3 tomato wedges, some haricot vert, the 2 pieces of hard-cooked egg, some shredded basil, and some of the olives on top of each serving and around the edges of each plate. You can also arrange it on a large platter to serve family-style. Serve immediately.

NOTES: To cook the eggs, bring enough water to cover them to a boil in a small saucepan. Add the eggs and simmer gently for about 10 minutes. Drain, place the eggs in ice-cold water until cool enough to handle, and then shell immediately. Cool the shelled eggs in the water until they are completely cold.

If you use tiny Niçoise olives, serve 12 olives per person; if using kalamatas, 6 per person.

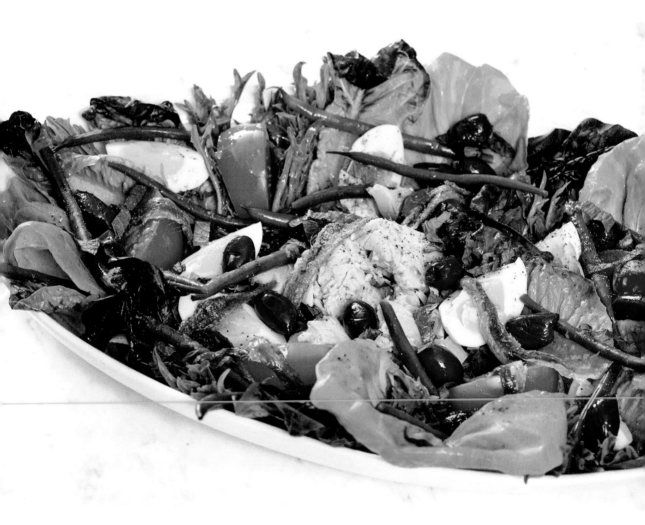

SALADE À L'AIL

∘ SERVES 4

1 head escarole (see Note)

Dressing

2 cloves garlic, peeled, crushed, and chopped fine (1 teaspoon)

1½ teaspoons Dijon-style mustard

⅛ teaspoon salt

⅛ teaspoon freshly ground black pepper

1½ teaspoons red wine vinegar

3 tablespoons virgin olive oil

Ail is the French word for garlic, which is used extensively in my cooking. Thick-ribbed and nutty, escarole has a slightly bitter taste that goes very well with the garlicky dressing in this winter salad. Unlike most green salads, this one can be seasoned up to half an hour before serving—the escarole will soften slightly in the dressing.

Remove and discard any wilted or damaged leaves from the escarole and cut the remainder into 2-inch pieces (you should have 5 to 6 cups). Wash and dry in a salad spinner. (This can be done ahead; the greens will keep in a plastic bag in the refrigerator for 4 or 5 days.)

Up to 30 minutes before serving, whisk the dressing ingredients together in your salad bowl. Add the greens and toss. Serve as you like; we usually serve it as a first course.

NOTE: Select escarole with as white a center as you can find; this indicates tenderness and a nutty flavor.

> **Unlike most green salads, this one tastes better if dressed half an hour before serving.**

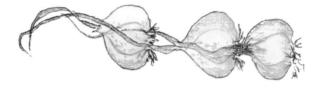

I prepare this salad often, especially when I am pressed for time or when unexpected guests drop in. It makes a great lunch.

If you keep frozen sausage in the freezer, it can be thawed quickly by sealing it in a plastic bag and submerging the bag in hot water for 10 to 15 minutes, or by microwaving it to defrost slightly. The sausage doesn't have to be completely defrosted before cooking.

Heat a charcoal or gas grill to medium heat. Prick the sausages, place them on the grill, cover, and grill for 10 to 12 minutes, turning them occasionally to brown on all sides.

While the sausages are cooking, cut the tomatoes into slices about ⅜ inch thick. Crumble the cheese into ½-inch pieces.

Toss the salad greens with the dressing in a large bowl and arrange on individual plates. Garnish with the tomato slices and scatter the cheese over the center. Sprinkle with the pepper.

When the sausages are cooked, cut each one into 4 pieces and divide them evenly among the plates, then serve.

GREEN SALAD WITH SPICY SAUSAGE

∘ SERVES 4

About 4 hot Italian-style sausages (12 ounces total)

1 large or 2 smaller very ripe tomatoes

4 ounces Manchego cheese

4 cups salad greens, preferably curly endive (called frisée), rinsed and thoroughly dried in a salad spinner

¼ cup Mustard Vinaigrette (page 12)

½ teaspoon freshly ground black pepper

CHICKEN-AVOCADO SALAD

∘ SERVES 4

Of course you can poach or sauté chicken breasts especially for this delicious main-course salad, but it's a great way to use leftover chicken. You can also use leftover turkey, roast pork, or veal. Shred the chicken (or other meat) rather than cutting it with a knife. It will absorb the dressing better.

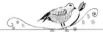

Dressing

1 tablespoon sherry vinegar

1 tablespoon dark soy sauce

1 teaspoon Worcestershire sauce

½ teaspoon Tabasco sauce

3 tablespoons safflower or corn oil

1 teaspoon sugar

½ teaspoon salt

3 scallions, cleaned and minced fine (about ½ cup)

2 cooked boneless, skinless chicken breasts (about 8 ounces; see Note)

1 small ripe avocado (about 7 ounces)

12 leaves lettuce or other greens

> **To save on time and cleanup, cut the avocado flesh into cubes while it's still in the skin.**

Prepare the dressing: Combine the vinegar, soy sauce, Worcestershire, Tabasco, oil, sugar, and salt in a large bowl and blend thoroughly. Stir in the scallions.

Shred the chicken by pulling it apart along the grain into narrow strips. Add it to the dressing and toss well.

Make an incision around the avocado lengthwise, cutting through to the pit, and twist the ends in opposite directions until the halves separate. Remove the pit. Using a sharp knife, slice through the flesh clear to the skin every ½ inch one way and then the other, creating a checkerboard pattern in both halves. Using a spoon, scoop out the cubes of avocado and add them to the bowl. Toss gently with the chicken and dressing.

Divide the lettuce leaves among individual plates, arrange the chicken-avocado salad on top, and serve.

NOTE: If the chicken has been refrigerated, heat it in a microwave oven for 20 to 30 seconds to take the chill off.

Leftover turkey is never very satisfying when it's reheated in its own gravy or in a sauce—try this flavorful salad instead. Or, if you want sandwiches for lunch, omit the tomatoes, add some Spicy Cucumber Relish (page 17), and fill pita breads with the mixture.

TURKEY SALAD

If the turkey is very cold, heat it in a microwave oven for 30 to 40 seconds to bring it to room temperature. Shred it into narrow strips (it will absorb the dressing better than if you cut it into cubes).

Place the shredded turkey in a bowl, add the remaining ingredients except the tomatoes and watercress, and mix well. Arrange the tomato slices on individual salad plates and mound the turkey salad on top. Garnish with watercress and serve.

> **If cooked meat is shredded rather than sliced or cubed, it will absorb a salad dressing better.**

> **This spicy salad will use up that leftover turkey—and it makes great sandwiches too.**

1 pound cooked turkey (white or dark meat)

¾ cup diced (¼-inch pieces) red onion

3 scallions, cleaned and minced fine (½ cup)

2 cloves garlic, peeled, crushed, and chopped fine (1 teaspoon)

¾ cup mayonnaise

2 tablespoons cider vinegar

1 tablespoon Dijon-style mustard, preferably "hot"

1 teaspoon salt

1 teaspoon freshly ground black pepper

1 teaspoon sugar

1 teaspoon Sriracha or other hot sauce

2 large ripe tomatoes (1 pound total), sliced thin (about 18 slices)

Watercress, for garnish

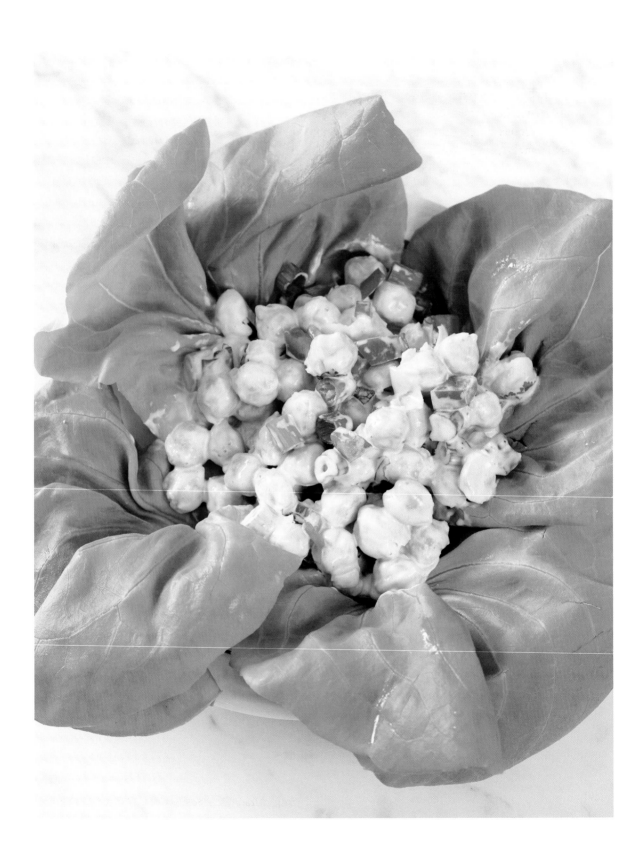

Canned chickpeas (also called garbanzo beans) are an excellent substitute for the dried version, which require a long cooking time. They do beg for seasoning, however—as in this highly flavored salad.

Mix all the ingredients together in a bowl. Serve at room temperature.

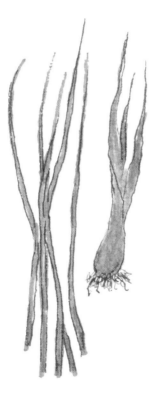

CHICKPEA SALAD

◦ SERVES 4

One 16-ounce can chickpeas, drained (2 cups)

3 tablespoons Spicy Red Salsa (page 13), or 1½ tablespoons Sriracha or other hot sauce

¼ cup mayonnaise

3 scallions, cleaned and minced fine (about ⅓ cup)

1 large clove garlic, peeled, crushed, and chopped (about 1 teaspoon)

¼ cup coarsely chopped cilantro

¼ teaspoon salt

RED PEPPER, ARTICHOKE, AND OLIVE SALAD

∘ SERVES 6

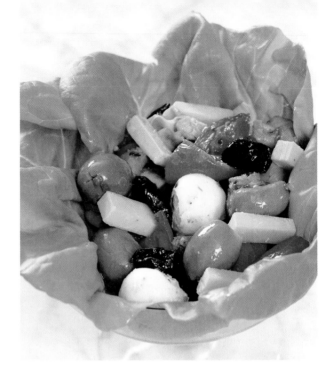

1½ cups marinated artichoke hearts in oil (6 ounces)

1 cup green olives, such as salad olives (sometimes stuffed with pimentos)

1 cup marinated mushrooms

1 cup sliced pimentos (6 ounces)

1 cup ½-inch pieces spicy cheddar cheese

½ teaspoon freshly ground black pepper

3 tablespoons virgin olive oil

2 tablespoons flat-leaf parsley leaves

1 teaspoon chopped hot chile pepper, such as jalapeño, or ½ teaspoon hot pepper flakes

1 head Boston lettuce, leaves separated

I often prepare this salad when I am pressed for time because all the ingredients except the cheese and parsley are available at the salad bar at most supermarkets. It can be made ahead or assembled at the last moment. Leftovers will keep, refrigerated, for more than a week and are great stuffed into sandwiches, with or without a meat filling.

Serve this with crusty country bread and a chilled red wine.

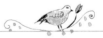

Mix all the ingredients together in a bowl. Serve the salad in the lettuce leaves.

> Most of the ingredients for this salad come from the salad bar or deli department at the supermarket, so it couldn't be easier to make.

I first made this salad when vacationing in a small town called Faro in the south of Portugal. It takes only a few minutes to combine all the ingredients for this salad, especially if you use the presliced, prewashed mushrooms that are available in most supermarkets. Do prepare it ahead so the mushrooms can marinate in the dressing. A terrific first course, it is also a great accompaniment for broiled or sautéed fish or meat.

Stir all the ingredients together in a bowl and let marinate for 30 minutes. Serve immediately, or set aside until serving time. This salad can be made up to 1 day ahead and refrigerated, but it should be served at room temperature.

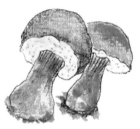

MUSHROOM SALAD FARO

◦ SERVES 4

About 2½ cups diced or sliced (½-inch) cremini mushrooms (8 ounces)

1 tablespoon white wine vinegar

2 tablespoons safflower or corn oil

2 teaspoons toasted sesame oil

1 tablespoon light soy sauce

1 teaspoon dry mustard

½ teaspoon sugar

¼ teaspoon salt

¼ teaspoon freshly ground black pepper

12 mint leaves, shredded

2 tablespoons toasted sesame seeds

MOZZARELLA AND CILANTRO SALAD

∘ SERVES 4

4 ounces best-quality mozzarella cheese, cut into ½-inch-thick slices and then into ½-inch-wide sticks

4 scallions, cleaned and cut into ½-inch pieces (¾ cup)

1 small sweet onion (like Vidalia), peeled and cut into ½-inch cubes

About 10 ounces yellow cherry tomatoes, halved (2 cups)

1 cup cilantro leaves

3 tablespoons virgin olive oil

1 tablespoon red wine vinegar

½ teaspoon salt

½ teaspoon freshly ground black pepper

This salad can be made up to an hour ahead, and in fact the flavor improves if you do so, since that gives the dressing time to penetrate the other ingredients and season them well. Serve as a first course with some crunchy bread.

I love the taste of fresh cilantro, also called coriander or Chinese/Japanese parsley. If you find it too assertive, try parsley, basil, chervil, or chives instead in this fresh-tasting salad.

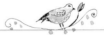

Up to 1 hour before serving, toss all the ingredients together in a salad bowl. Serve at room temperature.

> **For the best flavor, prepare this salad up to an hour ahead. Combine the ingredients right in your serving bowl.**

COLESLAW

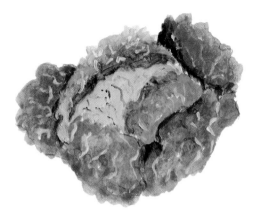

∘ SERVES 4

4 cups shredded savoy cabbage

1 cup shredded carrots (shredded on a box grater)

¼ cup sour cream

¼ cup mayonnaise

1½ tablespoons cider vinegar

1 tablespoon poppy seeds

1 teaspoon Tabasco sauce

1 teaspoon sugar

¾ teaspoon salt

Classic American coleslaw doesn't exist in France. I discovered it first when I was working at Howard Johnson's. It is certainly a standard at our house now, and Gloria wouldn't hear of having a steamed lobster without coleslaw.

This recipe duplicates somewhat, according to my memory, the coleslaw of the Howard Johnson restaurants. My preference is for savoy cabbage, but regular cabbage will work as well.

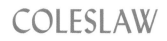

A few hours ahead of serving, mix all the ingredients together thoroughly in a large bowl and refrigerate. Serve cold.

WARM POTATO SALAD

◦ SERVES 4

1½ pounds cooked potatoes
(see Basic Boiled Potatoes,
page 170)

¼ cup mayonnaise

1½ tablespoons Dijon-style
mustard, preferably "hot"

2 teaspoons white wine vinegar
or rice vinegar

½ teaspoon Worcestershire sauce

½ teaspoon salt

½ teaspoon freshly ground
black pepper

4 scallions, cleaned and minced
(about ⅔ cup)

½ cup chopped mild onion,
such as Vidalia

This salad makes use of cooked potatoes. If the potatoes are cold, slice them and then reheat them slightly in a microwave oven for 20 to 30 seconds. The flavor is much better if the salad is not ice-cold.

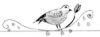

Scrape the skin from the potatoes and cut them into ¼-inch-thick slices. Rewarm them if necessary (see headnote) and place in a serving bowl. Mix in the mayonnaise, mustard, vinegar, Worcestershire, salt, pepper, scallions, and onion. Serve.

> **You can use leftover boiled potatoes
> in this tangy salad.**

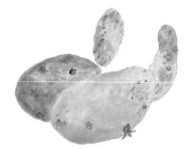

Moist smoked bluefish is available at many markets and is inexpensive. You could also use smoked salmon or another smoked fish. This salad is best served at room temperature. If you prepare it ahead and refrigerate it, reheat it for 45 seconds or so in a microwave or for a few minutes in a conventional oven to take the chill off.

Remove the eyes and any damaged parts of the potatoes. Wash the potatoes under cold running water, place in a pot, and cover with cold water. Bring to a boil and boil gently until tender, 20 to 25 minutes. Drain immediately, so the moisture remaining on the potatoes will evaporate because of their heat.

When the potatoes are cool enough to handle, cut them, with the skin, into ½-inch-thick slices, trying to keep the slices intact. As you slice them, spread the potatoes out in a large gratin dish or on a tray. (They are less likely to break and are easier to toss when arranged like this in a single layer.)

Remove the skin from the bluefish and peel off and discard the very dark flesh just under the skin. Flake the fish into ½-inch pieces (about 2 cups).

Add the fish to the potatoes. Add the scallions, garlic, chives, olive and peanut oils, vinegar, soy sauce, salt, and pepper. Toss lightly and cover with plastic wrap so that the wrap lies directly on the salad. Let stand for at least 30 minutes at room temperature or for 3 to 4 hours in the refrigerator.

Serve at room temperature. Place in a bowl to serve or serve in individual portions.

POTATO AND SMOKED BLUEFISH SALAD

∘ SERVES 6

2 pounds small round red or new yellow potatoes

12 ounces smoked bluefish

4 or 5 scallions, cleaned and minced (¾ cup)

2 cloves garlic, peeled, crushed, and chopped fine (about 1 teaspoon)

⅓ cup chopped chives

¼ cup olive oil

¼ cup peanut oil

3 tablespoons red wine vinegar

1 tablespoon dark soy sauce

1 teaspoon salt

1½ teaspoons freshly ground black pepper

CRABMEAT SALAD

∘ SERVES 4

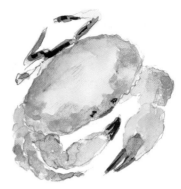

8 ounces cooked crabmeat, drained

1 rib celery from the heart (as white as possible), rinsed and cut into ¼-inch pieces (about ¼ cup)

1 clove garlic, peeled and chopped fine (about ½ teaspoon)

1 small mild onion, such as Vidalia, peeled and chopped (about ¼ cup)

¼ cup mayonnaise

1 teaspoon Sriracha or other hot sauce

1 tablespoon white rice vinegar

⅛ teaspoon freshly ground black pepper

8 small lettuce leaves, preferably Boston

This is an easy recipe, since cooked crabmeat is available from most fishmongers (try to get large lump crab). Serve this rich first-course salad at room temperature in lettuce-leaf cups.

Combine all the ingredients except the lettuce in a bowl and mix gently.

Arrange the lettuce leaves on four small plates and divide the salad among the plates, piling it on top of the lettuce. Serve immediately.

> Buy cooked crabmeat from your fishmonger for this simple but delicious salad.

For a change in texture, look, and bite, try this Asian-influenced pasta salad. You can prepare it ahead and keep it in the refrigerator for several days.

Bring 3 to 4 quarts water to a boil in a large pot. Drop the noodles into the water and stir well to separate the strands. Return the water to a boil and boil for just 3½ to 4 minutes. Immediately drain the noodles in a colander and sprinkle with cold water to stop the cooking. Allow the noodles to sit in the colander to dry for at least 10 minutes.

Using a slotted spoon, remove the solids from the mushroom, tomato, and nut mix. Coarsely chop, by hand or in a food processor, into ¼-inch pieces and place in a bowl. Add ⅓ cup of the oil from the mix and stir in the salt, chili oil, and cilantro. Add the rice noodles and toss until well coated. Serve immediately, or cover and set aside to serve later. The salad will keep for 2 to 3 days in the refrigerator; bring back to room temperature before serving.

TANGY RICE NOODLE SALAD

∘ SERVES 6

1 pound rice stick noodles

2 cups Mushroom, Tomato, and Nut Mix (page 19; do not drain)

1 teaspoon salt

1 teaspoon hot chili oil

½ cup shredded cilantro leaves

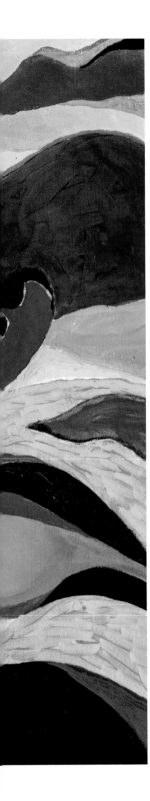

SOUPS

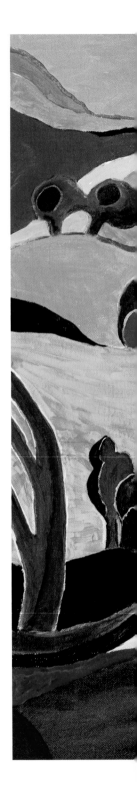

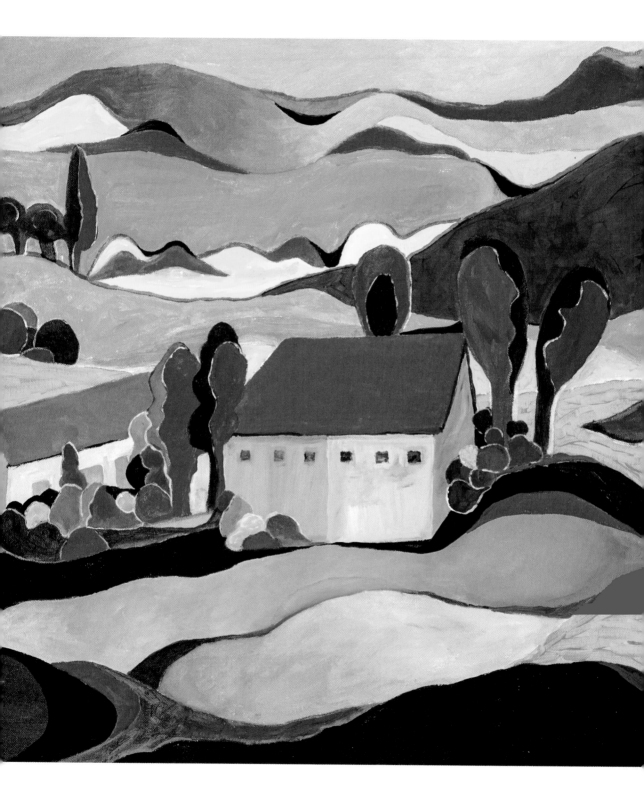

BORSCHT

SERVES 6 (MAKES 9 CUPS)

1 tablespoon unsalted butter

1 onion (4 ounces), peeled and sliced thin (about 1 cup)

4 cups shredded savoy cabbage (6 ounces)

1 carrot, peeled and shredded (about 1 cup)

6 cups Basic Chicken Stock (page 15) or canned chicken broth

One 16-ounce can sliced beets

1 cup sour cream

2 tablespoons grated fresh or bottled horseradish

1 teaspoon salt, or to taste

½ teaspoon freshly ground black pepper

1½ tablespoons cider vinegar

2 tablespoons chopped dill, for garnish

> **Cover your cutting board with plastic wrap to prevent it from becoming discolored when you cut the beets.**

Many people love borscht but don't often make it because it takes so long to cook the beets, the main ingredient in this classic Russian soup. To hurry things along, I use canned sliced beets, which are already cooked. I add shredded savoy cabbage to the borscht, and I especially like it served with sour cream mixed with a little grated horseradish. You can, of course, use fresh beets if you prefer, but instead of cooking them whole and unpeeled—the standard way—peel and shred them first so they'll cook faster.

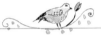

Melt the butter in a large stainless steel saucepan. Add the onion, cabbage, and carrot and sauté over high heat for about 5 minutes, until the vegetables have wilted but not browned. Add the chicken stock and bring to a boil, then reduce the heat and boil gently for 4 to 5 minutes.

Meanwhile, drain the beets, reserving the juice. Arrange the beets in stacks on a piece of plastic wrap spread out on a cutting board and slice into julienne strips about ¼ inch wide.

Add the beets, the reserved beet juice, the salt, pepper, and vinegar to the stock and return to a boil.

Stir together the sour cream and horseradish in a small bowl.

Divide the soup among six bowls. Garnish each with 1 tablespoon of the sour cream mixture and 1 teaspoon of the dill. Serve.

NOTE: This can also be served cold, with the garnish.

This is a family favorite. If you have homemade chicken stock or canned broth, a little leftover bread, and some good Gruyère on hand, it can be prepared in a matter of minutes.

I toast the bread and shred the cheese ahead, then arrange them in the soup bowls while I heat the stock. Pour the boiling stock over the toast and cheese, and the soup is ready!

Bring the chicken stock to a strong boil in a medium saucepan, then add the salt and pepper.

Meanwhile, break the toast into pieces and place the equivalent of 1 slice in each of four soup bowls. Divide the cheese among the bowls.

Pour the boiling stock on top of the toast and cheese and serve immediately.

> **With three basic items in your larder—chicken stock, bread, and cheese—you can make this delicious soup in a few minutes.**

BREAD AND CHEESE SOUP

○ SERVES 4 (MAKES 6 CUPS)

6 cups Basic Chicken Stock (page 15) or canned chicken broth

Salt to taste

½ teaspoon freshly ground black pepper

4 slices bread (4 ounces), toasted

4 ounces Gruyère cheese, shredded (1 cup)

BUTTERNUT SQUASH SOUP

○ SERVES 6 (MAKES 8 CUPS)

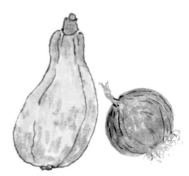

2 tablespoons unsalted butter

4 scallions, minced (⅔ cup)

1 onion, peeled and cut into
½-inch dice (¾ cup)

1 carrot (4 ounces), peeled and
cut into ¼-inch dice (¾ cup)

3 cups Basic Chicken Stock
(page 15) or canned chicken broth

2 cups apple cider, preferably
unfiltered

1 butternut squash (about
1½ pounds), halved lengthwise,
peeled, seeded, and cut into
½-inch dice (4 cups), or 1 pound
frozen cubed squash

1 teaspoon salt, or to taste

½ teaspoon freshly ground
black pepper

¼ teaspoon ground nutmeg

I usually make this soup with fresh butternut squash, but frozen cubed squash works quite well if you are in a hurry. The soup is cooked with apple cider, which gives it an appealingly sweet taste.

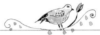

Melt the butter in a large saucepan. Add the scallions, onion, and carrot and sauté over high heat for about 3 minutes, then add the stock, cider, and squash. Bring the mixture to a boil, cover, reduce the heat, and simmer gently for 25 minutes.

Mix in the salt, pepper, and nutmeg and serve immediately.

▷ **If you're in a hurry, use frozen cubed squash from the supermarket.**

This is my daughter's and granddaughter's favorite soup, and Claudine always asked her grandmother to make it when she visited us from France. It is made with the very fine pasta called angel hair that comes in nestlike bundles. Once the stock has come to a boil, the pasta cooks very quickly, so the whole soup can be prepared in a little more than 10 minutes.

Pour the stock and water into a medium pot and bring to a boil over high heat. Add the scallions and cook for 1 minute. Break the pasta bundles into strings (so they don't form a block as they cook) and add to the boiling stock. Stir to separate the strands, and boil gently for 4 to 5 minutes.

Add the salt and pepper to the soup, and serve immediately, sprinkled with the cheese, if desired.

NOTE: This soup can be made ahead and reheated at serving time.

▷ **Most of the time required to make this soup is spent waiting for the chicken stock to come to a boil.**

SOUPE AU VERMICELLE

○ SERVES 4 (MAKES 5 CUPS)

4 cups Basic Chicken Stock (page 15) or canned chicken broth

1 cup water

5 scallions, cleaned and minced (about ¾ cup)

4 ounces capelli d'angelo (angel hair) pasta or vermicelli in bundles

Salt to taste

¼ teaspoon freshly ground black pepper

½ cup grated Swiss cheese

CHUNKY VEGETABLE SOUP

∘ SERVES 6 TO 8
(MAKES 10 CUPS)

1 onion (about 4 ounces), peeled

1 rib celery (about 2 ounces), rinsed

4 scallions, cleaned

2 tablespoons unsalted butter

1 tablespoon olive oil

2 carrots (about 4 ounces), peeled

1 zucchini (about 7 ounces), trimmed and rinsed

1 white turnip (about 3 ounces), peeled

A wedge of cabbage (about 4 ounces)

2 or 3 potatoes (8 ounces total), peeled

1½ teaspoons salt

7 cups water

3 cloves garlic, peeled

About ½ cup flat-leaf parsley or basil leaves, or a mixture

2 tablespoons extra-virgin olive oil

½ teaspoon freshly ground black pepper

This soup is made with water, which retains the flavors of the vegetables better than chicken stock would. I used onion, celery, scallions, carrots, zucchini, turnips, cabbage, and potatoes when I first made the soup because I had them on hand; you can use the same assortment or substitute other vegetables you have in your refrigerator or freezer.

After they are peeled or cleaned, the vegetables are thinly sliced in the food processor. The herbs and garlic are prepared in the processor as well, and there's no need to wash the bowl between uses. The herb-garlic garnish is added to the soup just before serving to give it a fresh flavor.

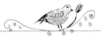

Fit a food processor with the 1-millimeter slicing blade and use it to slice the onion, celery, and scallions. Or coarsely chop by hand.

Heat the butter and oil in a large stockpot. When the mixture is hot, add the sliced vegetables and sauté for about 3 minutes.

Meanwhile, slice the remaining vegetables in the food processor or by hand. Add to the stockpot, along with the salt and water, and bring to a boil. Cover, reduce the heat, and boil gently for 20 minutes.

Meanwhile, fit the food processor with the chopping blade, combine the garlic, parsley, and olive oil in the bowl, and process to mince the garlic and parsley, or mince the garlic and herbs by hand, then stir in the oil.

Add the herb mixture to the soup and mix well, season with the pepper, and serve.

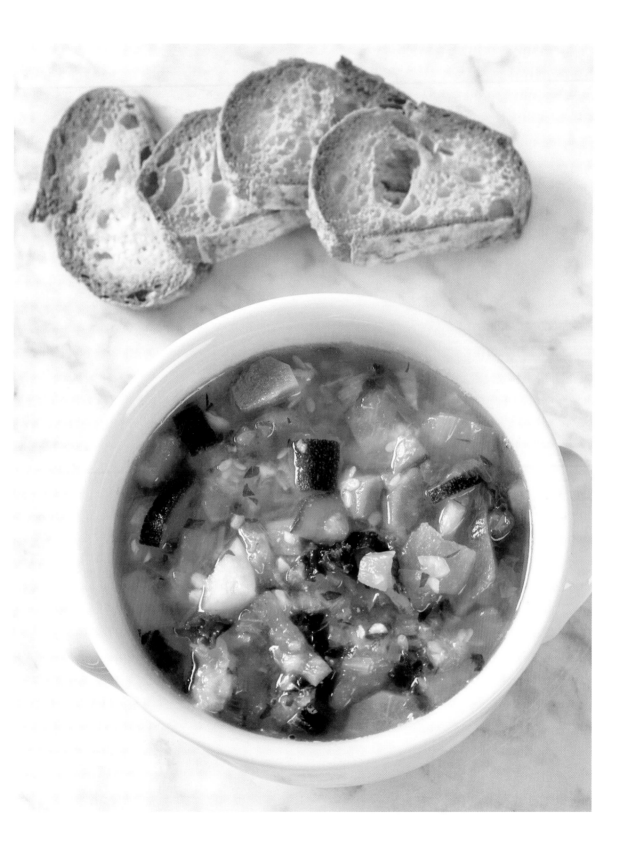

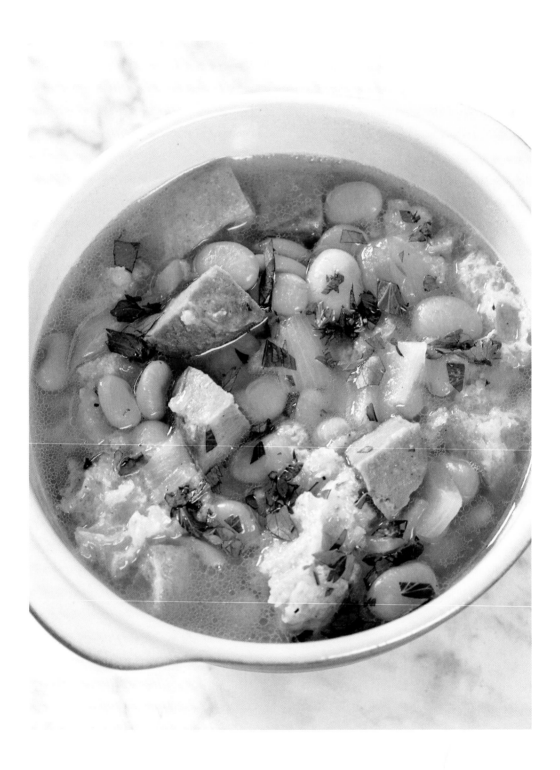

Lima beans are the main ingredient in this soup, but it can be made with another kind of canned bean if limas are not to your liking. It is quite flavorful, hearty, and filling—and the ingredients are common enough that you might even have them on hand for quick assembly when unexpected guests appear. I keep kielbasa sausage in the freezer specifically for soups such as this, and I usually have some stale leftover bread or rolls that I can use as a thickening agent.

Heat the oil in a large saucepan. When it is hot, add the sausage and onion and sauté, covered (to prevent splatters), over medium to high heat for about 3 minutes. Add the lima beans, with their liquid, the stock, bread pieces, pepper, and salt to taste and bring to a boil. Cover, reduce the heat, and boil gently for about 2 minutes.

Stir the soup well and serve sprinkled with the parsley.

> **Use stale leftover bread or rolls in this simple, hearty soup.**

LIMA BEAN, SAUSAGE, AND BREAD SOUP

◦ SERVES 4 (MAKES 6 CUPS)

1 tablespoon corn oil

5 ounces kielbasa sausage, cut into ½-inch pieces

1 onion (about 4 ounces), peeled and sliced thin (¾ cup)

One 16-ounce can lima beans

3½ cups Basic Chicken Stock (page 15) or canned chicken broth

2 ounces dried-out bread or rolls, broken into pieces (about 1½ cups)

Salt

¼ teaspoon freshly ground black pepper

1 tablespoon chopped flat-leaf parsley

BEAN AND HAM SOUP

∘ SERVES 6 (MAKES 5 CUPS)

1 tablespoon virgin olive oil

2 scallions, cleaned and minced
(⅓ cup)

½ cup chopped onion

½ teaspoon dried thyme

2 cups Basic Chicken Stock
(page 15) or canned chicken broth

One 16-ounce can white kidney
beans

1 slice cooked ham (about
2 ounces), cut into ½-inch pieces

⅛ teaspoon freshly ground
black pepper

Croutons (page 40), for garnish
(optional)

If you have a can of beans on your shelf and a piece of ham in your freezer or refrigerator, you can make this earthy, satisfying soup in just a few minutes. I use white kidney beans, but another type can be substituted. The soup has a chicken stock base and is flavored with scallions and thyme. Add some croutons for a heartier version.

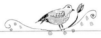

Heat the olive oil in a large saucepan. When the oil is hot, add the scallions, onion, and thyme and cook gently for about 30 seconds. Add the stock and bring to a boil.

Meanwhile, place the kidney beans and their liquid in a food processor and process for 5 to 10 seconds. The mixture will not be completely smooth; little pieces of bean should still be visible throughout.

Add the beans and ham to the stock and bring the mixture to a boil. Stir in the pepper, sprinkle with croutons, if desired, and serve.

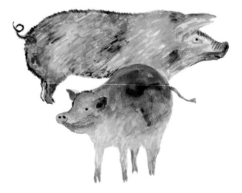

A very filling soup that makes a meal with the addition of a salad. I use codfish in this earthy, wholesome chowder because I like its thick white fillets, but if you don't like cod or can't find it at your supermarket, substitute fillets of haddock or another type of white fish.

Because this recipe involves a little work—dicing the pork, fish, and vegetables—I like to make enough to serve a large party at one sitting or a small group at two or three meals. (The chowder will keep, refrigerated, for 4 or 5 days.) If you use frozen hash-brown potatoes and frozen corn, you will eliminate much of the work and the soup can be prepared from start to finish in no more than 30 minutes.

Place the salt pork pieces in a large pot and cook over high heat for 5 to 6 minutes, until they are crisp and nicely browned and have rendered most of their fat. Add the onion and leek and sauté for 1 minute. Stir in the thyme, chicken stock, water, and potatoes and bring the mixture to a boil. Reduce the heat, cover, and boil gently for 15 minutes.

Add the corn kernels and fish to the pot and return to a boil. Cover, reduce the heat, and boil gently for about 1 minute. Add the cream, salt, and pepper and return to a boil, then remove from the heat. Serve immediately.

CORN, COD, AND POTATO CHOWDER

∘ SERVES 8 TO 10
(MAKES ABOUT 10 CUPS)

3 ounces salt pork, pancetta, or bacon, cut into ½-inch pieces

1 cup diced (½-inch pieces) onion

1 small leek, cleaned and cut into ¼-inch pieces (about 1 cup)

1 teaspoon dried thyme

5 cups Basic Chicken Stock (page 15) or canned chicken broth

1 cup water

12 ounces potatoes, peeled and cut into ½-inch dice, or 3 cups frozen hash-brown potatoes

1½ cups fresh or frozen corn kernels

1 pound codfish fillets, cut into 1-inch pieces

½ cup heavy cream

½ teaspoon salt, or to taste

½ teaspoon freshly ground black pepper

CLAM OR OYSTER AND CORN CHOWDER

∘ SERVES 6

2 tablespoons olive oil

3 cups thinly sliced leeks

½ cup water

1 teaspoon chopped garlic

5 cups milk

1 tablespoon potato starch, dissolved in 3 tablespoons water

1½ teaspoons salt

1½ teaspoons freshly ground black pepper

24 clams or oysters, shucked, juices reserved

2 cups fresh corn kernels (from 2 ears)

1 tablespoon chopped chives

I learned about New England clam chowder when I worked at Howard Johnson's. I make my recipe with milk, but for a richer version, some cream can be added.

This chowder can be made with either oysters or clams. The key is to make the base of the soup ahead and then cook the clams or oysters and corn kernels at the last moment, just before serving. This keeps the shellfish tender and moist.

I freeze the clams or oysters for about 15 minutes in the shell to make shucking easier. After shucking, I like to "wash" the clams or oysters in their own juices: I transfer them to a clean bowl and slowly pour the juices back over them after discarding any sediment or pieces of shell in the bottom of the first bowl.

Heat the olive oil in a large saucepan. Add the leeks and cook for 1 minute, then stir well, add the water, and cook, uncovered, over high heat until the water has boiled away. Add the garlic and mix well, then add the milk and bring to a boil. Add the dissolved potato starch, mix well, and the soup will thicken. Turn off the heat, then add the salt and pepper. If not serving immediately, remove from the heat. (Note: This can be done a few hours ahead.)

Place the clams in the freezer for 15 minutes to help in shucking, then shuck them, placing them in a bowl with their own juices. If the clams are large, they can be halved with scissors. "Wash" them in their juices, then transfer them to a clean bowl and slowly pour the juices over them, discarding any sediment at the bottom of the first bowl.

At serving time, bring the soup back to a boil and add the corn, clams, and the clams' juices. Mix well and bring the mixture barely to a boil, then remove from the heat. Serve immediately, sprinkled with the chives.

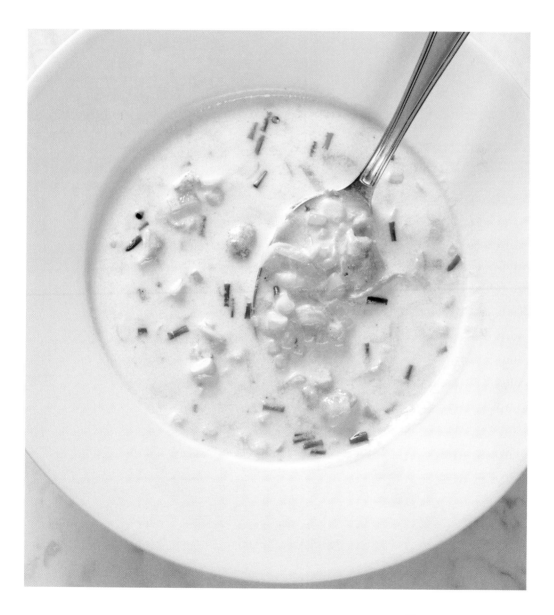

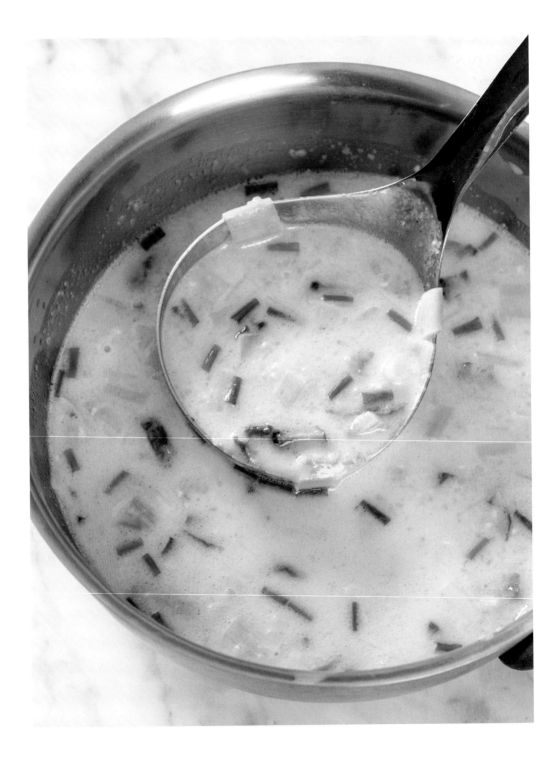

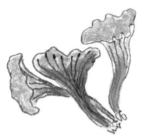

MUSHROOM SOUP

◦ SERVES 4 (MAKES 6 CUPS)

2 tablespoons unsalted butter

8 ounces cleaned mushrooms, coarsely chopped

1 small leek, cleaned and sliced thin (about 1 cup), or 1 cup thinly sliced scallions

4 cups Basic Chicken Stock (page 15) or canned chicken broth

¼ cup yellow cornmeal or yellow grits

1 cup light cream

1 teaspoon salt, or to taste

¼ teaspoon freshly ground black pepper

1 tablespoon chopped chives

If you use packaged sliced fresh mushrooms from the supermarket, this robust soup can be prepared in 10 minutes. The soup is thickened with cornmeal, which cooks quickly.

Heat the butter in a large saucepan. When the butter is hot, add the mushrooms and leek and cook over high heat for about 3 minutes. Add the stock and bring to a boil. Using a whisk, mix in the cornmeal. Cover, reduce the heat, and simmer for about 5 minutes.

Add the cream, salt, and pepper and bring to a boil, then remove from the heat. Serve immediately, sprinkled with the chives.

CREAM OF PUMPKIN SOUP

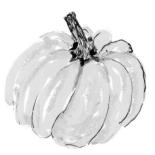

◦ SERVES 4 (MAKES 6 CUPS)

One 16-ounce can pure pumpkin puree

2½ cups Basic Chicken Stock (page 15) or canned chicken broth

1 cup light cream

1 tablespoon honey

1 teaspoon salt, or to taste

¼ teaspoon freshly ground black pepper

¼ teaspoon curry powder

Croutons (page 40), for garnish (optional)

The main ingredient in this elegant soup is a can of pumpkin puree. With some chicken stock and cream at hand, you can combine all the ingredients directly in the saucepan, and the soup will be ready in minutes. Serve with or without croutons, as you prefer.

Place all the ingredients in a saucepan, mix well, and bring to a boil. Divide the soup among four soup bowls, sprinkle with croutons, if desired, and serve immediately.

I make this delicious soup with the cooking liquid from Leeks Vinaigrette (page 160). Another vegetable stock or chicken stock can be substituted if you don't have leek cooking liquid. Each version will have its own distinctive flavor.

The soup is thickened with Cream of Wheat, but you can use tapioca, semolina, or even oat flakes instead. This easy, quick, comforting soup is also good reheated (you may want to dilute it with a little water or milk).

Bring the leek cooking liquid to a boil in a saucepan, then whisk in the chicken base and Cream of Wheat. Return to a boil and boil gently for about 3 minutes.

Stir in the cream and taste for seasonings. If the chicken base did not add sufficient salt for your taste, add a dash of salt, along with pepper. Ladle into soup bowls and sprinkle with the chives. Serve immediately.

CREAM OF LEEK SOUP

○ SERVES 4 (MAKES 5 CUPS)

4 cups cooking liquid from Leeks Vinaigrette (page 160) or vegetable or chicken stock

1 tablespoon organic chicken base (omit if using chicken stock)

½ cup Instant Cream of Wheat, semolina, or oat flakes

½ cup heavy cream

Salt and freshly ground black pepper

1 tablespoon chopped chives, for garnish

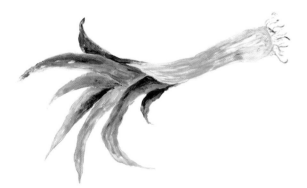

POTATO AND LEEK SOUP

○ SERVES 6 (MAKES 6½ CUPS)

2 leeks (about 6 ounces)

1 onion (about 4 ounces), peeled and cut into 4 to 6 pieces

2 cups water

3⅓ cups Basic Chicken Stock (page 15) or canned chicken broth

1 tablespoon unsalted butter

1 tablespoon olive oil

1 pound frozen hash-brown potatoes (about 3 cups), defrosted, or 3 cups diced, peeled potatoes

Salt

½ teaspoon freshly ground black pepper

1½ cups broken pita toasts (see page 106), for garnish

My favorite soup is made of potatoes and leeks, sometimes with the addition of onion. Now and then I make a coarser version, cutting the potato, leek, and onion into chunks and serving it as a chunky soup, but in its classic form, the soup is pureed. It is traditionally made with a combination of stock and water, although it could be made exclusively with one or the other.

Conventionally, for a cream soup like this one, the vegetables are cooked first and then pureed. In this easy version, puree the vegetables before cooking. I also use frozen hash-brown potatoes, which come already diced, eliminating another step.

Chilled, the soup can easily be transformed into the famous vichyssoise with the addition of cream and chives for another quick and satisfying dish.

Don't waste expensive leeks—use most of the leek, except one or two outside tough leaves.

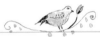

To clean the leeks, remove and discard the roots. Do not discard the entire green area: Instead, remove the outer dark green layer of leaves, which is often damaged and usually fibrous and tough, then cut away any dark or damaged inner leaves. Do not remove leaves that are lighter in color (an indication of tenderness). Preparing leeks this way enables you to use most of the leeks and avoids waste.

Cut the leeks into pieces and rinse thoroughly in a sieve. Place in a food processor, add the onion and ½ cup of the water, and process for 15 to 20 seconds, until pureed. Transfer the puree to a soup pot and add the chicken stock, butter, and olive oil. Bring to a boil.

Meanwhile, combine the potatoes with 1 cup of the water in the food processor and process until smooth. Add this to the mixture in the pot, along with the remaining ½ cup water and the pepper and salt to taste. Bring the mixture back to a boil, then cover the pot, lower the heat, and boil gently for about 15 minutes. The soup will be slightly grainy but creamy and a lovely light green color.

Divide the soup among six bowls and garnish with the pita toasts.

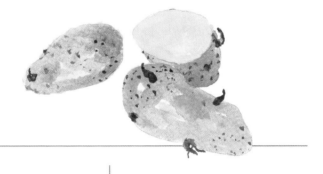

Vichyssoise

Stir the cream, salt to taste, and half the chives into the cold soup. Divide among six soup bowls, sprinkle the remaining chives on top, and serve.

• SERVES 6 (MAKES 7½ CUPS)

1 cup heavy cream

Salt

3 tablespoons chopped chives

Potato and Leek Soup (opposite), chilled

TOMATO SOUP WITH CHIVES

○ SERVES 6 (MAKES 7 CUPS)

2 tablespoons olive oil

2 tablespoons canola or safflower oil

3 onions (12 ounces total), peeled and cut into 1-inch pieces (2 cups)

1 teaspoon herbes de Provence (see Note, page 15)

3 large cloves garlic, peeled and crushed

1 rib celery, rinsed and diced (about ¼ cup)

3 pounds tomatoes, cut into 2-inch chunks, or 1½ (28-ounce) cans Italian plum tomatoes

1⅔ cups Basic Chicken Stock (page 15) or canned chicken broth

1 teaspoon sugar

½ teaspoon salt, or to taste

½ teaspoon freshly ground black pepper

3 tablespoons unsalted butter

2 tablespoons chopped chives, for garnish

2 cups Croutons (page 40)

As with most recipes that call for tomatoes, this soup is best made in a stainless steel pan; that prevents discoloration of the pan and ensures that the tomatoes retain their bright red color. Rather than puree the uncooked tomatoes in a food processor and then strain them through a sieve, I prefer to press the cooked soup through a food mill to remove the tomato seeds and skins. (The best food mills are plastic or stainless steel and have removable bottom screens. They are inexpensive and very useful.) You can substitute canned Italian plum tomatoes for fresh here with good results.

The soup is enriched by the addition of 3 tablespoons of butter just before serving. You can substitute an equal amount of olive oil, or a mixture of olive oil and butter, if you prefer, or eliminate this final addition altogether.

If you eliminate the stock in this recipe, you will have a good standard tomato sauce for pasta and other dishes.

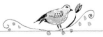

Heat the oils in a large stainless steel saucepan. When the oils are hot, add the onions, herbes de Provence, garlic, and celery and cook over medium to high heat for about 5 minutes. Stir in the tomatoes (with their liquid, if using), chicken stock, sugar, salt, and pepper and bring to a boil over high heat. Reduce the heat to medium, cover, and cook for about 10 minutes.

Remove from the heat. With a handheld immersion blender, puree the soup directly in the saucepan. Whisk in the butter. Divide the soup among six bowls, garnish with the chives, and serve topped with croutons.

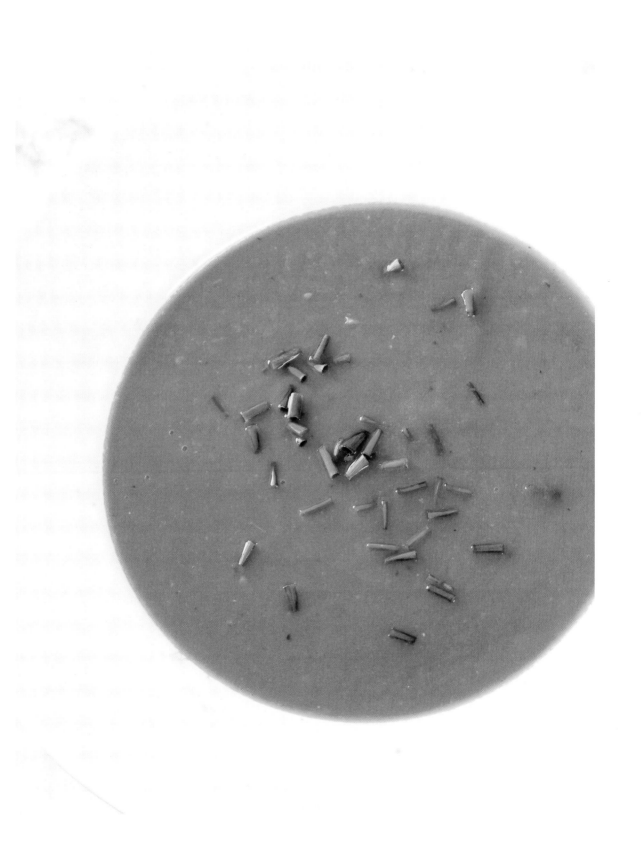

COLD RAW TOMATO SOUP

○ SERVES 6 (MAKES 5 CUPS)

3 pounds very ripe tomatoes

1 teaspoon thyme leaves (optional)

1 teaspoon Tabasco sauce

1½ teaspoons salt

½ teaspoon freshly ground black pepper

¼ cup extra-virgin olive oil

2 tablespoons red wine vinegar

¼ cup shredded basil leaves, plus 6 whole leaves for garnish

1 cup sour cream, for garnish

This is a favorite at our house. For best results, use very ripe, fleshy summer tomatoes. A food mill allows you to remove the skin and seeds from the pureed soup more easily than with a conventional sieve. This also makes a great base for Bloody Marys, and it can be used as a sauce for a cold pasta salad.

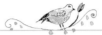

Cut the tomatoes into pieces and puree them in a food processor. If you object to a few seeds remaining in the mixture, strain the puree through a food mill fitted with a fine-mesh screen into a bowl (you should have about 5 cups).

Stir the thyme, Tabasco, salt, pepper, olive oil, vinegar, and shredded basil into the soup. If not serving immediately, set aside in a cool place or refrigerate.

At serving time, divide the soup among six bowls and garnish each with a dollop of sour cream and a whole basil leaf.

HOT CREAM OF TOMATO SOUP

Puree and strain the tomatoes as described, and pour the puree into a saucepan. Add the thyme, Tabasco, salt, pepper, oil, and vinegar, bring to a boil, and boil for 30 seconds. Stir in 1 cup heavy cream and heat through.

Divide the soup among six soup plates, sprinkle with ½ cup shredded basil, and serve.

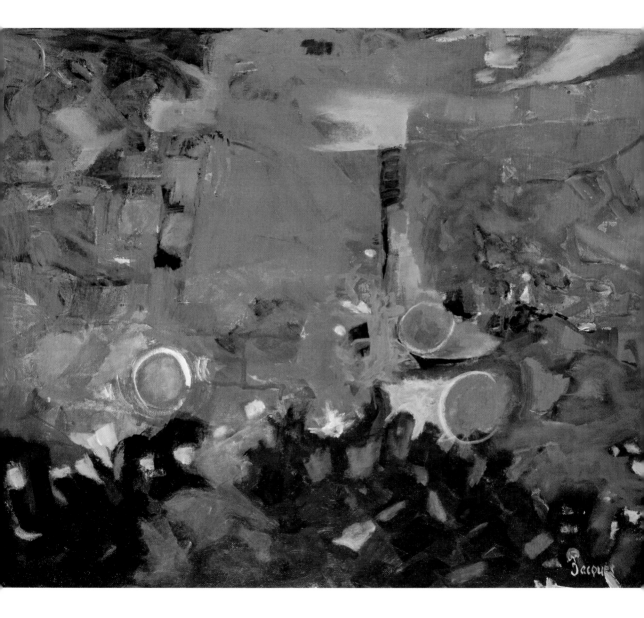

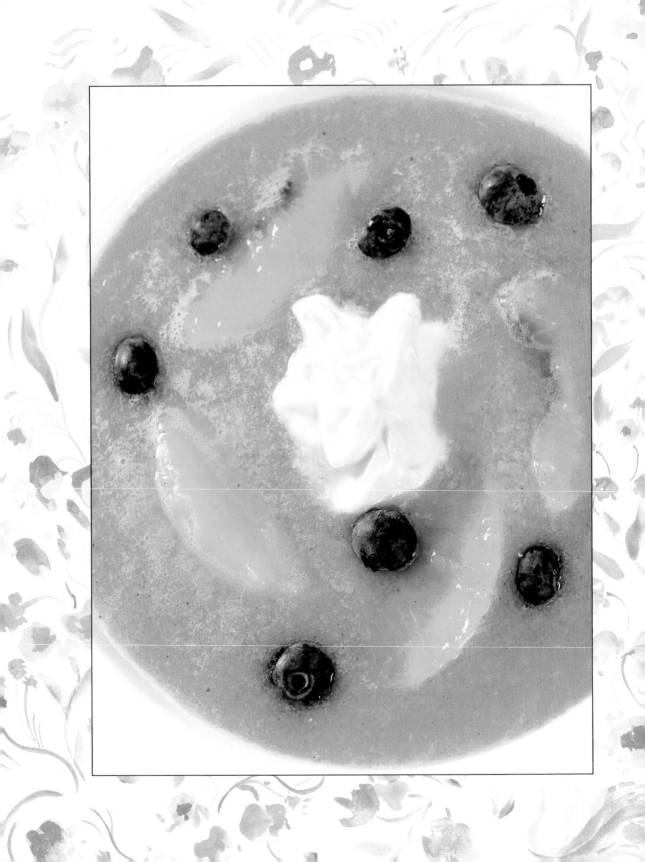

I used to make this soup at La Potagerie, a restaurant in New York City, where it was a great success in summer. Use fresh or unsweetened frozen peaches, if you are able to find them at your supermarket. Leftover peach soup is excellent mixed into plain hot or cold breakfast cereal.

Combine the sugar, water, cinnamon, nutmeg, and cloves in a saucepan, bring to a boil, and boil for 1 minute. Add the dissolved cornstarch and stir until the mixture boils (it will thicken). Stir in the wine and transfer to a bowl.

Puree the defrosted peaches in a food processor and stir them into the mixture in the bowl.

Peel the fresh peaches with a vegetable peeler (if they are very firm) or a knife (if they are soft). Or, if you don't object to the skin, leave them unpeeled. Cut the peaches into slices about ¼ inch thick (you should have about 2 cups). Add them to the soup, cover, and refrigerate until chilled.

At serving time, divide the soup among six bowls. Garnish each with a large dollop of sour cream and some blueberries and serve.

COLD PEACH SOUP WITH BLUEBERRIES

∘ SERVES 6
(MAKES ABOUT 6½ CUPS)

½ cup sugar

1 cup water

½ teaspoon ground cinnamon

⅛ teaspoon ground nutmeg

⅛ teaspoon ground cloves

1 tablespoon cornstarch, dissolved in 3 tablespoons water

1 cup dry fruity white wine, such as Chenin Blanc or Sauvignon Blanc

2 pounds fresh or frozen sliced peaches, defrosted if frozen

2 very ripe fresh peaches (12 to 14 ounces total)

1 cup sour cream, for garnish

1 cup fresh blueberries, for garnish

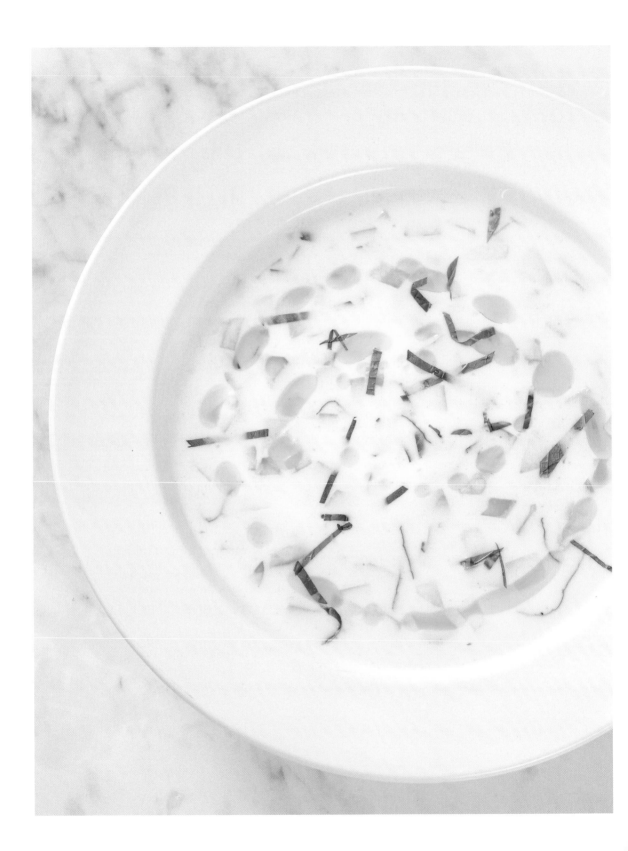

This is a good soup to make in the summer—it is fragrant and spicy, and the fresh mint complements it well. There is no cooking involved and assembly is quick and easy; the hardest part of the job is peeling and dicing the cucumber. Use the best yogurt you can find for this recipe. If you want to make the soup richer, replace some of the yogurt with sour cream.

Peel the cucumber, cut it lengthwise in half, and remove the seeds. Cut the flesh into long strips and then into ¼-inch dice (you should have about 2½ cups).

Put the yogurt in a serving bowl, add the cold water, and mix with a whisk until well combined. Add the olive oil, vinegar, Sriracha, salt, and garlic and mix well with the whisk. Stir in the cucumber and mint. If desired, sprinkle a dash of olive oil on top. Serve.

> **This cold soup is made right in the serving bowl.**

COLD YOGURT-CUCUMBER SOUP

° SERVES 6 (MAKES 5 CUPS)

1 English ("seedless") cucumber (about 1 pound)

One 16-ounce container plain Greek yogurt

1 cup cold water

¼ cup olive oil, plus more for serving, if desired

2 tablespoons cider vinegar

1 teaspoon Sriracha or other hot sauce

1 teaspoon salt

1 large clove garlic, peeled, crushed, and chopped fine (1 teaspoon)

About 18 mint leaves, piled together and cut crosswise into narrow strips

BEEF PELMENI IN CHICKEN BROTH

◦ SERVES 4

Filling

8 ounces ground beef, preferably sirloin

¼ cup chopped onion

About 2 cloves garlic, peeled and chopped (1 teaspoon)

1 slice bread, coarsely chopped

2 tablespoons chopped dill

2 teaspoons chopped mint

½ teaspoon ground coriander

½ teaspoon salt

¼ teaspoon freshly ground black pepper

¼ cup minced scallions

24 wonton wrappers (3 inches square)

6 cups Basic Chicken Stock (page 15) or canned chicken broth

1 teaspoon salt, or to taste

1 teaspoon freshly ground black pepper

2 tablespoons chopped cilantro

The beef filling for the dumplings in this classic Russian dish is flavored with ground coriander, mint, and dill. Wonton wrappers make it easy. The dumplings can be poached ahead and reheated at serving time.

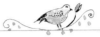

Prepare the filling: Mix together all the ingredients in a bowl.

Lay 12 of the wonton wrappers out on a work surface and moisten them lightly around the edges by brushing them with a little water. Divide the filling among the wrappers, mounding it in the center of each one. Cover with the remaining wrappers, aligning them with the bottom wrappers, and press gently around the edges to seal.

Bring 3 to 4 quarts water to a strong boil in a large saucepan. Carefully place the filled wontons in the boiling water, moving them gently at first so they don't stick to the bottom of the pan. After a minute or so, they will float to the top. Continue boiling gently for 5 to 6 minutes. Meanwhile, heat the chicken stock.

Lift the dumplings out of the water with a slotted spoon and arrange them, 3 per person, in four soup bowls. Pour about 1½ cups of the hot stock over the dumplings in each bowl and sprinkle the cilantro on top. Serve immediately.

▷ **Use packaged wonton wrappers to make the dumplings for this classic Russian dish.**

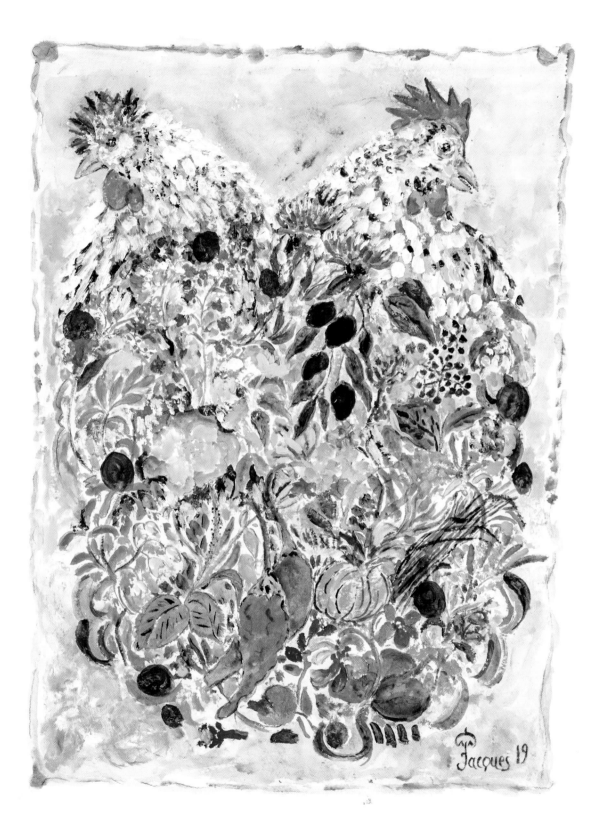

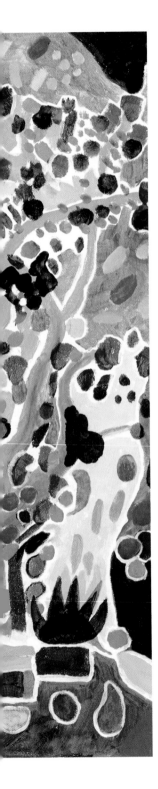

BREADS, PIZZAS & HOT SANDWICHES

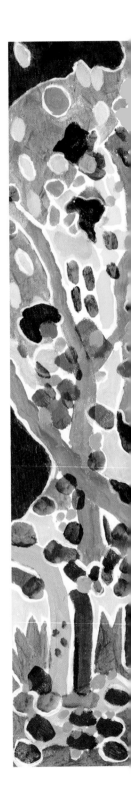

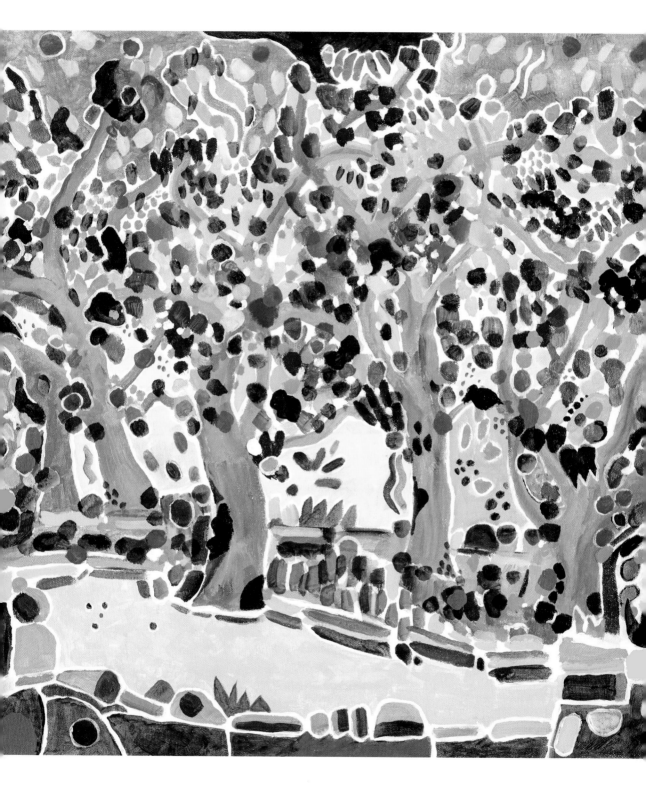

PROCESSOR BAGUETTES WITH BRAN

◦ MAKES 4 BAGUETTES

3 cups tepid water

Two ¼-ounce envelopes active dry yeast

1 teaspoon sugar

5 cups (1½ pounds) organic bread flour, also called strong or winter flour

1 cup (2 ounces) wheat bran

2 teaspoons salt

2 teaspoons peanut oil

2 tablespoons cornmeal

About ¼ cup water in a spray bottle

I love to make bread but sometimes don't have time to prepare it in the conventional way. This dough, made in a food processor, is easy and gives terrific results. The dough is not kneaded by hand and doesn't even touch the work table, so there isn't much cleanup involved, which suits me fine. I have a large plastic bowl with a tight-fitting lid that I use for letting the dough rise, and I use this same bowl beforehand for measuring the flour. So, when I finish this recipe, all I have to wash are the food processor bowl and steel blade, and the plastic bowl. I oil the bowl, which makes cleanup easier, and since the dough retains a little of that oil, it doesn't stick to the baking sheet.

If the air is dry, the dough will tend to form an outer skin or crust while it is rising, especially during the second rise. To prevent this, either spray the baguettes a few times with water while rising (I use a standard plant sprayer for this), or slide the baking sheet with the baguettes into a large plastic bag, taking care to prevent them from coming into contact with the bag and sticking to it as they rise.

In professional bread-baking ovens, steam is automatically injected into the oven at the beginning of the baking time; this gives the bread a thick, strong crust. To imitate this situation, I spray about 2 tablespoons of water into the oven when I first put the bread in, and then repeat this a few minutes later.

If you like, you can partially bake the baguettes—creating "brown and serve" loaves—and then finish baking them later. Securely wrapped in plastic, the partially baked loaves will keep in the refrigerator for 3 or 4 days or in the freezer for weeks. When you are ready to eat them, all you have to do is moisten them lightly and bake them until they are brown and crusty.

I added bran to this recipe to create a type of whole wheat bread; if you prefer, you can add cracked wheat instead.

Place the tepid water in a food processor and sprinkle the yeast and sugar over it. Let proof for 5 minutes.

Measure the flour, bran, and salt into a large bowl and add the mixture to the processor bowl. Process for 1½ to 2 minutes, holding the base of the machine to prevent it from "walking" on the counter. The dough should have formed a ball at this point.

Oil the bowl you used for the flour mixture with the peanut oil and transfer the ball of the dough to the bowl. Cover and allow to rise at room temperature for about 1½ hours, until the dough has doubled or tripled in bulk.

When the dough is ready, pull it away from the sides of the bowl and push it down into the bowl, forming it into a ball. Line a heavy aluminum cookie sheet that measures about 14 by 18 inches with nonstick aluminum foil. Place the ball of dough on the sheet and press down on it until it is about 8 inches wide and about the length of the cookie sheet. Cut the rectangle of dough into 4 lengthwise strips and arrange them on the cookie sheet so that they are equidistant from one another. Sprinkle the baguettes with half the cornmeal, then turn them over and sprinkle with the remaining cornmeal. Set

»—>

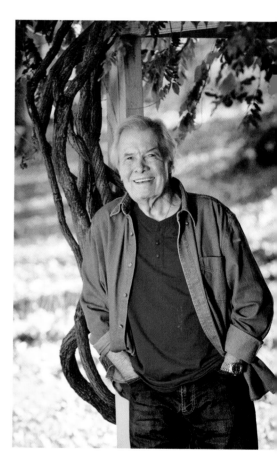

NOTE: Good bread dough is made with high-gluten (high-protein) flour, water, yeast, and salt. You can find good-quality packaged fresh or frozen pizza dough in most supermarkets. Fresh dough is ready to bake right away; frozen dough, which has a substantially longer storage life, is ready to use with very little advance notice—it thaws in a few hours in the refrigerator or in an hour or so at room temperature.

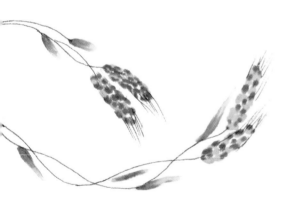

aside for about 45 minutes. Spray (or sprinkle or brush) the dough with water if it begins to form a dry crust as it rises.

Place a rack in the middle of the oven and preheat the oven to 425 degrees. Using a serrated knife, cut 4 or 5 gashes ¼ to ½ inch deep on a slight diagonal across the top of each baguette, or cut one long gash down the center of each. Place the cookie sheet on the middle oven rack and immediately spray about 2 tablespoons of water into the oven before closing the door. After 3 or 4 minutes, repeat the procedure.

If you are baking the bread completely, continue baking it for 30 to 35 minutes, until the loaves are brown and crusty. Remove and cool on wire racks. Serve warm or at room temperature.

If the bread is to be partially baked, remove the loaves from the oven after about 12 minutes, when they will have reached their ultimate size. (They will still be whitish at this point.) Cool completely, then wrap securely in plastic wrap and refrigerate for 3 or 4 days or freeze for up to 3 weeks. When you are ready to finish baking them, pass the frozen or refrigerated loaves under cool tap water to moisten them lightly all over. Arrange the loaves on a cookie sheet and bake in a 425-degree oven for 12 to 14 minutes, until nicely browned and crusty. Remove and cool on wire racks. Serve warm or at room temperature.

The dough for this classic bread from Provence is shaped to resemble a leaf.

Line a cookie sheet with nonstick aluminum foil. Place the dough on the cookie sheet, dampen your hands with water, and spread the dough out on the cookie sheet. The dough is elastic and will tend to shrink back and resist your efforts to extend it, but keep pressing and spreading until you have an oval approximately 12 inches long, 8 inches wide, and ¼ inch thick, with a slightly thicker edge.

Combine the olive pieces and olive oil and spread the mixture evenly over the surface of the dough, pressing the olives into the dough. Sprinkle with the herbes de Provence, salt, and pepper.

Cut the dough to resemble a leaf: Leaving a 2-inch-wide uncut strip down the center of the length of the oval, cut 4 angled slits, each 3 to 4 inches long, on either side of this strip to imitate the veins of a leaf; do not extend the slits to the edge of the dough—they should stop about 1 inch from the edge. Cut through the dough firmly and open each slit wide, or they will tend to close up when the dough is rising and/or baking. Allow the dough to rise at room temperature for 40 to 50 minutes.

Place a rack in the middle of the oven and preheat the oven to 425 degrees. Slide the dough into the oven and bake for 20 to 25 minutes, until the fougasse is nicely browned and very crusty. Set the fougasse aside to cool briefly, then remove it from

»—>

FOUGASSE

◦ MAKES 1 LOAF

1 pound packaged fresh or frozen bread or pizza dough, defrosted if frozen

¼ cup pitted olives (a spicy oil-cured variety or green kalamata), cut into ¼- to ½-inch pieces

2 tablespoons extra-virgin olive oil

1 teaspoon herbes de Provence (see Note, page 15)

½ teaspoon coarse salt

¼ teaspoon freshly ground black pepper

the cookie sheet with a large spatula and place it on a wire rack until completely cool.

Serve the bread at room temperature. Leftovers can be frozen and reheated (after lightly dampening the crust).

BREAKFAST ROLLS

◦ MAKES 12 ROLLS

1 pound packaged fresh or frozen bread or pizza dough, defrosted if frozen

2 tablespoons unsalted butter

¾ cup rolled oats

NOTE: These rolls freeze well: Let them cool completely on a wire rack, then wrap them individually in plastic wrap and pack in a plastic freezer bag. At serving time, moisten the frozen rolls lightly with water and place them in a 400-degree oven to recrisp for about 10 minutes.

These small rolls are flavored with butter and rolled oats. They can be served at any meal, but they are especially welcome at breakfast. One pound of packaged bread or pizza dough makes about twelve rolls, depending on how large you make them.

Cut the dough lengthwise in half, then cut each half crosswise into 6 equal pieces to form a total of 12 pieces. Melt the butter and pour it onto a plate. Spread the oats on another plate. Shape each piece of dough into a ball (they don't have to be perfectly round), roll them first in the butter and then in the oats, and arrange them on a cookie sheet lined with nonstick aluminum foil. Let the dough rise at room temperature for 45 minutes.

Preheat the oven to 425 degrees. Bake the rolls for 25 minutes, until brown and crispy. Serve warm.

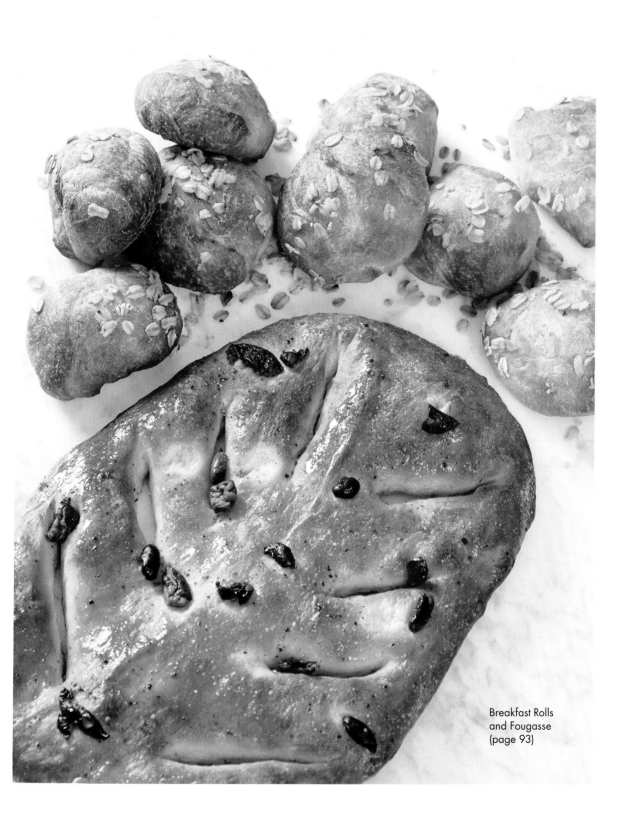

Breakfast Rolls
and Fougasse
(page 93)

CALZONE TWO WAYS

° MAKES 1 CALZONE (SERVES 2)

Brie Calzone

8 ounces packaged fresh or frozen bread or pizza dough, defrosted if frozen

4 ounces Brie or Camembert cheese

2 or 3 pickled hot chiles or cherry peppers, or to taste

About 3 scallions, cleaned and sliced (¼ cup)

1 tablespoon chopped cilantro

1½ tablespoons olive oil

Calzones are excellent eaten while still warm from the oven. You can cut this calzone into four slices and serve them with a meal, or enjoy for lunch, with a salad and a glass of wine.

Although I offer two different versions of calzone here, one with Brie and one with mozzarella, the bread can be stuffed with anything from Mushroom, Tomato, and Nut Mix (page 19) to fillings containing sausage meat, sliced cooked sausage or salami, mushrooms, or shrimp. Use your imagination and what you have on hand.

Defrost frozen bread dough overnight in the refrigerator or for about 1½ hours at room temperature.

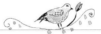

Line a cookie sheet with nonstick aluminum foil. Place the dough on the sheet and press to flatten it, then wet your hands and spread the dough out. It will tend to shrink and slide back, but keep pressing and spreading until you have formed the dough into a round about 10 inches in diameter. It should be about ½ inch thick but a bit thicker around the edge.

Cut the cheese into 7 or 8 slices and arrange them on half the dough, leaving a border of about 1 inch. Cut the peppers into pieces and arrange them on top of the cheese. Top with the scallions and cilantro. Sprinkle about 1 tablespoon of the olive oil over the top. Fold the unfilled half of the dough over to cover the filling and press firmly with your thumb all around the edges to seal well. Sprinkle the remaining ½ tablespoon oil on top and spread it evenly over the surface of the dough. Let the dough rise at room temperature for 40 to 50 minutes, until it has doubled in size.

Place a rack in the middle of the oven and preheat the oven to 425 degrees. Bake the calzone for 20 to 25 minutes. Some of the filling may seep out; if so, when you remove the calzone from the oven, allow it to cool and set for about 10 minutes, then push any filling that has spilled out back into the spot where it emerged. Transfer the calzone to a wire rack and let it cool to lukewarm before serving.

Line a cookie sheet with nonstick aluminum foil. Place the dough on the sheet and press to flatten it, then wet your hands and spread the dough out. It will tend to shrink and slide back, but keep pressing and spreading until you have formed the dough into a round about 10 inches in diameter. It should be about ½ inch thick but a bit thicker around the edge.

Shred the cheese or cut it into thin slices. Arrange it over half the dough, leaving a border of about 1 inch. Arrange the anchovy fillets on top of the cheese, then pour the oil from the can over the anchovies. Sprinkle the parsley evenly over the anchovies, then sprinkle with the pepper. Fold the unfilled half of the dough over to cover the filling

»—>

Mozzarella Calzone

2 teaspoons olive oil

8 ounces packaged fresh or frozen bread or pizza dough, defrosted if frozen

4 ounces mozzarella cheese

One 2-ounce can anchovy fillets in oil, undrained

2 tablespoons flat-leaf parsley leaves

½ teaspoon freshly ground black pepper

> Create your own tasty
> fillings for these meal-in-one
> turnovers.

and press firmly all around the edges with your thumb to seal well. Sprinkle the olive oil on top and spread it evenly over the surface of the dough. Let the dough rise at room temperature for 40 to 50 minutes, until doubled in size.

Place a rack in the middle of the oven and preheat the oven to 425 degrees. Bake the calzone for 20 to 25 minutes. Some of the filling may seep out; if so, when you remove the calzone from the oven, allow it to cool and set for about 10 minutes, then push any filling that has spilled out back into the spot where it emerged. Transfer the calzone to a wire rack and let it cool to lukewarm before serving.

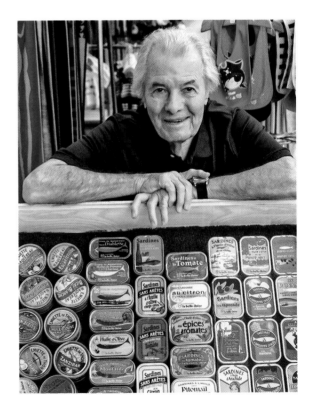

I garnish my version of this Italian flatbread with onions and garlic. It's delicious as a snack or as an accompaniment to soups and salads.

Focaccia is usually round, so use a round pan if you have one; otherwise, use a cookie sheet. Line the pan with nonstick aluminum foil. Place the dough on the cookie pan and press to flatten it, then wet your hands with cold water and press on the dough, extending it to form a circle 10 to 12 inches in diameter. The dough is elastic and will tend to shrink back, so press firmly until the circle holds its shape. Prick the dough about 10 times with a fork.

Combine the onion, garlic, olive oil, and oregano in a medium bowl and spread the mixture evenly over the dough. Sprinkle with the cheese and let the dough rise at room temperature for 40 to 50 minutes, or until doubled in size.

Place a rack in the middle of the oven and preheat the oven to 425 degrees. Bake the focaccia for 25 to 30 minutes, until the dough is nicely browned and the onions are cooked. Let the focaccia cool on the pan for a few minutes, then transfer it to a wire rack and cool completely. Cut into wedges to serve.

FOCACCIA

∘ MAKES 1 LOAF

1 pound packaged fresh or frozen bread or pizza dough, defrosted if frozen

1 onion, peeled and sliced very thin (about 1 cup)

3 cloves garlic, peeled and sliced thin (about 1 tablespoon)

3 tablespoons olive oil

2 teaspoons fresh oregano, or 1 teaspoon dried

2 tablespoons grated Pecorino Romano or Parmesan cheese

¼ teaspoon freshly ground black pepper

FRENCH BREAD STICKS GRATINEE

∘ SERVES 6

6 packaged brown-and-serve
French bread sticks (about
9 by 1½ inches each)

6 tablespoons olive oil

2 tablespoons grated Parmesan
cheese

½ teaspoon freshly ground
black pepper

I find French bread sticks at my supermarket, and these long, narrow rolls are handy to have in the freezer in case you run out of bread or have unexpected guests. Before browning them, coat the bread sticks with olive oil and sprinkle them with Parmesan cheese and black pepper—the added flavor and color transform them.

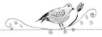

Preheat the oven to 425 degrees. Split the bread sticks lengthwise in half. Pour the olive oil onto a rimmed baking sheet or a jelly-roll pan and press the bread sticks, cut side down, into the olive oil so they are well moistened. Turn them over and sprinkle the cut sides with the Parmesan cheese and pepper.

Bake the bread sticks for 10 to 12 minutes, until crisp and brown. Serve warm.

> **The addition of olive oil, Parmesan cheese, and pepper turns these store-bought rolls into homemade.**

A great addition to a bread basket and good with soup, this bread takes little preparation time. I combine the ingredients in a food processor, but you can whisk them together by hand if you prefer.

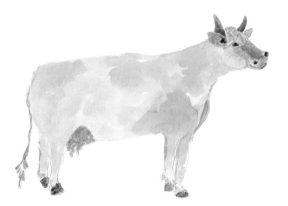

Preheat the oven to 400 degrees. Lightly grease a 6-cup (8½ by 4½-inch) loaf pan with the olive oil. Place all the remaining ingredients in a food processor and process for a few seconds to combine, or mix in a bowl with a whisk.

Pour the batter into the prepared loaf pan, set the pan on a cookie sheet, and bake for 45 minutes to 1 hour, until the loaf is well set and nicely browned. Cool in the pan on a wire rack for a few minutes, then unmold, slice, and serve warm.

▷ **If you use packaged grated cheese, the batter can be ready for the oven in minutes.**

CORNMEAL AND CHEDDAR BREAD

∘ MAKES 1 LOAF

½ teaspoon olive oil

1 cup all-purpose flour

1 cup yellow cornmeal

2 teaspoons double-acting baking powder

1 tablespoon sugar

½ teaspoon salt

⅛ teaspoon cayenne pepper

1 cup milk

¼ cup peanut oil

1 large egg

1½ cups grated cheddar cheese (about 6 ounces)

CHEESE STICKS

1 sheet frozen puff pastry
(about 8 ounces; ½ package)

2 tablespoons unsalted butter,
melted

⅓ cup grated Parmesan cheese

1 teaspoon paprika

¼ teaspoon salt

⅛ teaspoon cayenne pepper

▷ Rubbing a little melted
butter on packaged puff
pastry makes it richer.

Like the Cinnamon-Sugar Sticks (page 367), these are made with packaged puff pastry. They are excellent served with soup or with cheese, and they make an unusual addition to your bread basket.

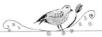

Preheat the oven to 400 degrees. Place the frozen pastry on a cookie sheet lined with nonstick aluminum foil and let sit at room temperature for 15 to 20 minutes.

While the pastry is still partially frozen, unfold the dough (it will tend to crack at the seams) and rub half the melted butter over the surface. Combine the Parmesan cheese, paprika, salt, and cayenne in a small bowl and sprinkle half of this mixture over the butter, spreading it with your fingers to distribute it evenly. Turn the pastry over and repeat, using the remaining butter and cheese mixture. Cut the pastry into ten 1-inch-wide strips, then cut the strips in half crosswise to yield 20 sticks, each about 1 inch wide and 5 inches long. Work quickly, because the pastry is easier to handle while it is still partially frozen. Or, for a different look, slit about 3 inches from the center of each stick. Bring one end of the stick throughout the slit and pull it through to give it a braided and twisted look.

Arrange the sticks evenly on the prepared cookie sheet and bake for 12 to 25 minutes, until the sticks are dark brown. Transfer to a wire rack and cool completely before serving.

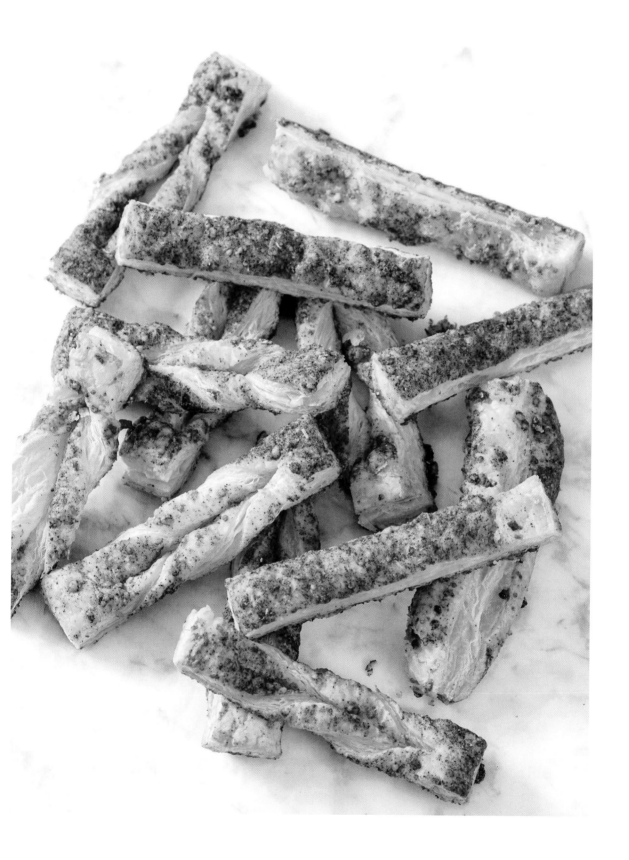

GARLIC AND HERB BREAD

◦ MAKES 1 LOAF (SERVES 4)

1 French-style baguette
(8 to 10 ounces)

3 tablespoons peanut oil

About 4 cloves garlic, peeled and
chopped fine (2 teaspoons)

1 teaspoon Italian seasoning

¼ teaspoon freshly ground
black pepper

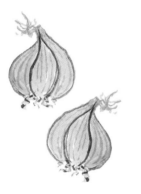

This bread is especially good with a hearty soup. I use a long, thin French-style baguette, but you can use another type of unsliced bread if you prefer. Although the bread can be prepared ahead, it is best to bake it at the last moment and serve it while it is still warm.

Split the baguette horizontally in half. Mix together the oil, garlic, Italian seasoning, and pepper in a small bowl. Spread this mixture on the cut side of each baguette half.

Preheat the oven to 400 degrees. Just before serving time, arrange the bread halves cut side up on a cookie sheet and bake for 12 to 15 minutes. Cut into pieces and serve while still warm.

> **Season the bread ahead, but bake it at the last minute and serve while it's still warm.**

You'll find this simple tart a life-saver when unexpected guests drop in. Although you can certainly use a homemade piecrust, a frozen pie shell works very well and saves time. To give the tart a more rustic look, fold the edges of the flattened pie shell back over the filling.

Remove the pie shell from its foil pan and place it on a cookie sheet lined with nonstick aluminum foil. Set it aside to defrost for about 30 minutes.

Preheat the oven to 400 degrees. Mix the remaining ingredients together in a bowl.

Flatten the softened pie shell against the cookie sheet, creating a flat circle of dough 10 to 12 inches across. Seal any cracks that develop by pressing the dough together gently with your fingers. Pour the ricotta mixture into the middle of the round of dough and spread it out to within 1 to 2 inches of the edge. Fold the border of dough back over the filling, lifting it with the help of the foil, pushing it against the cheese, and then peeling back the foil.

Bake the tart for 30 to 40 minutes, or until the filling is set and nicely browned. Cut into wedges and serve.

CHEESE TART

○ SERVES 4

One 9-inch frozen pie shell

1 cup ricotta cheese (8 ounces)

2 large eggs, lightly beaten

½ teaspoon salt

¼ teaspoon freshly ground black pepper

4 ounces Gouda or cheddar cheese, grated (1 cup)

2 teaspoons Spicy Red Salsa (page 13), or 1 teaspoon Sriracha or other hot sauce

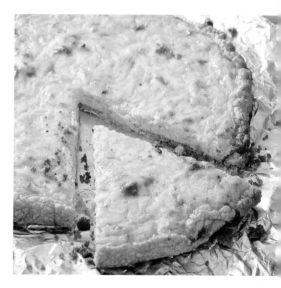

PITA CHEESE TOASTS

2 tablespoons unsalted butter

2 tablespoons peanut oil

4 pita breads (about 4 ounces each; 4 inches in diameter)

2 tablespoons grated Pecorino Romano cheese

These toasts are wonderful for serving with soups, salads, and main courses. They can also be broken into pieces and used as croutons, or even made into sandwiches. I top them with Romano cheese here, but you can make them without cheese. It is best to eat these within 24 hours.

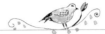

Preheat the broiler. Melt the butter with the oil and spread the mixture over one or two jelly-roll pans or rimmed baking sheets. Split the pita breads and press the halves, interior side down, into the butter-oil mixture, then turn them over and sprinkle with the cheese.

Place the pan (or one pan at a time) under the broiler, 5 to 6 inches from the heat source, and broil for about 3 minutes, until nicely browned. Cut into pieces and serve.

Wonton wrappers make terrific toasts. Wafer-like, they are ideal with spreads or dips (such as Red Pepper Dip, page 20) or can be served on their own as an hors d'oeuvre. They are an interesting addition to a bread basket and go particularly well with soups. I often cook them a few at a time in the toaster oven to eat as a snack.

Preheat the oven to 400 degrees. Arrange the wonton wrappers on a cookie sheet lined with nonstick aluminum foil and brush them with the olive oil. (You don't need to defrost them if they're frozen.) Bake for 7 to 8 minutes, until nicely browned and crusty. Serve warm.

> Fresh wonton wrappers, inexpensive and available in vacuum packs at most supermarkets, can be transformed quickly into delicious toasts. Leftover unbaked wrappers can be frozen for up to 2 weeks.

CRISPY WONTON WAFERS

∘ MAKES 6 WAFERS

6 wonton wrappers
(3 inches square)

1 teaspoon olive oil

PIZZA MAISON

○ SERVES 4

8 ounces packaged fresh or frozen bread or pizza dough, defrosted if frozen

2 tablespoons extra-virgin olive oil, plus for garnish, if desired

1 large ripe tomato (7 to 8 ounces), sliced

2 large cloves garlic, peeled and sliced thin

1 teaspoon herbes de Provence (see Note, page 15)

¼ teaspoon salt

¼ teaspoon freshly ground black pepper

5 ounces mozzarella cheese, grated (about 1½ cups)

Hot pepper flakes, for garnish (optional)

▷ **Create your own pizza quickly and easily by using frozen dough.**

Everyone loves pizza, but most people buy it ready-made because they think it's too hard to prepare themselves. Made with frozen bread dough, this pizza requires very little work and the result is spectacular and delicious. I top my pizza with tomato, garlic, herbes de Provence, and mozzarella, but you can create your own variations—try Swiss or Fontina cheese, zucchini, or onions.

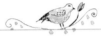

Place the dough on a pizza pan or cookie sheet. Dampen your hands and spread the dough out into a round about 11 inches in diameter. The dough will tend to shrink back; press it firmly with the tips of your fingers. (If you're adept at manipulating pizza dough, you can hold the dough on your closed fist and pull and extend it as pizza makers often demonstrate in pizza parlors.) The dough should be ¼ inch thick, with a slightly thicker edge.

Spread 1 tablespoon of the olive oil over the entire surface of the dough. Then lift the dough, turn it over, and spread it out again in the pan. Arrange the tomato slices evenly over the dough, leaving a 1-inch border. Sprinkle with the garlic, herbes de Provence, salt, pepper, and mozzarella, then drizzle with the remaining 1 tablespoon olive oil. Let rise at room temperature for 15 to 20 minutes.

Preheat the oven to 425 degrees. Bake the pizza for 25 to 30 minutes, until nicely browned and crusty on top. Cut into slices and serve sprinkled with pepper flakes and a little additional olive oil, if desired.

This makes a fast lunch. All you need are large flour tortillas, a can or two of red kidney beans, scallions, hot salsa, and cheddar cheese. One of these per person is sufficient. They go well with a crisp salad and beer or chilled white wine.

Line your cookie sheet with nonstick aluminum foil to eliminate a cleanup chore.

Place an oven rack in the middle of the oven and preheat the oven to 400 degrees. Line a large cookie sheet with nonstick aluminum foil. Sprinkle the tortillas with the oil on one side and place them oiled side down on the prepared cookie sheet.

Combine the beans, scallions, cilantro, and salsa in a bowl and stir well. Spread the mixture on the tortillas, dividing it evenly among them. Top evenly with the cheese. Bake the tortillas for 12 to 15 minutes, until the beans are heated through and the cheese has melted. Using two large spatulas, transfer each tortilla to a plate and serve.

SPICY BEAN TORTILLA PIZZAS

∘ SERVES 4

4 large flour tortillas
(about 7 inches in diameter)

4 teaspoons olive oil

Two 16-ounce cans red kidney beans, drained

About 5 scallions, cleaned and minced (¾ cup)

½ cup cilantro, coarsely chopped

¼ cup Spicy Red Salsa (page 13)

1½ cups shredded sharp cheddar cheese (about 6 ounces)

▷ **To catch cheese spills, line your cookie sheet with nonstick aluminum foil.**

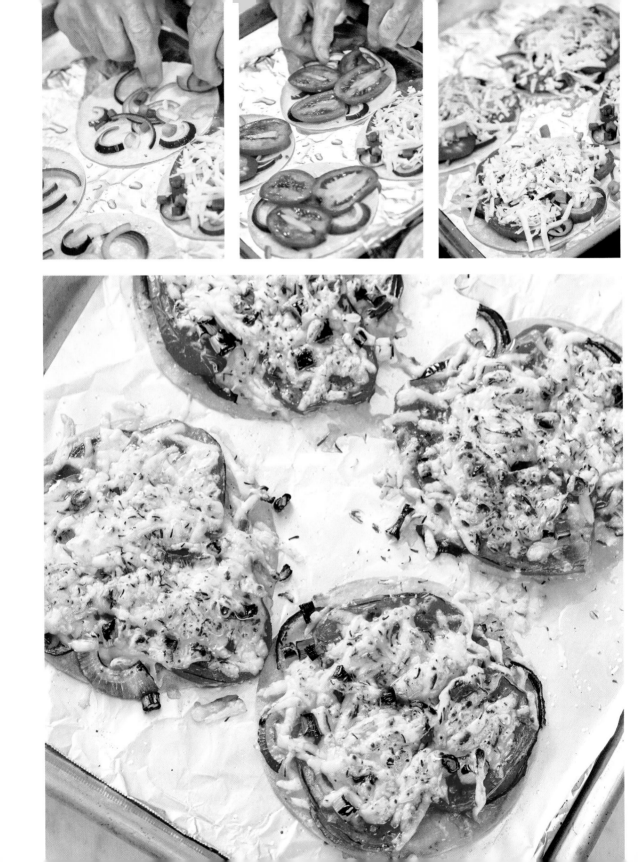

I love corn tortillas. I always have a package in my freezer—they defrost in a few minutes. These pizza-like open-face sandwiches are quick and easy to prepare for lunch and a guaranteed crowd-pleaser. You can vary the topping according to what you like and what you have on hand.

To make cleanup easier, line your cookie sheet with nonstick aluminum foil. If cooked just two at a time, these can be baked in a toaster oven.

Preheat the oven to 400 degrees. Line a large cookie sheet with nonstick aluminum foil. Arrange the tortillas on the prepared cookie sheet and place the onion slices, tomatoes, scallions, and cheese, in that order, on top of the tortillas. Sprinkle with the olive oil, oregano, and pepper.

Bake the tortillas for 12 to 14 minutes. Transfer the tortillas to individual plates and cut each into 4 wedges. Serve.

> **Keep a package of corn tortillas in the freezer—they defrost in minutes.**
>
> **Served one per person, these open-face sandwiches make a great lunch. Cut into smaller pieces, they make a delicious hors d'oeuvre.**

CHEESE AND TOMATO CORN TORTILLA PIZZAS

∘ SERVES 4

4 corn tortillas (5 to 6 inches in diameter)

8 thin slices red onion (1½ ounces)

3 plum tomatoes (6 ounces total), sliced thin (about 24 slices)

2 scallions, cleaned and minced (2 tablespoons)

8 slices Monterey Jack, Port Salut, or mozzarella cheese (6 ounces)

1½ teaspoons olive oil

1 teaspoon dried oregano

½ teaspoon freshly ground black pepper

SPICY SAUSAGE AND MUSHROOM CORN TORTILLA PIZZAS

◦ SERVES 4

4 corn tortillas (5 to 6 inches in diameter)

6 ounces kielbasa sausage, sliced thin

1 cup thinly sliced mushrooms (4 ounces)

2 tablespoons Spicy Red Salsa (page 13)

1 cup grated Fontina or mozzarella cheese (about 3 ounces)

I use garlicky Polish kielbasa sausage here, preferring it to pepperoni for these open-face tortilla sandwiches. If you don't want to make the salsa, substitute a good bottled hot salsa. I use Fontina or mozzarella, but Leicester or raclette cheese would also work well.

Preheat the oven to 400 degrees. Line a large cookie sheet with nonstick aluminum foil. Arrange the tortillas on the prepared cookie sheet and top with the kielbasa, mushrooms, salsa, and cheese, in that order.

Bake the tortillas for 12 to 15 minutes, until the cheese is bubbling. Transfer the tortillas to individual plates, cut each into 4 wedges, and serve.

▷ **Using packaged cleaned and sliced mushrooms is a real time-saver here.**

A traditional croque-monsieur is a thin ham and cheese sandwich that is browned in butter in a skillet. For this adaptation, I use large flour tortillas instead of bread, filling them with blue or Brie cheese and ham. The sandwiches, which can be made in just a few minutes, are terrific for lunch with a salad.

Arrange 4 tortillas on the counter, and place half of the cheese on each of them, making sure to spread it to the outer edge of the tortilla. Place a slice of ham on top of the cheese, and sprinkle with the pepper. Cover with the remaining cheese, again making sure to spread it to the edge, and then place the remaining tortillas on top and press on them gently to make them adhere well.

Heat 1½ teaspoons of the butter in each of the two nonstick skillets. When it is hot, add a tortilla to each skillet, and cook over medium to low heat for 2 to 3 minutes on each side. Set aside and let rest for 4 to 5 minutes before removing from the skillet, so the cheese can set up a little. Remove to a plate and keep warm. Repeat with the two remaining filled tortillas.

Cut each of the tortilla sandwiches into four wedges and serve.

> **Flour tortillas replace the bread in this variation of the classic Croque-Monsieur.**

BLUE CHEESE TORTILLA CROQUE-MONSIEUR

∘ SERVES 4

8 flour tortillas (about 7 inches in diameter)

6 ounces blue cheese, such as Gorgonzola or Stilton, crumbled, or Brie cheese, cut into pieces

4 slices cooked ham (about 3 ounces)

¼ teaspoon freshly ground black pepper

2 tablespoons unsalted butter

RED PEPPER AND CHEESE TARTINE

∘ SERVES 4

1 French-style baguette
(about 10 ounces)

1 red bell pepper, cored, seeded,
and sliced thin (about 2 cups)

¼ cup sunflower seeds or
pignoli nuts

7 to 8 cloves garlic, peeled and
sliced thin (2 to 3 tablespoons)

½ teaspoon freshly ground
black pepper

¼ cup virgin olive oil

8 ounces Muenster or Gruyère
cheese, sliced thin

½ teaspoon herbes de Provence
(see Note, page 15)

This is a delicious open-face sandwich created with
an unusual assortment of ingredients. The finishing
touch, Muenster cheese, melts nicely in the oven and
lends a delicate flavor.

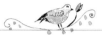

Preheat the oven to 400 degrees. Line a cookie
sheet with nonstick aluminum foil. Split the baguette
lengthwise in half. Place the bread halves cut side
up on the prepared cookie sheet. Lay the bell
pepper slices on top of the bread, dividing them
evenly. Sprinkle the sunflower seeds and garlic on
top, then season with the black pepper and drizzle
with the olive oil. Arrange the cheese slices on top
and sprinkle with the herbes de Provence.

Bake the sandwiches for 10 to 12 minutes, until
the bread is crisp, the cheese has melted, and the
sandwiches are heated through. Cut each half in
half and serve.

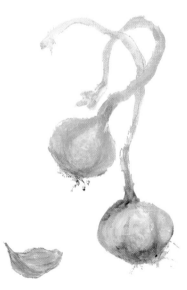

I love Stilton cheese and often use it in this sandwich, although I have also made it with Gorgonzola, another favorite. I use a baguette here, but the sandwiches can also be made on large slices of country bread. A great luncheon dish, the sandwiches can be cooked quickly, a few at a time in a toaster oven or all together in a conventional oven.

Serve these with cold white wine.

Preheat the oven to 400 degrees. Line a cookie sheet with nonstick aluminum foil. Place the pieces of bread cut side up on the prepared cookie sheet. Drizzle 1 tablespoon of the olive oil over each piece of bread, then cover with the onion, olives, tomatoes, salt, pepper, and cheese, in that order.

Bake the sandwiches for 12 to 14 minutes, until the cheese has melted and the bread is hot and crusty. Serve immediately.

NOTE: To pit olives, press gently on them with your thumb until they open up and the pits pop out.

WARM FRENCH BREAD AND STILTON TARTINE

∘ SERVES 4

1 French-style baguette (8 to 10 ounces), split lengthwise in half and then cut crosswise in half to make 4 pieces total

4 tablespoons extra-virgin olive oil

1 onion (about 4 ounces), peeled and sliced thin (about 1 cup)

24 oil-cured olives, pitted (see Note)

About 4 plum tomatoes (8 ounces total), sliced thin

⅛ teaspoon salt

¼ teaspoon freshly ground black pepper

4 ounces Stilton cheese, cut into 4 equal slices

FONDUE AU FROMAGE

◦ SERVES 4

2 tablespoons unsalted butter

3 cloves garlic, peeled, crushed, and chopped (1 tablespoon)

2 cups dry white wine

1¼ teaspoons salt

1½ teaspoons freshly ground black pepper

5 cups packed shredded Gruyère, Emmenthaler, or Beaufort cheese (about 1 pound)

About 40 bread cubes, each about 2 inches square, from a crusty country-style loaf (12 ounces)

Cheese fondue is a popular dish in the French part of Switzerland, not far from where I grew up in France. We ate it often in Bourg-en-Bresse, where I was born, calling it *ramequins*. The quality of the cheese you use is essential in this recipe.

Requiring only a few ingredients and quickly assembled, fondue is a dish to be enjoyed with friends. The cheese is melted in white wine flavored with garlic and then the pot is placed over a burner on the table so the fondue stays hot and melted. In Switzerland the ingredients are conventionally boiled together, thickened slightly with flour or cornstarch, and finished with kirsch, but I don't thicken the mixture here. As a result, the cheese tends to stay in the bottom and the clearer liquid rises to the top, but that is the way it should be—you mix the ingredients together by stirring them with the bread as you dip it into the pot.

Unlike meat fondue, which requires special forks, here you can hold the pieces of bread easily with a regular table fork. I use a crusty country-type French bread for dipping, cutting it into 2-inch cubes. The bread pieces are impaled soft part first on the forks, so they don't fall off and drop into the fondue. (When I ate fondue in cafés in France as a young man with my friends, anyone losing a bread chunk in the fondue had to buy a round of drinks for everyone in the party!) This dish is one of my daughter's favorites, high on her list of requests when she is home.

Fondue is great followed by a plate of charcuterie, a green salad, and a fruit dessert. The amounts listed here usually serve four. People unaccustomed to the taste may eat timidly at first, but the flavor grows on you—two people can consume this amount of fondue as a main course.

Heat the butter in a small enameled cast-iron pot. When it is foaming, add the garlic and sauté, stirring, for about 30 seconds. Add the wine, salt, and pepper and bring to a boil, then add the cheese and mix gently with a wooden spoon or spatula over medium heat until the mixture returns to a boil and all the ingredients are well incorporated. Remove the pot from the heat and place it on the table over a butane burner or Sterno set on low heat.

To eat, impale one piece of bread at a time, soft side first, on a fork and stir the mixture gently in a circular way until the bread is coated with cheese. When only about 1 cup of the cheese mixture remains, make the "soup": Add a dozen pieces of bread to the pot and mix them in well. Encourage your guests to enjoy the last pieces coated with the cheesy liquid, along with the crusty bits sticking to the bottom of the pot.

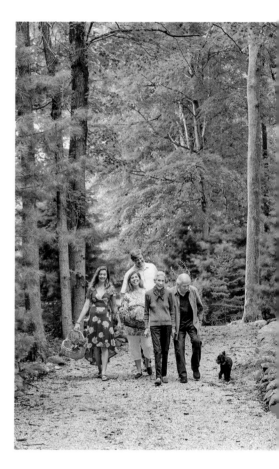

PAN BAGNAT

1 avocado (7 to 8 ounces)

1 round or oval loaf French- or Italian-style bread (1 pound)

2 tablespoons chopped basil, flat-leaf parsley, or chervil (optional)

6 tablespoons virgin olive oil

2 tablespoons red wine vinegar

2 ripe tomatoes (about 10 ounces total), cut into ¼-inch-thick slices

½ teaspoon salt

½ teaspoon freshly ground black pepper

One 5-ounce can tuna in olive oil

Pan bagnat translates as "bathed bread." This sandwich is a specialty of Provence and tastes great with a cold rosé wine from that region. It makes an ideal summer lunch. You can make individual pan bagnat or one large one, as I've done here.

My filling consists of sliced tomato, avocado, and tuna, but you can use a different combination. With olive oil as the one standard ingredient, other popular additions include anchovy fillets, olives, peppers, and sardines. The sandwich can be assembled the night before, wrapped, and refrigerated, with a 2- to 3-pound weight on top to make it hold together well when sliced.

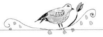

Cut the avocado in half, remove the pit, and scoop out the flesh; rinse under cold water to prevent discoloration. Cut the flesh into slices.

Cut the loaf of bread horizontally in half and sprinkle the cut sides with the basil, olive oil, and vinegar. Arrange the tomato slices on the bottom half of the loaf and sprinkle with half the salt and pepper. Cover with the avocado slices and the tuna, crumbling it over the bread, and sprinkle the remaining salt and pepper on top. Position the top half of the loaf over the filling, wrap the sandwich tightly in plastic wrap or a plastic bag, and refrigerate with a 2- to 3-pound weight on top for a few hours or as long as overnight.

At serving time, cut the sandwich into wedges.

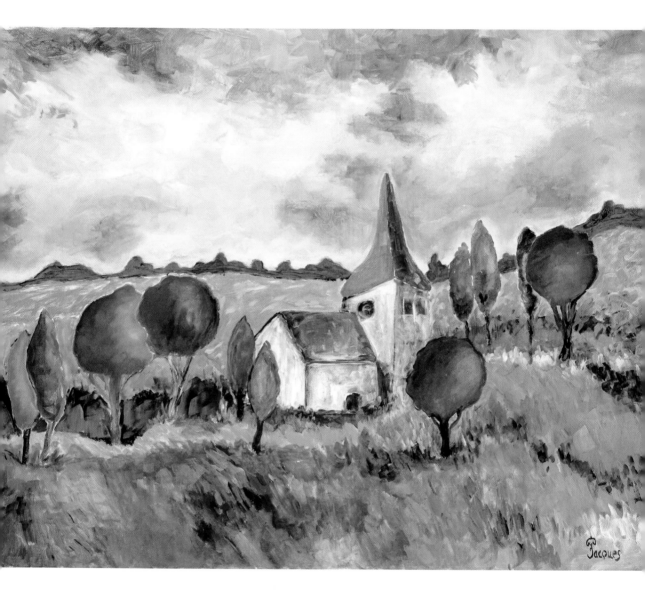

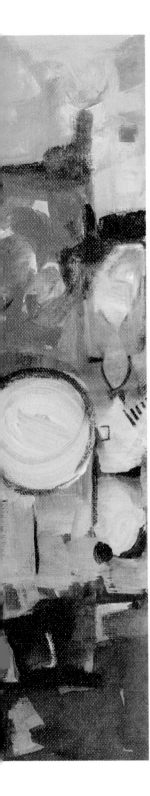

PASTA & RICE

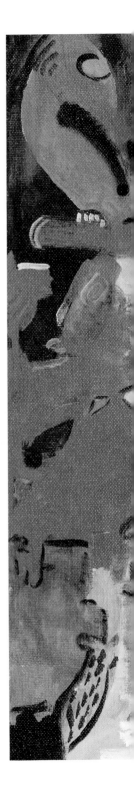

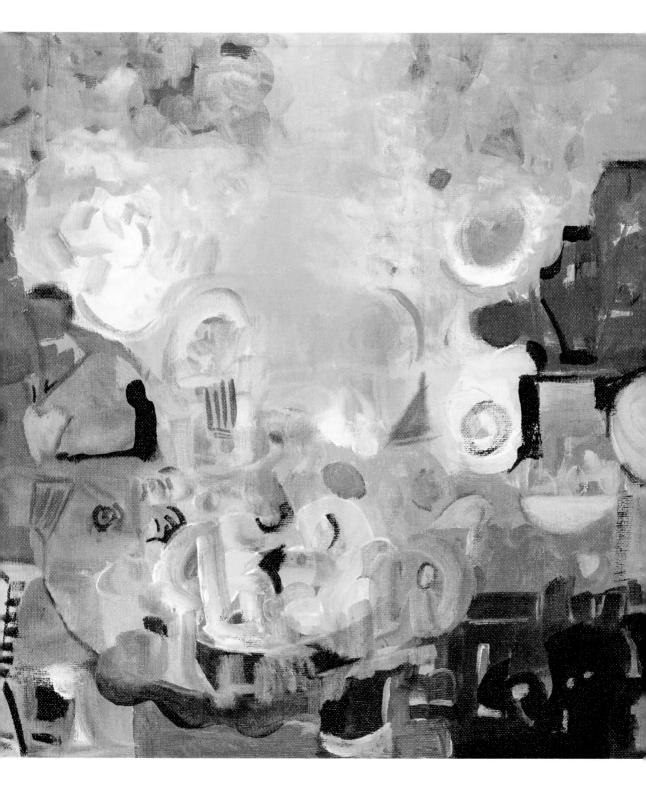

PASTA PRIMAVERA ED

∘ SERVES 4

Tomato Sauce

2 to 3 very ripe tomatoes
(1 pound)

1 mild onion, such as Vidalia
(about 3 ounces), peeled and
chopped fine (about ⅔ cup)

2 cloves garlic, peeled, crushed,
and chopped (1 teaspoon)

½ teaspoon salt

½ teaspoon freshly ground
black pepper

¼ cup extra-virgin olive oil

½ cup shredded basil leaves

1 pound spaghetti

2 tablespoons virgin olive oil

¼ teaspoon salt

½ teaspoon freshly ground
black pepper

3 to 4 tablespoons grated
Parmesan cheese, plus more
for serving, if desired

Pasta primavera (*primavera* means "spring" in Italian) was conceived by my friend Ed Giobbi at New York's Le Cirque restaurant in the 1970s. Although various vegetables have been used in the numerous adaptations that have evolved since then, at home Ed makes the dish with raw tomatoes only, flavoring them with olive oil, basil, onion, and garlic. The simple tomato-and-herb taste of this delightful first course does bring to mind a fresh spring day.

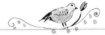

Prepare the sauce: Cut the tomatoes crosswise in half, squeeze out the seeds, and cut the flesh into ¼-inch dice (you should have about 2 cups).

Place the chopped onion in a sieve and rinse it under warm tap water (this removes the strong smell and acidic taste). Drain well.

Combine the tomatoes, onion, garlic, salt, pepper, olive oil, and basil in a bowl. Toss well and set aside.

When ready to serve, bring 3 to 4 quarts of salted water to a boil in a large pot. Add the pasta and push it below the surface of the water with a fork, stirring gently to separate the strands. Bring the water back to a boil and cook for about 10 to 12 minutes, or until as tender as you like.

When the pasta has finished cooking, remove about 1 cup of the cooking liquid and pour it into your serving bowl. Stir in the olive oil, salt, and pepper. Drain the pasta, add it to the bowl, and toss to mix well. Place the tomato mixture in the microwave for 1 minute to make it tepid.

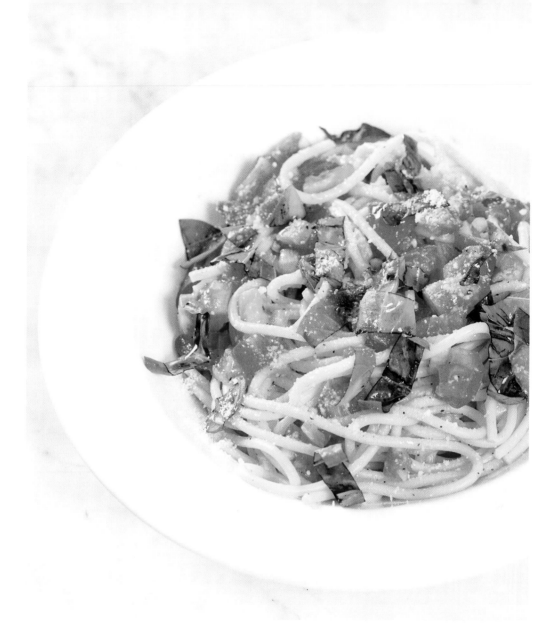

Divide the pasta among four plates and sprinkle with the grated cheese (or pass it at the table). Spoon the sauce over the pasta and serve immediately, with extra cheese if desired.

> **Reserving 1 cup of the pasta cooking liquid and tossing the drained pasta with it before adding the tomato sauce adds moisture and flavor.**

LINGUINE WITH STEWED TOMATO SAUCE

◦ SERVES 4

1 pound thin linguine

¼ cup virgin olive oil

1 teaspoon salt

¼ teaspoon freshly ground
black pepper

¾ cup shredded good-quality
Swiss cheese, preferably Gruyère,
or ¼ cup grated Parmesan cheese

2½ generous cups Quick Tomato
Sauce (page 16)

Hot pepper flakes

There are many different types of pasta at the market, of course, but I prefer linguine for this dish with Quick Tomato Sauce (page 16). The French often serve grated Gruyère with pasta, and I like it this way, but you can substitute the more familiar Parmesan.

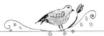

Bring 3 to 4 quarts water to a strong boil in a large pot. Add the pasta to the boiling water and push it under the water with a spoon or fork to submerge it completely. As the water returns to the boil, stir gently to separate the strands of linguine, and cook for 10 to 12 minutes, or until the pasta is as tender as you like. Scoop ½ cup of the cooking liquid into a large stainless steel bowl and drain the pasta.

Add the olive oil, salt, pepper, cheese, and the pasta to the reserved cooking liquid into the bowl. Toss until well combined. Divide among four plates and top each serving with ½ cup of the hot tomato sauce and some pepper flakes if desired. Serve immediately.

▷ **Leftover pasta reheats perfectly in a microwave oven.**

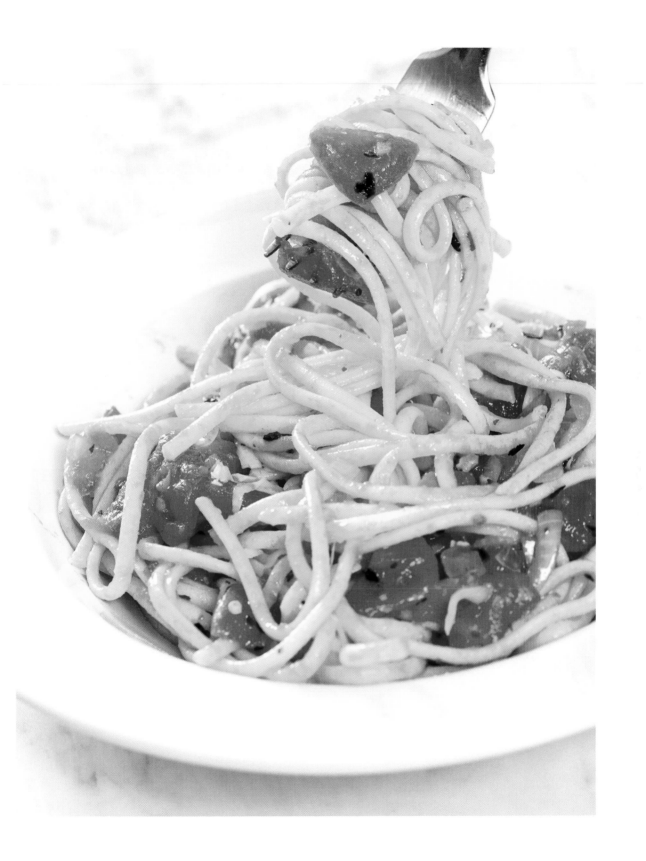

LINGUINE WITH CLAM SAUCE GLORIA

○ SERVES 6

Sauce
───────

8 cloves garlic, peeled

1 small jalapeño pepper, halved and seeded, or 1 teaspoon hot pepper flakes

3 dozen cherrystone clams, shucked, juices reserved, cut into halves with scissors, or two 10-ounce cans whole baby clams

One 8-ounce bottle clam juice (optional, if using canned clams)

1 cup loosely packed flat-leaf parsley leaves

½ cup virgin olive oil

1⅓ cups diced (¼-inch pieces) onion

1 cup dry fruity white wine

1 teaspoon Italian seasoning

Salt (optional)

1½ pounds thin linguine

Salt and freshly ground black pepper

Grated Parmesan cheese, for serving (optional)

Gloria, my wife, makes a linguine with clam sauce that is my favorite in the summer, when she uses fresh clams and fresh clam juice. Sometimes, however, she doesn't have access to fresh clams, so she opts for the canned baby clams that are always stocked in our pantry. Although they may not produce the same result, they still make a delicious dish. If using fresh clams, use cherrystones, cut into halves with scissors, and their juices.

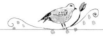

Bring 4 to 5 quarts water to a boil in a large pot over high heat.

Meanwhile, prepare the sauce: Place the garlic and jalapeño pepper halves in a mini-chop and pulse a few times to coarsely chop. Add enough of the clam juice to provide a little moisture, then add the parsley, pushing it down on top of the other ingredients. Starting and stopping the machine a few more times, coarsely chop the parsley; the liquid will help it become incorporated. (This can also be done by hand.)

Heat the olive oil in a shallow saucepan. When it is hot, add the onion and sauté for 2 to 3 minutes. Add the garlic-parsley mixture and stir for 15 to 20 seconds, then add the remaining clam juice. Rinse out your mini-chop with the white wine, then add it to the saucepan, along with the Italian seasoning. Bring to a boil and add salt if desired (depending on how salty the clams and clam juice are). Reduce the heat, cover, and simmer for 3 minutes. Add the clams and bring to a boil. Set aside.

Add the linguine to the boiling water, stir well, return to a boil, and boil for about 10 to 12 minutes, until as tender as you like. Drain in a colander and return to the cooking pot. Add about ½ cup of the liquid from the sauce and mix it into the linguine to prevent it from sticking together. Add a dash each of salt and pepper if needed.

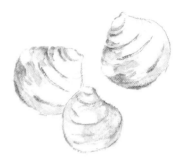

Divide the linguine among six plates and season some clam sauce over each serving. Serve with Parmesan cheese if desired, although conventionally Italians do not put Parmesan on seafood pastas.

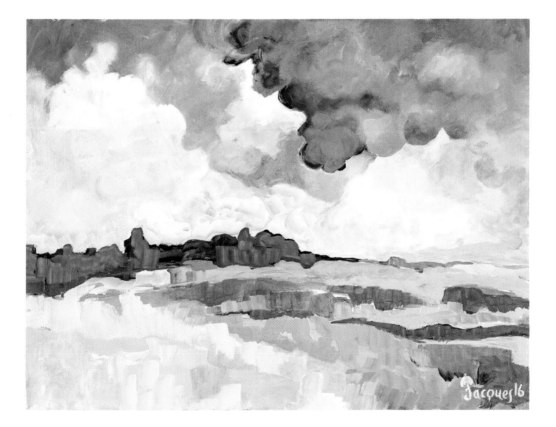

PENNE WITH MUSHROOM, TOMATO, AND NUT SAUCE

∘ SERVES 2

8 ounces penne

¾ cup Mushroom, Tomato, and Nut Mix (page 19), with about ¼ cup oil from the mix (see Note)

¼ teaspoon salt

About 3 tablespoons grated Pecorino Romano cheese

I like to serve this delicious sauce over penne because the tube-shaped pasta absorbs the flavors so well.

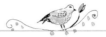

Bring 3 quarts of water to a strong boil in a large pot. Add the pasta, bring the water back to a boil, and cook for 12 to 14 minutes, or until as tender as you like. Near the end of the cooking time, remove ½ cup of the cooking liquid and place it in a large bowl. To this, add the mushroom-tomato mix with its oil and the salt and mix well.

Drain the cooked pasta, add it to the bowl, and toss well. Divide between two plates, top with the grated cheese, and serve.

NOTE: If you like, cut the tomatoes into ½-inch pieces.

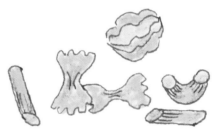

Red Pepper Dip is delicious and can be made ahead, and if transformed into a sauce, it goes particularly well with rigatoni, whose tube shape holds it so well. This recipe serves four as a first course but can be doubled for a main course.

Bring 3 quarts water to a boil in a large pot over high heat. Add the pasta, stir well, return the water to a boil, and boil for 12 to 14 minutes, or to your liking. Near the end of the cooking time, remove ½ cup of the cooking liquid from the pot and place it in your serving bowl. Drain the pasta.

Add the red pepper dip to the reserved liquid in the bowl, then stir in the oil, salt, and pepper. Mix well and add the pasta. Toss to combine, divide between two plates, and serve with the cheese sprinkled on top.

RIGATONI WITH RED PEPPER SAUCE

◦ SERVES 4 AS A FIRST COURSE

8 ounces rigatoni

1½ cups Red Pepper Dip (page 20)

2 tablespoons virgin olive oil

⅛ teaspoon salt

¼ teaspoon freshly ground black pepper

2 tablespoons grated Parmesan cheese

BOW-TIE PASTA WITH MUSHROOMS

○ SERVES 4 AS A FIRST COURSE

8 ounces bow-tie (butterfly or farfalle) pasta

¼ cup virgin olive oil

4 cloves garlic, peeled and chopped fine (1 tablespoon)

4 scallions, cleaned and chopped fine (about ⅔ cup)

4 ounces mushrooms, washed and coarsely chopped (1½ cups)

½ teaspoon salt

¼ teaspoon freshly ground black pepper

3 tablespoons grated Parmesan or Pecorino Romano cheese

This delicious pasta sauce is composed of fresh mushrooms sautéed with garlic and scallions. Save time by using the presliced prewashed mushrooms found in most supermarkets. Bow-tie pasta makes it a decorative first course.

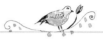

Bring 3 quarts of water to a strong boil in a large pot. Add the pasta, bring the water back to a boil, and cook for 10 to 12 minutes, or to your liking. Near the end of the cooking time, remove ½ cup of the cooking liquid and set it aside.

Drain the cooked pasta in a colander and return the pot to the stove. Add the oil, garlic, scallions, and mushrooms and cook over high heat for about 2 minutes. Return the pasta and the reserved cooking liquid to the pot, season with the salt and pepper, and toss to mix well.

Divide the pasta and sauce among four plates and serve with the grated cheese sprinkled on top.

> **Adding a little of the pasta cooking liquid extends and enriches the sauce.**

I follow the same procedure here as for the Shrimp Wonton Ravioli (page 132), but fill the ravioli with a ricotta cheese mixture and serve them with a light, dressing-like sauce. These make an excellent first course.

🐦

Prepare the ravioli: Mix the ricotta, egg, Romano, salt, pepper, and chives together in a bowl.

Lay 12 of the wonton wrappers out on a work surface and moisten them lightly around the edges by brushing them with a little water. Divide the cheese mixture among the wrappers, mounding it in the centers. Cover with the remaining wrappers, aligning them with the squares beneath, and press gently around the edges to seal.

Bring 3 to 4 quarts of water to a strong boil in a large saucepan Carefully place the filled wontons in the boiling water, moving them gently around at first so they don't stick to the bottom of the pan. After a minute or so, they will float to the top. Continue boiling gently for about 5 to 6 minutes, until the wrappers are tender.

Meanwhile, prepare the sauce: Combine the olive oil, lemon juice, salt, pepper, and chicken stock in a bowl and stir well.

Drain the ravioli and divide among small bowls or plates. Drizzle the sauce on top.

> It only takes a minute to prepare the delicious dressing-like sauce served with this ravioli.

RICOTTA CHEESE WONTON RAVIOLI

◦ SERVES 4

Ravioli

1 cup ricotta cheese (8 ounces)

1 large egg

2 tablespoons grated Pecorino Romano cheese

¼ teaspoon salt

¼ teaspoon freshly ground black pepper

2 tablespoons minced chives

24 wonton wrappers (3 inches square)

Sauce

2 tablespoons extra-virgin olive oil

2 teaspoons lemon juice

⅛ teaspoon salt

⅛ teaspoon freshly ground black pepper

¼ cup Basic Chicken Stock (page 15) or canned chicken broth

SHRIMP WONTON RAVIOLI

◦ SERVES 4

Ravioli

1 slice white bread

8 ounces uncooked shrimp, peeled

1 scallion, cleaned and trimmed

1 clove garlic, peeled and crushed

1 large egg

¼ teaspoon salt

⅛ teaspoon freshly ground black pepper

1 tablespoon minced chives

24 wonton wrappers (3 inches square)

Wonton wrappers, which are available in most supermarkets, are inexpensive and very useful. The wrapper dough is usually rolled out on cornstarch—that is the white powder you see coating packaged wrappers.

In this recipe the wonton wrappers are used to create ravioli, which are stuffed with a shrimp puree. You can find shrimp in various forms—fresh or frozen, shelled or unshelled—at most supermarkets. If they are frozen, defrost them before processing in the food processor.

This recipe can be prepared quite quickly—a few seconds for processing the filling, and a few minutes for poaching the ravioli. It makes an elegant first course.

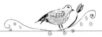

Prepare the ravioli: Tear the slice of bread into pieces, put in a food processor, and process for a few seconds (you should have ½ to ¾ cup crumbs). Transfer the crumbs to a dish and set aside.

Add the shrimp, scallion, garlic, egg, salt, and pepper to the processor bowl and process for 10 to 15 seconds, just until the mixture is smooth and well combined. Transfer to a bowl and gently fold in the bread crumbs and chives.

Lay 12 of the wonton wrappers out on a flat work surface and moisten them lightly around the edges by brushing them with a little water. Divide the shrimp mixture among the wrappers, mounding approximately 1½ teaspoons in the center of each. Cover with the remaining wrappers, aligning them with the squares beneath, and press gently around the edges to seal.

Bring 3 to 4 quarts water to a strong boil in a large saucepan. Carefully place the filled wontons in the boiling water, moving them around at first so they don't stick to the bottom of the pan. After a minute or so, they will float to the top. Continue boiling gently for about 5 to 6 minutes, until the wrappers are tender.

Meanwhile, prepare the sauce: Combine the clam juice, cream, salt, pepper, and chili paste in a saucepan and bring to a boil. Add the dissolved potato starch and return to a boil, stirring. Remove from the heat.

Drain the ravioli and divide among small bowls or plates. Coat them with the sauce and serve.

▷ **Wonton wrappers, available at most supermarkets, can be used to make ravioli and dumplings and can even be shredded or used as a garnish in soups.**

Sauce

One 8-ounce bottle clam juice

½ cup heavy cream

¼ teaspoon salt

1 teaspoon freshly ground black pepper, or more to taste

1 teaspoon Chinese chili paste with garlic, or to taste

2 teaspoons potato starch, dissolved in ⅓ cup water

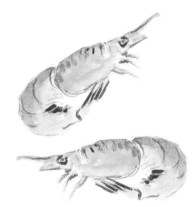

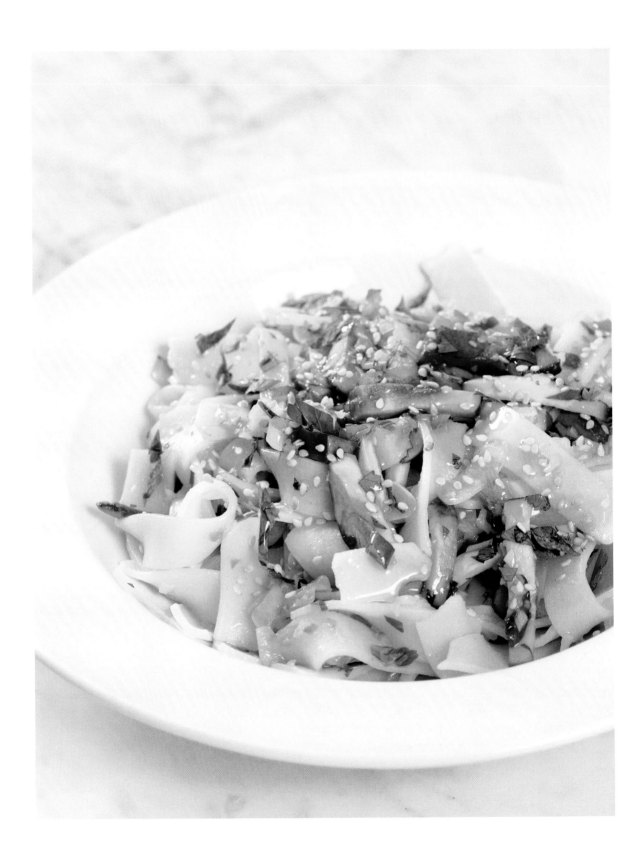

Rice noodles have an absolutely wonderful texture when properly prepared. I prefer those that are at least ¼ inch wide—they're very easy to handle. For this recipe, the rice noodles are soaked in hot water and then drained. When the sauce is ready, the noodles are stir-fried at the last moment, just before serving

Place 3 quarts hot water (about 170 degrees) in a bowl, add the rice noodles, and soak for about 15 minutes.

Meanwhile, wash the mushrooms and cut into julienne strips, or slice them in a food processor using the 2-millimeter blade (you should have about 4 cups).

Heat the oil in a large nonstick saucepan. When it is hot, add the onions and cook over medium heat for about 3 minutes. Add the garlic, mix well, and stir in the mushrooms. Cook for about 5 minutes, until all the juices from the mushrooms has released and evaporated. Add the salt and Sriracha and set aside.

Drain the rice noodles and let them sit in the colander until they are somewhat cool to dry them out a little.

A few minutes before serving, combine the noodles and hot mushroom mixture in a wok or in two nonstick skillets and sauté over high heat for 2 to 3 minutes to warm the noodles and finish cooking them. Sprinkle with the parsley, sesame oil, and sesame seeds and serve immediately.

RICE STICK NOODLES WITH MUSHROOMS

○ SERVES 6

1 pound rice stick noodles (about ¼ inch wide)

12 ounces mushrooms

⅓ cup virgin olive oil

2 cups chopped onions

5 cloves garlic, peeled and chopped (about 1 tablespoon)

1 teaspoon salt

1 tablespoon Sriracha or other hot sauce

¾ cup coarsely chopped flat-leaf parsley

2 tablespoons toasted sesame oil

2 tablespoons sesame seeds

▷ **Keep rice stick noodles, available in most supermarkets, on hand. They're quick and easy to prepare.**

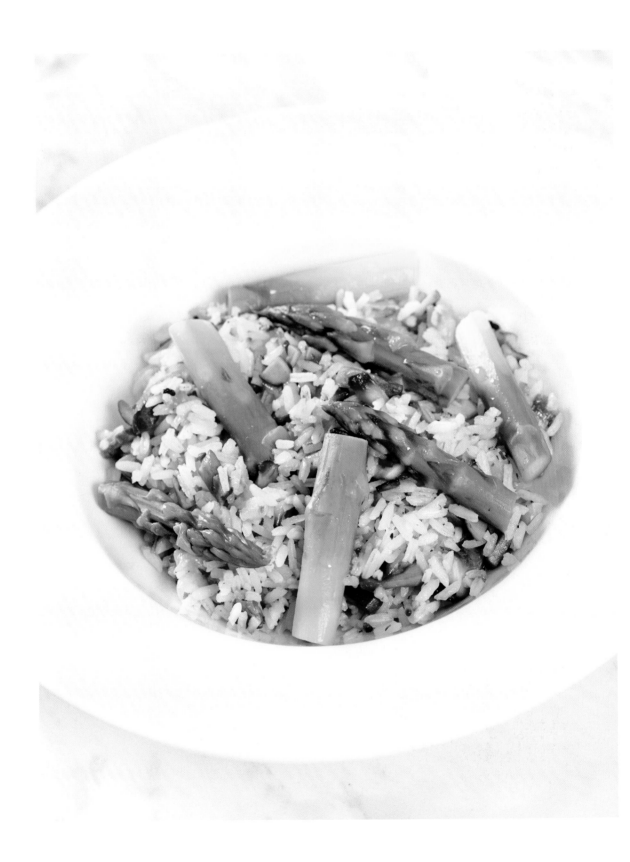

For this unusual recipe, rice is cooked until almost done and then asparagus is laid on top of the rice to cook in the steam rising from it. Just remember to use a saucepan that is large enough to accommodate the asparagus.

Heat the oil and butter in a large saucepan and sauté the onion for about 2 minutes, until it is almost transparent. Add the mushrooms and herbes de Provence and cook for another 2 minutes. Stir in the rice, chicken stock, salt, and pepper and bring to a boil, stirring occasionally. Cover tightly, reduce the heat to very low, and cook for about 15 minutes, until most of the liquid has been absorbed.

While the rice is cooking, using a vegetable peeler, peel the lower third of the stalks or cut them off and discard.

After the rice has cooked for 15 minutes, lay the asparagus on top of it and continue cooking for another 10 minutes, or until the asparagus is cooked but still firm.

Serve the asparagus with the rice on individual plates.

> **Cooking rice and a vegetable together in one pan is a time- and work-saver.**

RICE WITH MUSHROOMS AND STEAMED ASPARAGUS

◦ SERVES 6

2 tablespoons extra-virgin olive oil

1 tablespoon unsalted butter

1¼ cups coarsely chopped onion (about 6 ounces)

2 cups coarsely chopped cremini or portobello mushrooms

1 teaspoon herbes de Provence (see Note, page 15)

2 cups Carolina rice (about 12 ounces)

4 cups light chicken stock, Basic Chicken Stock (page 15), or canned chicken broth

½ teaspoon salt

¼ teaspoon freshly ground black pepper

18 stalks asparagus with firm tips

BROWN RICE RAGOUT

∘ SERVES 6

8 ounces salt pork or pancetta, as lean as possible, in one piece

1 onion (about 3 ounces), peeled and coarsely chopped (1 cup)

6 scallions, cleaned and cut into ½-inch pieces (about 1 cup)

1 tablespoon chopped crushed fresh ginger

2 teaspoons chopped jalapeño or serrano pepper

About 2 cups brown rice (1 pound), preferably Wehani (see Note)

5 cups water, Basic Chicken Stock (page 15), or canned chicken broth

This dish is basically a highly flavored, spicy rice. The pork gives it richness, and the ginger and jalapeño pepper give it zip. I use Wehani rice, available at most health food stores. It is a dark, very-long-grain rice with thick hulls and a strong, nutty, delicious taste, and it has to cook longer than regular rice.

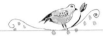

Cut the salt pork into ½-inch-thick slices and then into ½-inch-wide strips. Place in a saucepan and cook over medium heat for 10 to 12 minutes, stirring occasionally. The fat should be rendered and the pork (lardons) nicely browned.

Add the onion, scallions, ginger, and hot pepper, mix well, and cook for 2 to 3 minutes. Then add the rice, stir well, and add the water. Bring to a boil, stirring occasionally, reduce the heat to very low, cover tightly, and cook for about 1 hour, testing the rice for tenderness after about 30 minutes. Serve.

NOTE: Wehani rice, which comes from California, cooks in about 1 hour and absorbs 2½ times its volume in liquid. Other brown rices will vary, taking from 30 minutes to an hour and using from 1½ to 3 cups of liquid per cup of rice.

Cornmeal grits is basically the same as polenta, a variety of yellow cornmeal that is also the name of the mush-like Italian dish, made with this cornmeal. Here I cook the cornmeal in a light chicken stock and flavor it with Parmesan cheese. It is easy, takes only about 20 minutes to make, and tastes great with roasted meat—especially if some of the meat juices are spooned over it.

Bring the stock, chicken base, and pepper to a boil in a large saucepan, then add salt to taste. Pour in the cornmeal in a slow, steady stream, whisking continuously. Bring the mixture back to a boil, then reduce the heat to very low and cook, partially covered to avoid splattering, for about 20 minutes, stirring with your whisk (especially in the corners) every now and then to prevent sticking.

Add the cheese and butter, mix well, and serve immediately.

CORNMEAL MUSH WITH CHEESE

◦ SERVES 4

3½ cups Basic Chicken Stock (page 15) or canned chicken broth

1 tablespoon organic chicken base

¼ teaspoon freshly ground black pepper

Salt to taste

1 cup yellow cornmeal

¼ cup grated Parmesan cheese

1½ tablespoons unsalted butter

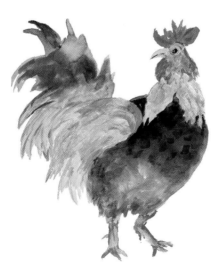

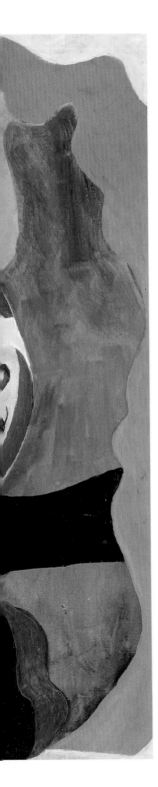

LEGUMES & VEGETABLES

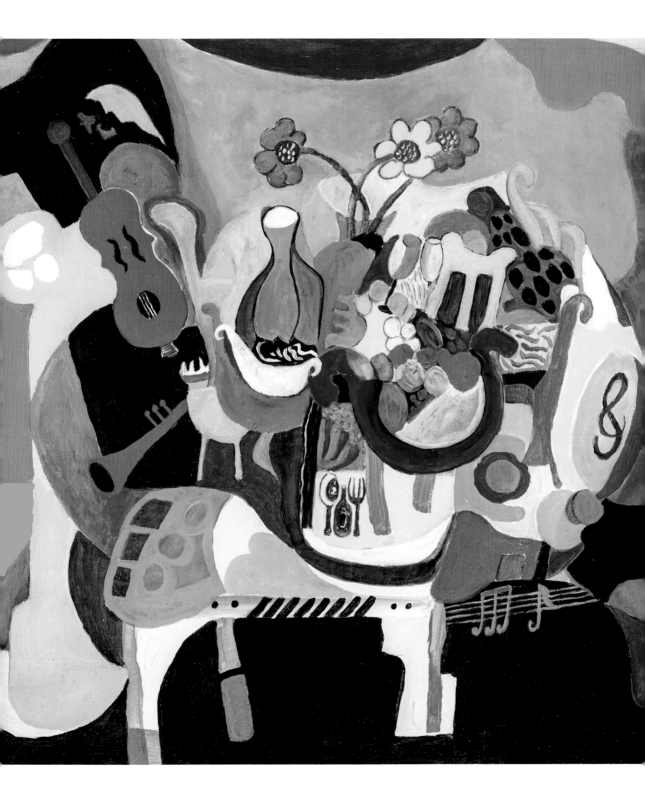

BLACK-EYED PEAS AND HAM

○ SERVES 6

2 tablespoons peanut oil

2 onions, peeled and chopped coarsely (about 2 cups)

2 carrots, peeled and cut into ½-inch pieces (1 cup)

2 teaspoons chili powder

1 teaspoon dried thyme

½ teaspoon hot pepper flakes

1 pound dried black-eyed peas

4 cloves garlic, peeled and sliced (about 2 tablespoons)

1½ teaspoons salt

6 cups water

12 ounces fully cooked ham, cut into 1-inch pieces

2 ripe tomatoes (about 10 ounces total), halved, seeded, and cut into 1-inch pieces (about 2 cups)

Tabasco sauce, for serving (optional)

▷ **This earthy stew can be served directly from the pot.**

Black-eyed peas are one of my favorite legumes. (Black-eyed beans are the same thing—just more oval in shape.) This earthy one-pot dish does not involve much work and can be served family-style, directly from the pot. Any leftovers freeze well.

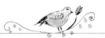

Combine the oil, onions, carrots, chili powder, thyme, and pepper flakes in a sturdy pot or large casserole. Stir well, and cook over medium heat for about 5 minutes.

Meanwhile, put the black-eyed peas in a sieve, rinse thoroughly under cold running water, and drain. Add them to the pot, along with the garlic, salt, and water. Bring to a boil, cover, and boil gently over very low heat for about 1 hour, or until the peas are cooked through.

Mix in the ham and tomatoes and cook for another 10 minutes. Serve as is or with Tabasco sauce to taste.

NOTE: Depending on the dryness of the beans, the cooking time can vary a great deal.

CREAMY BLACK-EYED PEA SOUP

Leftovers can be turned into a delicious soup: Simply puree the stew in a food processor, adding enough water to thin it to the desired consistency. Season with salt and pepper. Reheat and serve with croutons.

I love Boston baked beans and so does my wife, Gloria. They take time to cook but involve only about ten minutes of actual work when prepared this way. Canned small white beans are combined with seasonings, bacon, and onion in an earthenware crock. The ingredients are stirred together and then the dish is baked for several hours.

The earthenware crock I use is 9 inches in diameter and 3 inches high. It will take more than an hour for the bean mixture to come to a boil in the oven. If you want to speed up the process, bring the mixture to a boil on the stovetop before putting it in the oven.

The beans are delicious reheated.

Preheat the oven to 350 degrees. Place the beans, with their liquid, in an earthenware crock or casserole and stir in all the remaining ingredients. The mixture should be at least ½ inch from the top of the crock. Set the crock uncovered on a baking sheet and bake for 2 hours.

Stir the crust that has formed on top of the beans down into the mixture. Cook for 1 hour longer.

Again stir in the crust, and cook for 1 hour longer (4 hours total), or until the mixture is glossy and most of the liquid has been absorbed. Serve.

NOTE: These beans are not as sweet as those in most traditional recipes. If you like your beans sweeter, add more brown sugar or molasses.

BOSTON BAKED BEANS

∘ SERVES 8

Three 16-ounce cans small white beans

6 slices bacon (about 4 ounces), cut into 1-inch pieces

1 large onion, peeled and chopped coarsely (about 1¼ cups)

¼ cup ketchup

2 tablespoons molasses

2 teaspoons dry mustard

¼ teaspoon cayenne pepper

1 teaspoon dried oregano

¼ teaspoon salt

¼ cup packed dark brown sugar

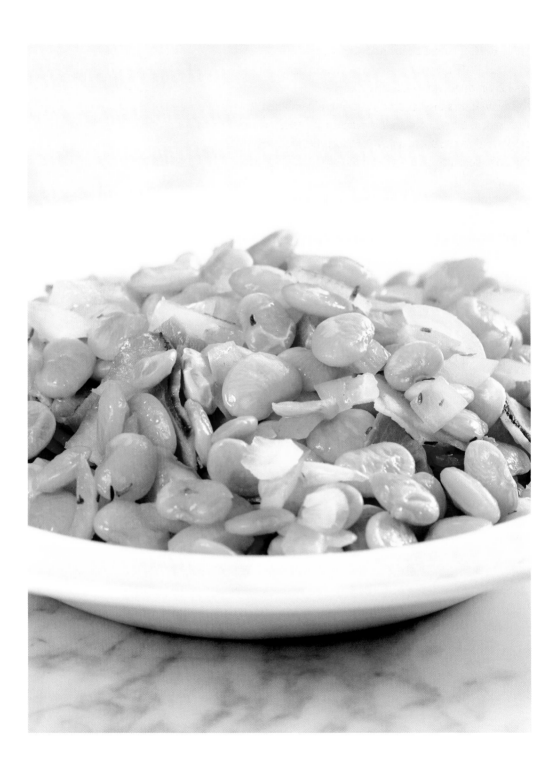

I always have packaged frozen lima beans on hand for use in quickly prepared fricassees like this one. The dish is ready to eat in about 15 minutes.

The beans are flavored with Canadian bacon, but ham would be good too. Canadian bacon tends to be salty, so don't add any salt to the dish until you've tasted it near the end of the cooking period.

Heat the butter and oil in a large saucepan. Add the Canadian bacon and onion and sauté over medium-to-high heat for 3 to 4 minutes, until the bacon is nicely browned.

Meanwhile, place the frozen lima beans in a sieve and run them under warm tap water to thaw them slightly and to remove any ice particles. Add the beans to the mixture in the saucepan, cover, and bring to a boil, stirring occasionally. Reduce the heat and cook, covered, over low heat for 8 to 10 minutes. Add salt if needed, and the pepper and serve.

> **Made with frozen lima beans, this dish is ready to eat in 15 minutes.**

FRICASSEE OF LIMA BEANS

○ SERVES 4

1 tablespoon unsalted butter

1 tablespoon olive oil

3 ounces Canadian bacon, cut into ½-inch pieces (about ¾ cup)

1 onion (4 ounces), peeled and cut into ½-inch dice

½ teaspoon herbes de Provence (see Note, page 15) or Italian seasoning

One 10-ounce package frozen baby lima beans

Salt to taste

¼ teaspoon freshly ground black pepper

WHITE BEAN PUREE

○ SERVES 4

1 tablespoon olive oil

1 onion (about 3 ounces), peeled and sliced thin (1 cup)

1 large clove garlic, peeled and crushed

One 16-ounce can small white beans, drained

½ teaspoon salt

¼ teaspoon freshly ground black pepper

1 tablespoon unsalted butter

½ teaspoon Tabasco sauce

You can make this creamy, delicious puree on short notice with canned white beans. It is a great side dish with sautéed chicken, roast veal, roast beef, and especially lamb. It also makes a good dip!

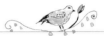

Heat the oil in a large skillet, then add the onion and sauté over medium-to-high heat for about 1 minute. Add the garlic and cook, stirring, for 5 to 6 seconds. Add the beans and cook for 2 to 3 minutes, until they are hot.

Transfer the mixture to a food processor and process for 8 to 10 seconds, until smooth. Add the salt, pepper, butter, and Tabasco and process briefly to incorporate.

Serve immediately, or keep warm in a double boiler until ready to serve.

NOTE: You can make this puree ahead of time and then reheat it in a microwave oven.

This vegetable stew is seasoned with pancetta, which is unsmoked lean Italian bacon.

You can use a mixture of fresh vegetables, from carrots to turnips to peas to string beans, or use frozen mixed vegetables as a time-saver. If you keep a 20-ounce bag of frozen mixed vegetables in your freezer and have pancetta on hand, you can prepare this dish on the spur of the moment. It is hearty enough to serve as a brunch dish with a salad, or it can be a vegetable accompaniment for roasted meats.

JARDINIERE OF VEGETABLES

° SERVES 4

One 20-ounce bag frozen mixed vegetables or the same amount of diced fresh vegetables, such as carrots, potatoes, onions, and/or peas, along with garlic

3 ounces pancetta in one piece, cut into ½-inch pieces (about ½ cup)

1 onion (about 5 ounces), peeled and cut into ½-inch dice (1 cup)

1 tablespoon all-purpose flour

1 cup water

¼ teaspoon salt

¼ teaspoon freshly ground black pepper

1 tablespoon chopped flat-leaf parsley, for garnish

If using frozen vegetables, place them in a sieve and run them momentarily under hot water to partially defrost them. Set aside to drain.

Place the pancetta in a saucepan and cook over medium heat for 6 to 8 minutes, until the pieces are brown and crisp. Add the onion and cook for 2 minutes. Mix in the flour and cook, stirring, for about 30 seconds. Add the water and bring to a boil, stirring. Mix in the vegetables, salt, and pepper and bring to a boil, stirring. Mix well again, cover, reduce the heat, and boil gently for 8 to 10 minutes. Or, if using fresh vegetables, cook for about 20 minutes, until tender.

Serve immediately, or cool and then reheat at serving time. Sprinkle with the parsley before serving.

> **Keep a few 20-ounce bags of frozen mixed vegetables in your freezer for vegetable stews and soups.**

 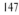

STEAMED CAULIFLOWER WITH LEMON BUTTER

◦ SERVES 6

1 head cauliflower (2 pounds), trimmed of green and root end

Sauce
—
¼ cup water

4 tablespoons (½ stick) unsalted butter, cut into pieces

1 tablespoon lemon juice

1 tablespoon virgin olive oil

½ teaspoon salt

¼ teaspoon freshly ground black pepper

2 tablespoons chopped chives, for garnish

A firm white head of cauliflower looks handsome when you serve it whole. This quick, delicious recipe goes well with grilled meat, fish, or stew. Try the lemon butter sauce with other steamed vegetables as well, or with steamed or broiled fish.

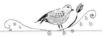

Rinse the cauliflower under cold water and place it whole in a saucepan that is tall enough to hold it in an upright position. Add 2 cups water and bring to a boil over high heat, then cover and cook for 10 to 12 minutes, until the cauliflower is tender but still somewhat firm and most of the water has evaporated. Place the cauliflower on a round serving platter or in a gratin dish and set aside in a warm place.

Meanwhile, make the sauce: Bring the water to a boil in a small saucepan (preferably stainless steel). Stir in the butter, lemon juice, olive oil, salt, and pepper and bring to a strong boil. When the mixture emulsifies, pour it over the cauliflower.

Sprinkle with the chives and serve in wedges, cutting the cauliflower as you would a pie.

> This easy-to-make lemon butter sauce goes well with other steamed vegetables as well as with steamed or broiled fish.

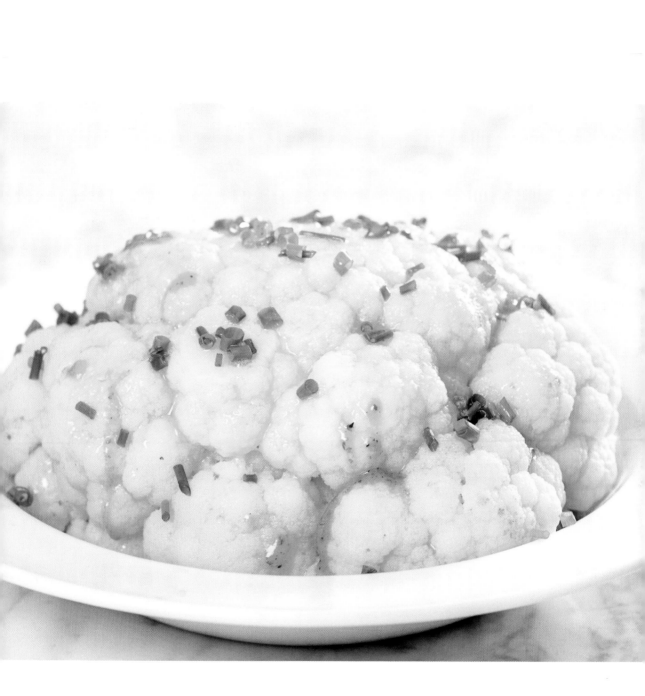

PUREE OF CARROTS AND POTATOES

○ SERVES 6

4 cups diced (1-inch pieces) peeled potatoes

1 pound baby carrots (4 cups)

4 tablespoons (½ stick) unsalted butter, cut into pieces

1 teaspoon salt

¼ teaspoon freshly ground black pepper

For this recipe, just enough water is added to cook the vegetables, leaving no excess moisture to be drained away at the end of the cooking time. That way, all the flavor is retained.

This is great with grilled or roasted meat or fish.

Place the potatoes, carrots, and 2 cups water in a stainless steel saucepan and bring to a boil, then cover, reduce the heat, and boil gently for about 10 minutes. The water should be almost gone; if there is still some remaining, remove the lid and cook over high heat for a few minutes, until almost all the moisture has evaporated except for about ⅓ cup.

Transfer the potatoes and carrots to a food processor and add the rest of the ingredients. Process for 10 to 15 seconds, or longer of if you'd like it very smooth. Serve.

▷ If you don't have time to peel fresh potatoes for this puree, use frozen ones; they work beautifully.

Although you can use larger carrots cut into 1-inch pieces here, I like the baby carrots that come already peeled. Cooked with honey, butter, and a dash of pepper, these carrots have a wonderful flavor.

Place all the ingredients in a saucepan (preferably stainless steel), stir, and bring to a boil. Cover, reduce the heat, and boil gently for 6 to 8 minutes, until the carrots are cooked through but still firm. Serve immediately.

> **Frozen baby carrots work well here— they don't require peeling and cook in just a few minutes.**

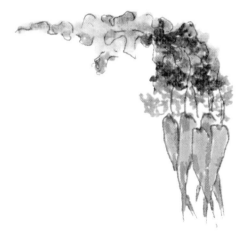

BLACK PEPPER– HONEYED CARROTS

◦ SERVES 4

1 pound baby carrots (4 cups)

½ cup water

2 tablespoons unsalted butter

¼ teaspoon salt

¼ teaspoon freshly ground black pepper

2 tablespoons honey

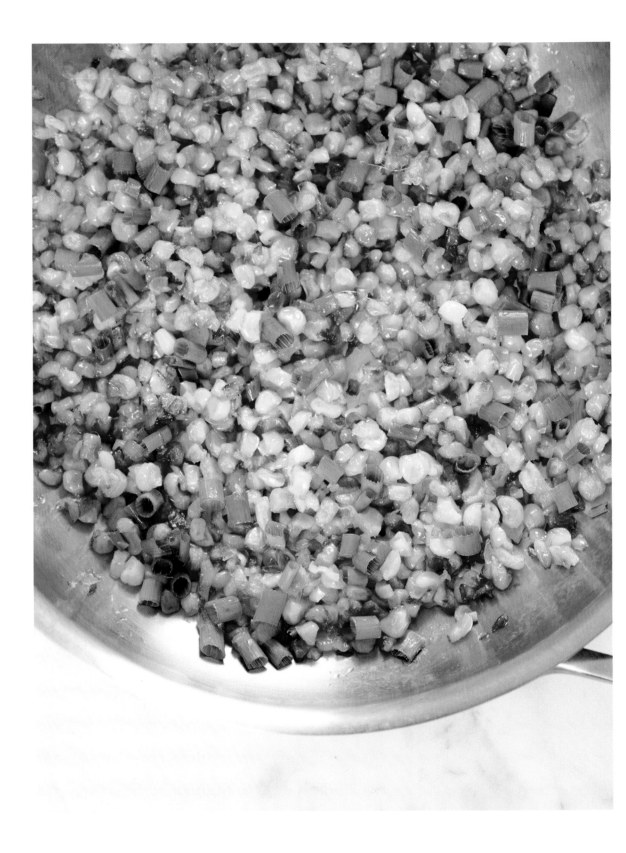

This tasty dish can be made with either fresh or frozen corn kernels, both of which take only a few minutes to sauté. Some of the kernels become slightly caramelized and candied as they cook, resulting in an intense flavor. This is a perfect last-minute addition to a meal when you find you need another vegetable.

Heat the oil and butter in a large nonstock skillet over medium to high heat. When the mixture is hot, add the scallions and the corn kernels and cook, covered, for 3 to 4 minutes. Remove the lid and cook for 1 to 2 minutes, shaking the pan (be careful, as the corn tends to splatter), until the mixture is practically dry and some of the kernels are starting to brown a little. Add the salt and pepper and serve.

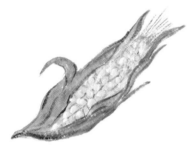

CORN POELE

○ SERVES 4

2 tablespoons corn oil

1 tablespoon unsalted butter

2 scallions, minced

4 cups fresh corn kernels (from 4 ears), or one 1-pound package frozen corn kernels

¼ teaspoon salt

¼ teaspoon freshly ground black pepper

▷ **Either fresh or frozen corn can be used in this flavorful dish.**

CORN FRITTERS IN BEER BATTER

∘ SERVES 6

¾ cup all-purpose flour

1 cup beer

2 cups fresh corn kernels
(from 2 ears)

¼ teaspoon salt

About ½ cup corn oil

Sour cream and caviar,
for garnish (optional)

I use corn here, but any type of vegetable from spinach to zucchini to carrots to peas—or even a mixture of vegetables—can be coarsely chopped and used in these delicious little fritters. These can be served with aperitifs, as a first course, or as a garnish for meats. Although they are good eaten plain, they are especially flavorful topped with a dollop of sour cream and a spoonful of caviar.

This recipe takes only a few minutes to prepare. The fritters should be small—2 to 2½ inches in diameter—as they are best when very thin. If you cook them ahead, place them on a wire rack so the undersides don't get soggy, and then reheat in a very hot oven just before serving or recrisp under a hot broiler (5 or 6 inches from the heat source) for a few minutes.

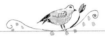

Place the flour in a medium bowl. Pour about ¾ cup of the beer over the flour and mix well with a whisk until smooth. Add the remaining beer and mix again. Add the corn kernels and the salt and mix gently.

Heat 1½ to 2 tablespoons of the oil in each of two large skillets. When the oil is hot, spoon about 2 tablespoons of the batter into each skillet and spread it out with a spoon; don't be concerned about a few holes here and there. Add more spoonfuls of batter to the skillets to make 3 or 4 fritters at a time in each pan, spreading the batter out for each fritter. Cook over high heat for about 3 minutes per side, until the fritters are brown and

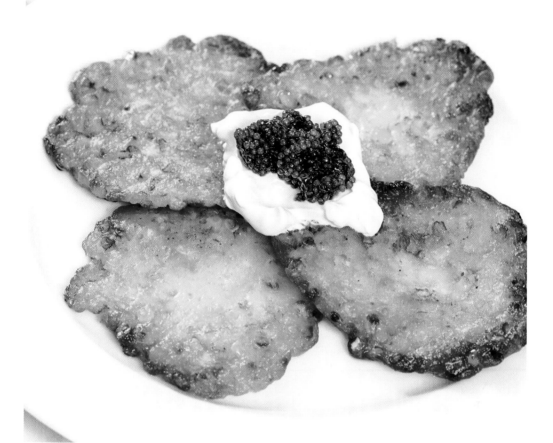

crisp, and transfer to a wire rack. Continue making fritters, adding a little more oil to the skillets as needed, until you have used all the batter.

Serve the fritters immediately, or reheat them later in a hot oven or under the broiler (see headnote). Serve topped with sour cream and caviar, if desired.

> If you don't plan to eat the fritters immediately, place them on a wire rack so they don't get soggy on the undersides.

CREAM OF CORN PUDDING

∘ SERVES 4

1 tablespoon unsalted butter, plus more for the gratin dish

2 cups fresh or frozen corn kernels

3 large eggs

½ cup milk

¼ cup all-purpose flour

½ teaspoon salt

¼ teaspoon freshly ground black pepper

1 tablespoon sugar

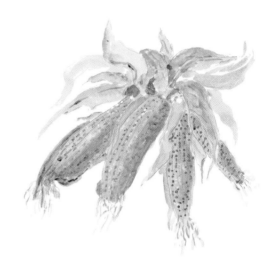

Made with fresh or frozen corn kernels, this custardy pudding goes well with sautéed meats and with stews.

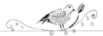

Preheat the oven to 375 degrees. Butter a 5- or 6-cup gratin dish. Place all the ingredients in a food processor and process for 10 seconds. Pour the pudding mixture into the prepared gratin dish.

Bake for about 45 minutes, until the pudding is golden, puffy, and set. Serve.

This was inspired by a Russian recipe that features eggplant seasoned with cinnamon, coriander, and dill. Easy to do, it can be prepared ahead and then reheated at serving time.

Preheat the oven to 400 degrees. Arrange the eggplant and onion slices in a large gratin dish, alternating between eggplant and onion and overlapping the slices. Season with the cinnamon, coriander, dill seeds, salt, and pepper. Then sprinkle on the oil, vinegar, and water.

Cover with aluminum foil and place on a foil-lined cookie sheet. Bake for about 25 minutes. Remove the foil cover and bake for about 15 minutes longer, until tender and lightly brown. Serve immediately, or set aside and reheat, covered with plastic wrap, in a microwave oven, just before serving.

> **You can prepare this dish ahead and reheat it in a microwave oven at serving time.**

EGGPLANT BORANI

◦ SERVES 4

1 eggplant (12 ounces), peeled and cut lengthwise into ½-inch-thick slices (about 10 slices)

1 onion (4 ounces), peeled and sliced thin

½ teaspoon ground cinnamon

½ teaspoon ground coriander

¼ teaspoon dill seeds

½ teaspoon salt

½ teaspoon freshly ground black pepper

3 tablespoons safflower or olive oil

1 tablespoon cider vinegar

⅓ cup water

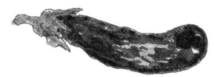

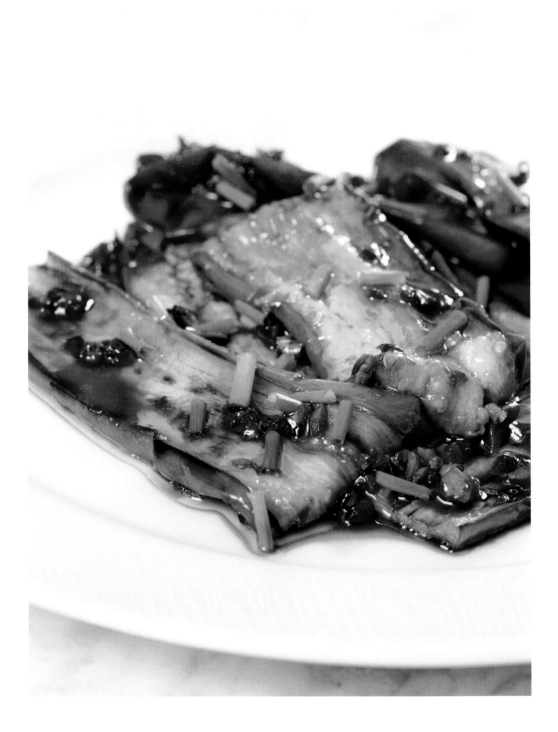

Make this quick, flavorful dish in the summer, when freshly picked eggplant is plentiful. Select long, narrow Japanese or Chinese eggplants. This makes a good first course, and it can also be served with broiled or roasted meat or fish in place of a salad.

Preheat the broiler. Line a cookie sheet with nonstick aluminum foil and spread the oil onto it. Press the eggplant slices into the oil, turning them so they are coated on both sides, and arrange them in one layer on the cookie sheet. Sprinkle with the salt.

Place the eggplant under the broiler, 5 to 6 inches from the heat source, and broil for 5 minutes, until the surface is bubbly and brown spots have appeared. Turn the eggplant slices and broil for 5 minutes on the other side.

While the eggplant is broiling, prepare the sauce: Mix all ingredients together in a bowl.

Transfer the broiled eggplant to a platter and immediately pour the sauce over it. Set aside to cool, then serve at room temperature.

NOTE: The sauce is also good on salads, or with sushi or poached fish.

BROILED EGGPLANT JAPONAISE

◦ SERVES 4

2 tablespoons peanut oil

2 small Japanese or Chinese eggplants (1 pound total), unpeeled, cut lengthwise into ½-inch-thick slices (about 8)

¼ teaspoon salt

Sauce
———

1 clove garlic, peeled, crushed, and chopped fine (½ teaspoon)

1 teaspoon sugar

1½ tablespoons light soy sauce

1 tablespoon olive oil

1 tablespoon toasted sesame oil

¼ teaspoon Tabasco sauce

LEEKS VINAIGRETTE

○ SERVES 6

6 leeks (1½ pounds), trimmed of roots and fibrous dark green outer leaves

5 cups water

Vinaigrette

1½ tablespoons Dijon-style mustard, preferably "hot"

2 tablespoons red wine vinegar

⅓ cup olive oil

¼ teaspoon salt

¼ teaspoon freshly ground black pepper

Although in modern cuisine most vegetables are cooked only briefly, leeks are most flavorful when cooked until very tender. People tend to trim leeks too much, discarding any part of the vegetable that is green. However, the leeks we buy at the supermarket are already trimmed. I remove the roots and the first layer of tough, fibrous leaves, then I trim selectively, removing only damaged or dark green leaf ends from the second layer and keeping all the tender center leaves. The trimmed leek has a shingled look, with the outer leaves closely cropped and the taller inner leaves intact.

After the leeks are cooked, they are removed from the pan and the excess liquid is pressed out of them. The vinaigrette is added while the leeks are still warm, so they can absorb it. Serve them with some crusty French bread, or cover tightly and refrigerate—they will keep for a couple of days. Then warm the leeks briefly in a microwave oven to bring them back to room temperature before serving.

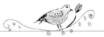

Beginning about 1½ inches above the root end of the trimmed leeks, split each leek lengthwise into 4 sections, leaving them attached at the root end. Open the sections and wash thoroughly to remove the sand inside the leaves.

Bring the water to a boil in a 9- to 10-inch saucepan. Add the leeks in a bunch, all facing the same direction, bending the extending leaves back in so they fit in the saucepan. Press down to position the leeks in one layer. Bring back to a boil, cover, and boil over medium to high heat for 10 minutes, or until the leeks are tender when pierced with the

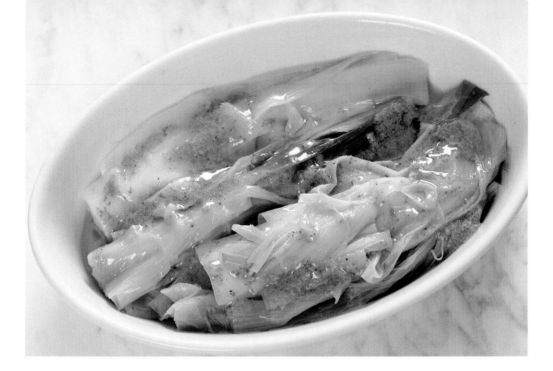

point of a knife. Using a slotted spoon, remove the leeks to a gratin dish suitable for serving. (Reserve the cooking liquid for Cream of Leek Soup, page 75, or Chunky Vegetable Soup, page 64, adding water as needed to make about 4 cups.)

When the leeks have cooled to room temperature, press on them with a spoon, a few at a time, to remove additional liquid (add this to the reserved cooking liquid). Place the leeks on a cutting board and cut them into 2-inch pieces. Return the leeks to the gratin dish, alternating white and green pieces.

Prepare the vinaigrette: Mix together the mustard, vinegar, olive oil, salt, and pepper in a small bowl. Pour the vinaigrette over the leeks, then lift the leeks gently with a fork so the vinaigrette can flow between the pieces and flavor them completely. Serve at room temperature.

▷ **As a bonus, Cream of Leek Soup (page 75) can be made with the delicious cooking liquid obtained here.**

MARINATED MUSHROOMS

1½ pounds button mushrooms (prewashed, if available)

5 tablespoons extra-virgin olive oil

1 teaspoon coriander seeds

½ teaspoon fennel seeds

1 teaspoon salt

1 teaspoon coarsely ground black pepper

¼ cup dry white wine

¼ cup water

1 tablespoon lemon juice

4 bay leaves

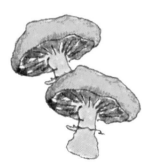

This is a dish that you can prepare ahead in just a few minutes and keep on hand in the refrigerator. It can be served as a first course or as part of a buffet, added to salads, or eaten with cold cuts or other types of meat. The mushrooms will keep in the refrigerator for up to 2 weeks.

Fresh button mushrooms often come prewashed, so you need only cook them briefly with the other ingredients. Frozen button mushrooms can be used as well.

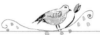

Place all the ingredients in a stainless steel saucepan and stir gently. Bring to a boil, cover, and boil over medium to high heat for 4 to 5 minutes. Pour into a crock or jar and let cool.

Serve the mushrooms warm, cold, or at room temperature.

> **These will keep in the refrigerator for up to 2 weeks—good to have on hand for unexpected guests.**

When you can't think what to serve as a first course, try this simple dish—it is always satisfying. Just be sure to make the toasts at the last minute so they are crunchy, not soggy.

To simplify the preparation, use presliced prewashed fresh mushrooms, available at most supermarkets.

Heat the olive oil in a large skillet. When the oil is hot, add the mushrooms and sauté over high heat for about 5 minutes, until the liquid released by the mushrooms has evaporated and there is just a little moisture remaining around them. Add the salt, pepper, salsa, and sour cream and bring to a boil. Remove from the heat. Stir in the parsley and keep warm.

Toast the bread and cut the slices into quarters. Arrange the quarters on individual plates, forming 1 whole slice per serving. Top with the mushroom mixture and serve.

SPICY MUSHROOM TOASTS

∘ SERVES 4

2 tablespoons olive oil

6 cups sliced mushrooms

½ teaspoon salt

¼ teaspoon freshly ground black pepper

About 2 tablespoons Spicy Red Salsa (page 13) or Sriracha or other hot sauce

½ cup sour cream

2 tablespoons coarsely chopped flat-leaf parsley

4 (¾-inch-thick) slices country bread

PEAS AND PEARL ONIONS IN CREAM SAUCE

∘ SERVES 6

One 10-ounce package frozen pearl onions

One 10-ounce package frozen petite peas

¾ cup Basic Chicken Stock (page 15) or canned chicken broth

⅓ cup heavy cream

½ teaspoon salt

¼ teaspoon freshly ground black pepper

⅛ teaspoon ground nutmeg

1 teaspoon potato starch, dissolved in 2 tablespoons cold water

For this and the next three pea recipes, fresh peas are best when in season. But out of season, frozen peas are a good choice. This recipe is made with frozen tiny peas, which are of excellent quality, and frozen pearl onions.

Place the onions in a sieve and run warm tap water over them to partially defrost. Repeat with the peas.

Combine the onions and chicken stock in a saucepan and bring to a boil over high heat. Reduce the heat to low, cover, and simmer for about 3 minutes, until the onions are cooked through. Add the peas, cream, salt, pepper, and nutmeg. Mix well, return to a boil, and cook, covered, for about 1 minute. Add the dissolved potato starch and bring to a boil, then remove from the heat and serve.

▷ **When a recipe calls for fresh peas, you can use frozen petite peas instead, which are of excellent quality.**

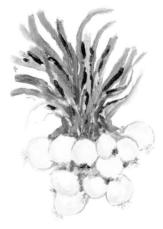

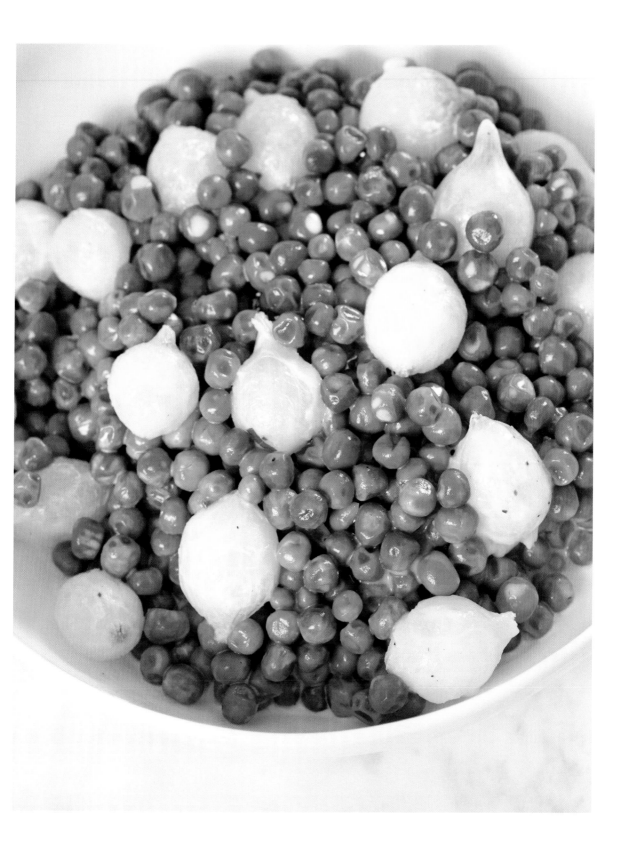

FRICASSEE OF PEAS WITH HAM

∘ SERVES 4

One 10-ounce package frozen petite peas

2 tablespoons olive oil

1 tablespoon unsalted butter

1¼ cups diced carrots (½-inch dice)

1 cup diced (¼-inch pieces) onion

4 ounces cooked ham, cut into ½-inch dice (¾ cup)

¼ teaspoon dried savory

2 teaspoons all-purpose flour

1 cup water

½ teaspoon salt

¼ teaspoon freshly ground black pepper

Frozen tiny peas are one of the best vegetables on the market. They are selected according to a procedure involving gravity: Freshly picked peas are dumped into a vat of salted water. The heavy ones drop to the bottom and the small, lighter ones, higher in sugar, float to the top. These are the tiny sweet peas, often labeled "petite," "tiny," or "tender," that you find in the freezer section of most supermarkets.

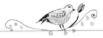

Defrost the peas by placing them in a sieve and running hot tap water over them.

Heat the olive oil and butter in a saucepan. When the mixture is hot, add the carrots, onion, ham, and savory and sauté over medium heat for 3 to 4 minutes, until the vegetables are soft. Add the flour, mix well, and cook for about 30 seconds. Add the water, salt, and pepper and bring the mixture to a boil. Cover, reduce the heat, and cook for 3 to 4 minutes.

Add the peas and bring the mixture back to a boil. Cover and boil gently for 2 minutes, then remove from the heat. Serve.

> This flavorful dish, which is ready to eat in less than half an hour, goes well with most roasts or grilled meat.

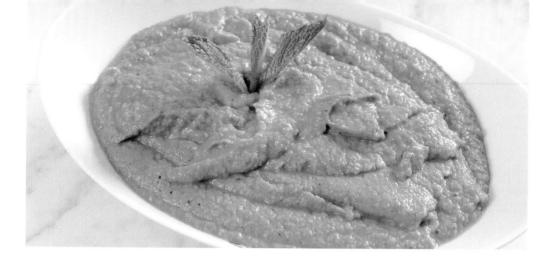

This delicious puree is made with fresh mint and frozen petite peas—the smallest, sweetest peas. Make sure that after you drain them, the hot peas go directly into the blender. If left longer before pureeing, their skins will shrivel and toughen, and consequently the puree will not be smooth. A blender does a better job than a food processor for this recipe.

PUREE OF PEAS WITH MINT

∘ SERVES 6

Bring 3 cups water to a boil in a large saucepan. Add the peas, return the water to a boil, and cook for 2 minutes.

Drain the peas in a colander and immediately place them in a blender. Blend for about 20 seconds. Using a rubber spatula, push any peas clinging to the sides down to the bottom. Add the mint and blend for another 20 seconds. Add the remaining ingredients and process for 10 to 15 seconds. The mixture should be smooth and bright green. Serve.

Two 10-ounce packages frozen petite peas

1 tablespoon chopped mint

1 teaspoon sugar

½ teaspoon salt

¼ teaspoon freshly ground black pepper

3 tablespoons unsalted butter

▷ **This makes a great garnish for poultry, fish, or roast veal.**

BUTTERY PEAS AND LETTUCE

◦ SERVES 4

One 10-ounce package frozen petite peas or same amount of fresh peas

1 small head Boston lettuce (5 ounces)

2 tablespoons virgin olive oil

3 cloves garlic, peeled and sliced thin (1 tablespoon)

½ teaspoon salt

½ teaspoon freshly ground black pepper

¼ teaspoon sugar

1 tablespoon unsalted butter

Use fresh peas in season or frozen peas for this recipe, being careful to select the type marked "petite" or "tiny" peas.

Boston lettuce is the best choice for this recipe. At our house, we often serve this vegetable dish—or Zucchini Flan (page 193), Sautéed Spinach with Nutmeg (page 187), or Corn Fritters in Beer Batter (page 154)—as the first course for a simple family dinner.

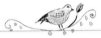

If using frozen peas, place them in a sieve and run hot tap water over them to defrost them.

Cut the lettuce into 2-inch pieces and wash it thoroughly. Drain.

Heat the olive oil and garlic in a large skillet or saucepan (preferably stainless steel). When the oil is hot, sauté for about 1 minute, taking care not to burn the garlic. Add the drained lettuce, cover, and cook for about 1 minute, until the lettuce is wilted. Uncover, add the peas, and cook for 2 to 3 minutes, until most of the moisture has evaporated. Remove from the heat.

Stir in the salt, pepper, sugar, and butter and serve.

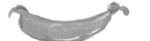
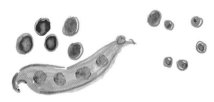

I like iceberg lettuce raw in salads because of its crunchy, cool taste, but I also like it cooked. In this recipe, I sauté the lettuce with garlic, olive oil, and pepper flakes. Although the ultimate goal is to remove the moisture from the lettuce, I do add some water at the beginning of the cooking time so the garlic doesn't burn; eventually, however, moisture emerges from the lettuce so it cooks in its own liquid. Prepared in a few minutes, this is a very simple, light vegetable dish that goes well with roasted and stewed meats.

Heat the olive oil in a large skillet with a tight-fitting lid. When the oil is warm, add the garlic and pepper flakes and cook for 15 to 20 seconds. Place 2 handfuls of the lettuce on top and mix well so the garlic doesn't stick to the bottom of the pan. Add the rest of the lettuce and the water, cover, and cook over medium to high heat for 2 to 3 minutes. Mix well, add the salt, and cook, covered, for 2 minutes longer, or until the lettuce is completely wilted. Uncover, and if there is too much moisture, cook over high heat for 1 to 2 minutes, until most of the moisture has evaporated. There should be only enough moisture remaining so that the lettuce is moist.

Serve immediately, sprinkled with the chives.

ICEBERG AND GARLIC SAUTE

∘ SERVES 4

2 tablespoons virgin olive oil

3 cloves garlic, peeled and chopped (about 2 teaspoons)

¼ teaspoon hot pepper flakes

1 head iceberg lettuce (about 1 pound), cut into 2-inch pieces and layers separated

¼ cup water

½ teaspoon salt

1 tablespoon chopped chives, for garnish

▷ **Iceberg lettuce, which keeps for a long time in the refrigerator, is good cooked as well as raw.**

BASIC BOILED POTATOES

∘ SERVES 4

About 12 small boiling potatoes, such as Red Bliss or Yukon Gold (1½ pounds total)

When I boil or steam potatoes, I usually make extra, since I have several recipes that call for precooked potatoes—among them Potatoes Persillade (page 176) and Ragoût of Potatoes (page 175). Boiled potatoes will keep, refrigerated, for a few days and are delicious in salad as well. This recipe calls for 1½ pounds of potatoes, but you can make double or triple this amount and use the remainder later in the week.

Wash the potatoes thoroughly and place them in a saucepan. Add enough water to cover the potatoes by about 1 inch. Cover the pan, bring the water to a boil, and boil gently for 18 to 22 minutes, until the potatoes are tender when pierced with the point of a sharp knife.

Pour out the water and set the potatoes aside in the pan to dry. (The residual heat in the potatoes will draw more moisture from them, making them firmer and creamier than if they were cooled in the water.) When they are cool enough to handle, peel the potatoes for immediate use in another recipe, or cool completely and refrigerate (unpeeled) for later use.

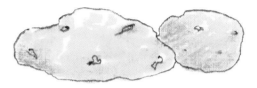

PARSLEY POTATOES WITH BUTTER

These go well with poached, steamed, or grilled fish, as well as with lighter meats like veal.

∘ SERVES 4

Place the potatoes in a skillet with the butter and salt, cover, and heat over high heat for 3 to 4 minutes, until the potatoes are hot. Sprinkle with the parsley and serve.

1½ pounds small Yukon Gold or Red Bliss potatoes, cooked (see Basic Boiled Potatoes, opposite) and peeled

2 tablespoons unsalted butter

⅛ teaspoon salt

2 tablespoons chopped flat-leaf parsley

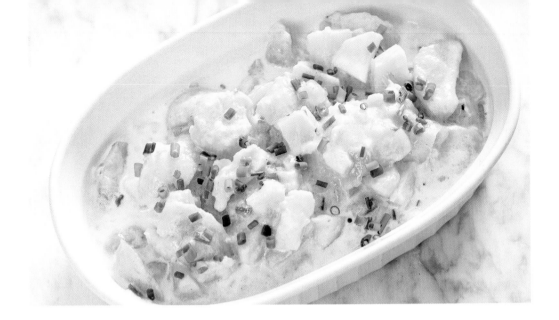

CREAMY STEWED POTATOES

∘ SERVES 4

4 cups diced (½-inch) peeled cooked potatoes (see Basic Boiled Potatoes, page 170)

1½ cups half-and-half

2 cloves garlic, peeled, crushed, and chopped fine (about 1 teaspoon)

½ teaspoon salt

¼ teaspoon freshly ground black pepper

1 tablespoon chopped chives, for garnish

In this recipe, I use half-and-half, but this could be replaced with cream if you want the dish to be very rich, or with milk if you want it less rich. Either way, it is delicious with grilled meat or fish.

Place the potatoes in a saucepan and add the half-and-half, garlic, salt, and pepper. Bring to a boil, partially cover, reduce the heat to low, and cook for 8 to 10 minutes, until most of the liquid has been absorbed and the potatoes are just moist. Sprinkle with the chives and serve.

When I was a child in France, whenever my aunt made mashed potatoes, she put a few cloves of unpeeled garlic in the cooking water. After the potatoes were cooked, she pushed them—garlic and all—through a food mill to eliminate the skin, and the resulting potato mixture had a delicate garlic flavor, which I recall fondly and have tried to recapture in this recipe. Unlike my aunt's smooth mashed potatoes, though, these aren't pressed through a food mill after cooking, so the garlic should be peeled.

MASHED POTATOES WITH GARLIC

○ SERVES 6

1¾ pounds Red Bliss potatoes, peeled and cut into 2-inch cubes

4 large cloves garlic, peeled

4 tablespoons (½ stick) unsalted butter

½ teaspoon salt

½ teaspoon freshly ground black pepper

1 cup milk

Place the potatoes and garlic in a saucepan, cover with water, add ¼ teaspoon of the salt, and bring to a boil. Boil gently for 20 to 22 minutes, until the potatoes are tender, then drain and return the potatoes and garlic to the pan.

Add the butter, remaining ¼ teaspoon salt, and the pepper and crush with a potato masher into a coarse puree. Add the milk and mix with a whisk until the mixture is as smooth as you desire. Serve immediately.

NOTE: To prepare the potatoes ahead, cover the whisked mixture with 2 or 3 tablespoons milk so the top remains moist and to keep a skin from forming. Set aside, then reheat at serving time.

OVEN-ROASTED POTATOES AND ONIONS

◦ SERVES 4

3 Yukon Gold potatoes (about 1¼ pounds total), peeled

1 large onion (about 10 ounces), peeled

½ teaspoon salt

½ teaspoon freshly ground black pepper

½ teaspoon herbes de Provence (see Note, page 15)

¼ cup olive oil

3 tablespoons minced chives

I like to make dishes that can be prepared ahead and cooked with a minimum of fuss. This simple potato dish can be roasted in a hotter oven (375 to 400 degrees) in less than half the time given below, but I happened to be braising a piece of meat in a low-temperature oven the first time I made it, so I took advantage of the opportunity to cook the potatoes and onions in the low oven at the same time.

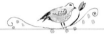

Preheat the oven to 275 degrees. Cut the potatoes lengthwise into 3 slices each. Cut the onion into 4 slices about ¾ inch thick.

Lay all the potato and onion slices in a large gratin dish and sprinkle with the salt, pepper, herbes de Provence, and olive oil. Place in the oven and cook for 2 hours, or until the potato and onion slices are soft and lightly browned.

Turn the potatoes and onions in the oil, sprinkle with the chives, and serve.

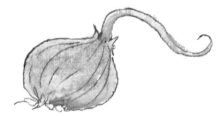

This potato dish can be prepared ahead and then rewarmed, preferably in a microwave oven, at the last minute.

Heat the oil in a large skillet. When the oil is hot, add the onions and sauté for 3 to 4 minutes, until they begin to soften and brown. Add the garlic, potatoes, chicken stock, salsa, herbes de Provence, and salt, cover, and bring to a boil. Reduce the heat and simmer gently for 10 minutes, until the potatoes are tender and most of the liquid has evaporated but the mixture is just slightly moist. Serve sprinkled with the chives.

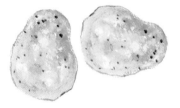

RAGOUT OF POTATOES

○ SERVES 4

2 tablespoons vegetable oil

2 medium onions (about 10 ounces total), peeled and cut into ½-inch dice

4 cloves garlic, peeled and sliced (about 2 tablespoons)

1½ pounds Yukon Gold potatoes, peeled and cut into 1-inch pieces (about 4 cups)

1 cup Basic Chicken Stock (page 15) or canned chicken broth

1 tablespoon Spicy Red Salsa (page 13) or hot sauce

1 teaspoon herbes de Provence (see Note, page 15)

¼ teaspoon salt

2 tablespoons chopped chives, for garnish

POTATOES PERSILLADE

○ SERVES 4

3 tablespoons peanut oil

1½ pounds small Yukon Gold potatoes, cooked (see Basic Boiled Potatoes, page 170), peeled or unpeeled as you like, and cut into ¼-inch-thick slices

3 cloves garlic, peeled, crushed, and chopped (1½ teaspoons)

3 tablespoons chopped flat-leaf parsley

¼ teaspoon salt

1 tablespoon unsalted butter

Persillade, a signature of Provençal cooking, is a mixture of equal amounts of chopped parsley and garlic that is added at the end to vegetable dishes as well as meat and fish dishes.

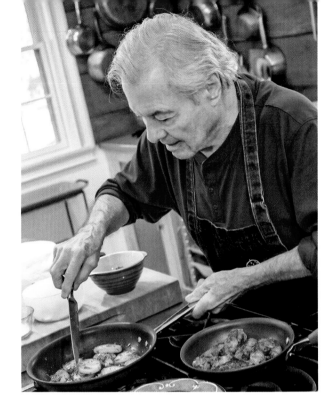

This recipe is ready in a few minutes if made with cooked potatoes. It goes well with everything from poached fish to sautéed meats and roasts.

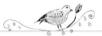

Heat the oil in an 8-inch skillet (preferably nonstick), then add the potatoes and sauté over medium to high heat for 6 to 8 minutes, turning halfway through, until browned.

Add the garlic, parsley, salt, and butter and cook, stirring, for 5 to 6 seconds. Serve immediately.

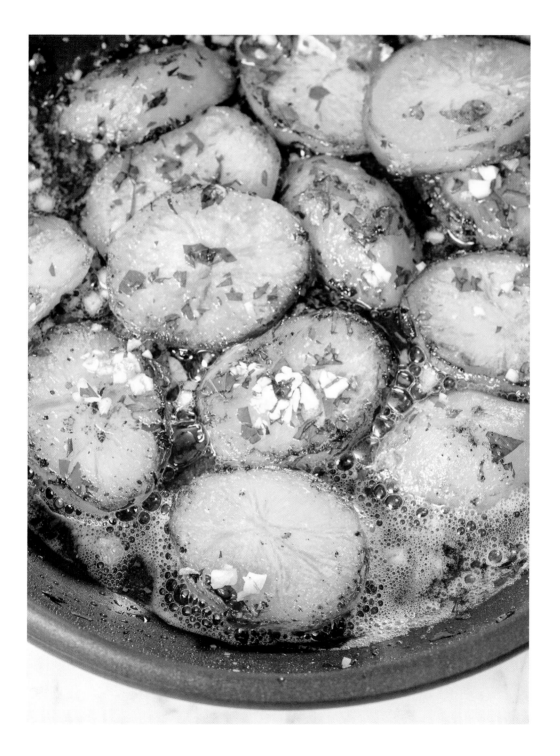

HASH-BROWN POTATO CAKE

◦ SERVES 4

2 tablespoons unsalted butter

2 tablespoons peanut oil

3 cups diced (½-inch pieces) peeled potatoes or frozen hash-brown potatoes

¼ teaspoon salt

¼ teaspoon freshly ground black pepper

⅛ teaspoon ground nutmeg

Here hash-brown potatoes (you can use frozen hash-browns) are pressed down to form a large beautiful patty that is crisp and brown on the bottom. If you are proficient or daring enough, you can turn the patty and brown it on the other side. The potatoes are just as good, however, when cooked on one side only, as here, and then inverted onto a plate so they are presented brown side up.

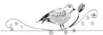

Heat the butter and oil in a 9-inch nonstick skillet. When the mixture is hot, add the potatoes, salt, pepper, and nutmeg, and sauté, stirring occasionally, over medium to high heat for about 3 minutes, until the potatoes begin to brown. Cover, reduce the heat to medium, and cook for about 5 minutes.

Press on the potatoes with a spatula to compact them into a ½-inch-thick layer. Cover and cook over low heat for another 5 minutes. Press down on the potatoes again, re-cover, and cook for 5 more minutes, or until the underside is nicely browned.

Invert the potato cake onto a serving platter, cut into wedges, and serve.

NOTE: A nonstick skillet is essential for making this dish.

This interesting combination—potatoes, walnut (or other nut) pieces, and croutons—is made with cubes of cooked potato. An easy dish to prepare, it is delicious with fish or meat, or just a salad.

Heat the olive oil in a large nonstick skillet. When the oil is hot, add the potatoes and sauté over high heat, stirring every few minutes for 6 to 8 minutes, until lightly browned. Add the nuts and bread cubes and cook, stirring every few seconds, for 3 to 4 minutes, until the nuts and bread have browned. Add the butter and allow it to melt into the mixture.

Transfer to a serving platter, sprinkle with the salt and chives, and serve immediately.

> **Walnut pieces should be stored in the freezer so they don't get rancid.**

POTATOES WITH WALNUTS AND CROUTONS

∘ SERVES 4

6 tablespoons olive oil

4 cups peeled and diced (1-inch pieces) cooked potatoes (see Basic Boiled Potatoes, page 170)

⅔ cup walnut, pecan, or other nut pieces

2 to 3 slices bread, cut into ½-inch cubes (about 1½ cups)

1 tablespoon unsalted butter

¼ teaspoon salt

2 tablespoons chopped chives or flat-leaf parsley

POTATO OMELET

° SERVES 4

2 to 3 Idaho potatoes (1 pound),
peeled and sliced thin (about
3 cups)

3 tablespoons olive oil

1 tablespoon unsalted butter

½ small leek, trimmed, washed,
and sliced thin (about 1 cup)

8 large eggs, preferably organic

½ teaspoon salt

¼ teaspoon freshly ground
black pepper

2 tablespoons chopped chives,
for garnish

> **You probably already have
the basic ingredients—eggs
and potatoes—on hand for
this great last-minute dish.**

This is an ideal recipe for a last-minute meal when
unexpected guests arrive. I always have potatoes and
eggs on hand, so all I need to make this delicious omelet
is a bit of leek, which lends taste and color to the dish
and enhances its flavor. Served with a salad, the omelet
makes a perfect main dish for an informal meal.

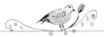

Wash the potatoes in cool water, drain, and pat dry
with paper towels.

Heat the olive oil and butter in a 10-inch nonstick
skillet. When hot, add the potatoes, cover (they tend
to splatter), and cook over medium to high heat for
10 minutes, stirring every 3 to 4 minutes. Add the
leek and cook, covered, for another 3 minutes, until
cooked through and lightly browned.

Meanwhile, break the eggs into a bowl and add the
salt and pepper. Mix well with a fork.

When the potatoes and leek are cooked, add the
egg mixture to the skillet and, using a silicone or
wooden spatula, stir from the sides toward the center
of the pan for about 1 minute, allowing the eggs to
move between the potatoes and cook. Keep stirring
until most of the egg is set, but still be wet in the
center. Cover, reduce the heat to medium to low,
and cook for about 2 minutes, until a nice crust has
formed on the underside. (There will still be some
moisture on top.)

Loosen the omelet around the edges by sliding the
spatula underneath it and invert onto a serving
plate. Cut into 6 wedges and serve sprinkled with
the chives.

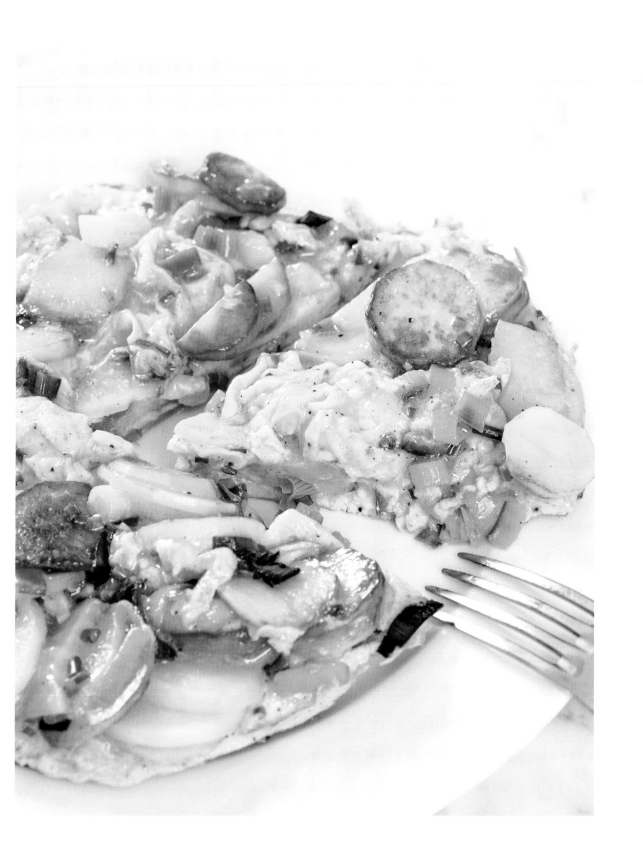

HASH-BROWN POTATOES BOULANGERE

○ SERVES 4

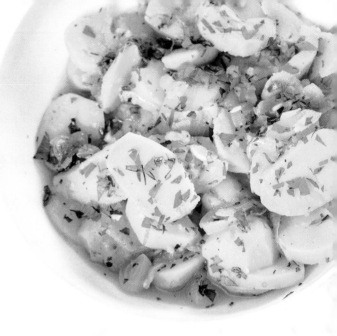

4 cups sliced (¼-inch-thick) peeled potatoes (about 20 ounces)

1 onion (about 5 ounces), peeled and sliced thin (1¼ cups)

1½ cups homemade beef stock or canned beef broth

½ teaspoon herbes de Provence (see Note, page 15) or Italian seasoning

1 tablespoon chopped garlic

2 tablespoons virgin olive oil

¼ teaspoon freshly ground black pepper

2 tablespoons chopped flat-leaf parsley

Boulangère refers to a classic dish of sliced potatoes smothered with onions and stock. If you have a little beef stock and an onion on hand, you can prepare this gratin in a few minutes. Serve with roast lamb, veal, or beef.

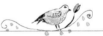

Preheat the oven to 400 degrees. Mix all the ingredients together in a 6-cup gratin dish. Set the dish on a cookie sheet and bake for about 45 minutes, until the potatoes are very tender.

Remove the dish from the oven and let rest for about 15 minutes, then serve.

You can use yams or sweet potatoes for this recipe. The sweetness and rich texture of the yams makes this a great accompaniment for roast turkey or capon over the holidays.

Preheat the oven to 400 degrees. Arrange the yams cut side up in a single layer in a gratin dish and sprinkle the rest of the ingredients over them.

Bake for 30 minutes, then turn the yams cut side down and bake for another 10 minutes, until browned and tender. Serve.

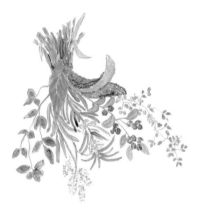

YAMS WITH MAPLE SYRUP AND BUTTER

∘ SERVES 4

4 small yams or sweet potatoes (about 1 pound), peeled and halved lengthwise

¼ teaspoon salt

¼ teaspoon freshly ground black pepper

3 tablespoons maple syrup

2 tablespoons unsalted butter, cut into small pieces

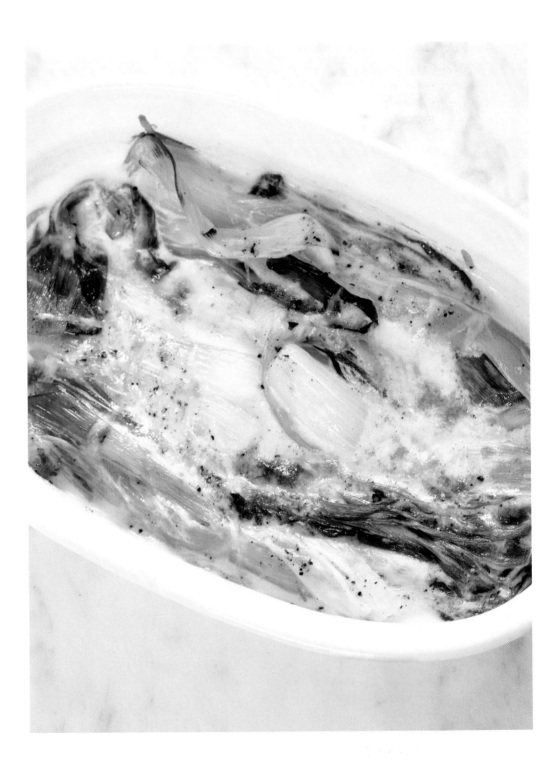

This flavorful gratin goes well with roasted or grilled meat, and it is elegant enough to serve as a first course for a dinner party or as the main dish for a special lunch. The dish can be assembled several hours ahead or even the night before and refrigerated until you are ready to bake and serve.

Preheat the oven to 400 degrees. Cut off and discard the top 3 inches of the scallion greens and any damaged outer leaves. Wash the scallions thoroughly under cool tap water and pat dry.

Place the scallions in a stainless steel skillet, add 1½ cups water, and bring to a boil over high heat. Cover and boil for about 4 minutes, until the water has evaporated. If necessary, cook uncovered to evaporate the water. Remove from the heat.

Arrange the scallions in one layer in a 6-cup oval gratin dish. Sprinkle with the salt and pepper, then pour the cream over and sprinkle with the Parmesan. (At this point, the dish can be covered and refrigerated until ready to cook.)

Place the gratin in the oven and bake for about 15 minutes. Then, to lightly brown the top, turn on the broiler, place the dish under the broiler, about 4 inches from the heat source, and cook for about 2 minutes. Serve immediately.

SCALLIONS AU GRATIN

∘ SERVES 4

4 bunches scallions (about 36)

⅛ teaspoon salt

⅛ teaspoon freshly ground black pepper

½ cup heavy cream

2 tablespoons grated Parmesan cheese

> **You can cook the scallions and assemble the dish a few hours ahead, or even the night before, and refrigerate it until ready to cook and serve.**

GRATIN OF PUMPKIN WITH CHEESE

◦ SERVES 4

One 16-ounce can pure pumpkin puree

2 large eggs

1 cup light cream

¾ teaspoon salt

½ teaspoon freshly ground black pepper

¼ teaspoon ground nutmeg

1 teaspoon unsalted butter

2 ounces Swiss cheese, preferably Gruyère or Emmenthaler, grated (about 1 cup)

I use canned pure pumpkin puree, the type used for pumpkin pie, combining it in the French style with salt, pepper, cream, and cheese to make this vegetable gratin. It can be assembled hours ahead and refrigerated, but it should be baked just before serving.

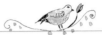

Preheat the oven to 375 degrees. Place all the ingredients except the butter and cheese in a food processor and process for a few seconds, until combined, or whisk together in a bowl.

Grease a 4-cup gratin dish with the butter and pour the pumpkin mixture into the dish. Top with the cheese. (At this point, the gratin can be covered and refrigerated until about half an hour before serving.)

Place the dish in the oven and bake for 30 minutes, or until set and browned on top. Serve as needed.

> **Canned pumpkin puree is prepared French-style here for a vegetable dish.**

In this dish, nutmeg-flavored spinach is stirred into a browned butter-and-oil mixture, giving it a wonderfully nutty taste.

Combine the butter and oil in a large skillet and cook over medium to high heat until the mixture turns light brown. Pile some of the spinach in the hot butter and press on it so it wilts. Keep adding more spinach until you have added and wilted it all. Sprinkle with the nutmeg, salt, and pepper. Using a fork, spread out the spinach so that the flavorings are distributed evenly. Cook for 1 to 2 minutes, then serve.

> **Nutmeg and browned butter give this quick, easy dish its nutty flavor.**

SAUTEED SPINACH WITH NUTMEG

○ SERVES 6

4 tablespoons (½ stick) unsalted butter

1 tablespoon olive oil

1 pound baby spinach

¼ teaspoon ground nutmeg

½ teaspoon salt

¼ teaspoon freshly ground black pepper

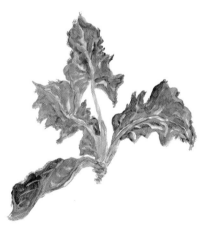

TOMATOES PROVENÇALE

○ SERVES 4

4 large ripe fleshy tomatoes
(about 2 pounds)

3 tablespoons virgin olive oil

Crumbs
2 cloves garlic, peeled

½ cup loosely packed flat-leaf
parsley leaves

1 teaspoon thyme leaves

1½ slices bread, torn into
2-inch pieces

½ teaspoon salt

¼ teaspoon freshly ground
black pepper

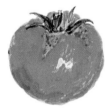

This recipe is good in late summer, when large
beefsteak tomatoes are ripe and very fleshy. The
tomatoes can be partially cooked ahead of time in a
gratin dish that can go directly from the oven to the
table, so it takes only a few minutes to complete the
dish just before serving.

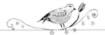

Preheat the broiler. Cut the tomatoes crosswise
in half and arrange them in a gratin dish that is
attractive enough to bring to the table. Oil the tops
of the tomatoes with 1 tablespoon of the olive oil.

Place the tomatoes under the broiler, about 4 inches
from the heat source, and broil for 6 to 8 minutes,
until the tomatoes are firm but tender when pierced
gently with the point of a knife and look slightly
crusty and lightly brown on top. Remove from the
broiler but keep the broiler on.

Meanwhile, prepare the bread crumb mixture: Place
the garlic, parsley, and thyme in a food processor
and pulse for about 10 seconds. Add the bread and
process for another 10 seconds, until the mixture is
combined. Transfer it to a bowl, add the remaining
2 tablespoons oil and the salt and pepper, and toss
gently. Spoon evenly over the tomatoes.

Return the tomatoes to the broiler, about 8 inches
from the heat source, and broil for 5 to 6 minutes,
until they are heated through and brown on top.
Serve immediately.

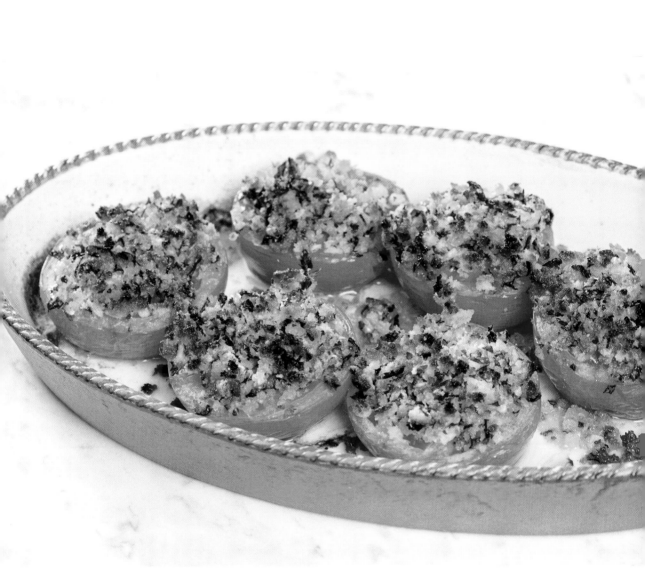

NOTE: To prepare this ahead of time, broil the tomatoes
for 6 to 8 minutes, then let them cool to room temperature
and refrigerate. When ready to serve, bring the tomatoes
to room temperature. About 10 minutes before serving,
prepare the bread crumb mixture and finish the tomatoes.

MUSHROOM-AND-ANCHOVY-STUFFED TOMATOES

◦ SERVES 6

6 tomatoes (about 2½ pounds total), of about equal size and as ripe as possible

½ teaspoon salt

Filling

3 tablespoons olive oil

2 onions (about 6 ounces total), peeled and chopped fine (1½ cups)

1 teaspoon dried oregano

1 pound mushrooms, washed and sliced (or use presliced prewashed mushrooms)

One 2-ounce can anchovy fillets in oil, chopped, oil reserved

1½ cups fresh bread crumbs

¾ teaspoon salt

½ teaspoon freshly ground black pepper

2 tablespoons grated Parmesan cheese

I love to make stuffed tomatoes at the end of summer, when tomatoes are ripe, flavorful, and inexpensive. This is the time when I also freeze or can tomatoes, or make tomato sauce or soup and freeze it for later use.

Here the tomatoes are stuffed with a mixture of mushrooms, anchovy fillets, and onion. A substantial amount of juice is released by the tomatoes as they cook—spoon some of these natural juices over them and serve hot or cold. The dish can be served as a first course, but it also makes an excellent luncheon entrée with a salad and a piece of cheese.

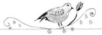

Preheat the oven to 400 degrees. Cut a thin (½-inch) slice from the stem end of each tomato. Then, holding each tomato cut side down over a bowl, press to extract most of the juice and seeds. (This can be reserved and used for stock.)

Arrange the tomatoes cut side up in a gratin dish that holds them snugly. With your thumb, press around the inside of each tomato to smooth it and create a nice cavity. Sprinkle the inside of the tomatoes with the salt.

Prepare the filling: Heat the olive oil in a large saucepan. When it is hot, add the onions and oregano and cook for about 1 minute. Add the mushrooms and cook for 5 minutes, or until they render their liquid. Add the chopped anchovies and their oil (there will still be a lot of liquid in the pan at this point), then add the bread crumbs and stir in the salt and pepper.

Stuff the tomatoes with the filling, dividing it evenly and mounding it so you use all of it. Sprinkle with the Parmesan. Place the gratin dish in the oven and bake for about 35 minutes, until the tomatoes are well cooked and soft. Allow them to cool to lukewarm, basting them with the natural juices released during cooking, then serve warm or cool.

NOTE: The tomatoes can be reheated by placing them in a microwave oven for 1 to 2 minutes.

> **Note that there's a difference in volume in bread crumbs made from fresh versus dried bread. One slice of fresh bread makes ¾ cup crumbs, while 1 slice of dried or toasted bread makes less than ¼ cup crumbs.**

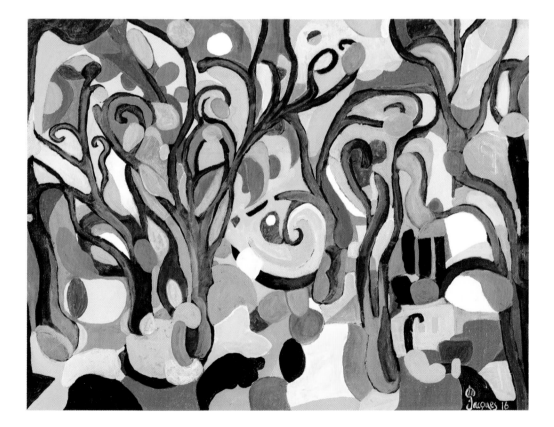

BROILED HEIRLOOM TOMATO WITH BREAD-AND-SCALLION CRUST

○ SERVES 2

2 ripe tomatoes, preferably heirloom (10 to 12 ounces each)

½ teaspoon salt

½ teaspoon freshly ground black pepper

3 tablespoons olive oil

1 cup diced (about ¼-inch pieces) French-style baguette

½ cup diced (about ¼-inch pieces) scallions (about 4)

As with all recipes using tomatoes, the result depends on the quality and ripeness of the tomatoes. Very often, I buy heirloom tomatoes at my market as far ahead as a week before I plan to use them. They stay in a bowl in the kitchen, and when I am ready to use them, they are ripe and flavorful. Here I cook halved tomatoes under the broiler with just a touch of salt until they are cooked and blistered, with some black spots on top. Just before serving, I cover them with a diced-bread-and-scallion mixture.

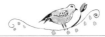

Preheat the broiler. Remove the stems from the tomatoes and cut them crosswise into halves. Arrange them cut side up in a gratin dish and sprinkle with the salt. Place under the hot broiler, 5 to 6 inches from the heat source, and cook for 5 to 6 minutes, until the tomato halves are soft and the tops are blistered. (The tomatoes can be cooked ahead and set aside at room temperature.)

When ready to serve, heat the olive oil in a large saucepan. Add the diced bread and scallions and cook, stirring occasionally, until the bread is lightly browned and the scallions are soft, about 3 minutes. Spread the mixture on top of the tomatoes and serve.

My mother used to make a lot of gratins, flans, and other custard-like dishes, and this was one of her favorites. I prepare it often in the summer when I have an abundance of zucchini in the garden, although pumpkin or another type of squash could be used as well. It is an easy recipe because all the preparation is done in a food processor.

The flan can be served by itself or as an accompaniment to roasted or grilled meat or fish.

Preheat the oven to 400 degrees. Arrange the zucchini slices on a cookie sheet lined with nonstick aluminum foil. Sprinkle with ½ teaspoon of the salt and bake for 10 minutes, until softened. Reduce the oven temperature to 375 degrees.

Transfer the zucchini to a food processor and process for a few seconds to puree. Using a rubber spatula, push down any zucchini clinging to the sides of the bowl and process again until very smooth (you should have about 4 cups). Add the cream, eggs, cornstarch, the remaining 1 teaspoon salt, and the pepper. Process for 10 seconds.

Grease a 7-cup gratin dish (2 inches deep) with the butter. Pour the zucchini mixture into the dish and sprinkle with the cheese. Place the dish on a cookie sheet lined with nonstick aluminum foil and bake for about 45 minutes, until the flan is nicely set. If you want the top of the flan to be browner, place it under the broiler for a few minutes. Serve.

ZUCCHINI FLAN

○ SERVES 6

4 medium zucchini (2½ pounds total), rinsed and cut crosswise into ¾-inch-thick slices

1½ teaspoons salt

½ cup heavy cream

4 large eggs

2 tablespoons cornstarch

½ teaspoon freshly ground black pepper

1 tablespoon unsalted butter

¼ cup grated Parmesan or Pecorino Romano cheese

> **All the work here is done by the food processor.**

NOTE: To prepare this dish ahead, assemble the ingredients in the gratin dish and refrigerate for up to 24 hours. Stir the mixture lightly just before baking.

ZUCCHINI AND EGGPLANT GRATIN

○ SERVES 6

2 Japanese or Chinese eggplants
(the long narrow type; about
1¾ pounds total)

2 or 3 small zucchini (about
1¾ pounds total), as close
to the eggplants in diameter
as possible

1 teaspoon salt

½ teaspoon freshly ground
black pepper

⅓ cup olive oil

2 slices country bread

¼ cup grated Pecorino Romano
cheese

In summer, when zucchini and eggplant are plentiful,
I often make this gratin. It only takes a few minutes to
prepare, and the recipe can be varied by adding other
vegetables, such as slices of tomato and garlic.

I arrange the slices of eggplant and zucchini
alternately in the gratin dish, standing them almost
upright, like a deck of cards. As they cook, the slices
sink down into the dish.

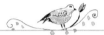

Preheat the oven to 400 degrees. Wash the
eggplants and zucchini (do not peel) and cut them
crosswise into ½-inch-thick slices (you should have
about 20 slices of each). Sprinkle with the salt and
pepper. Arrange slices of eggplant and zucchini in
a large gratin dish, alternating between eggplant
and zucchini and standing the slices almost upright
in the dish. Pour all but 1 tablespoon of the oil over
the slices. Bake for 30 minutes.

While the gratin is cooking, process the bread in a
food processor to make crumbs (you will have about
1 cup). Mix the bread crumbs with the cheese and
the remaining 1 tablespoon oil in a small bowl.

Remove the gratin from the oven (keep the oven on)
and press down on the vegetable slices so that they
are flat in the dish. Sprinkle the bread crumb mixture
evenly over the top, and bake for about 20 minutes
longer. Serve immediately.

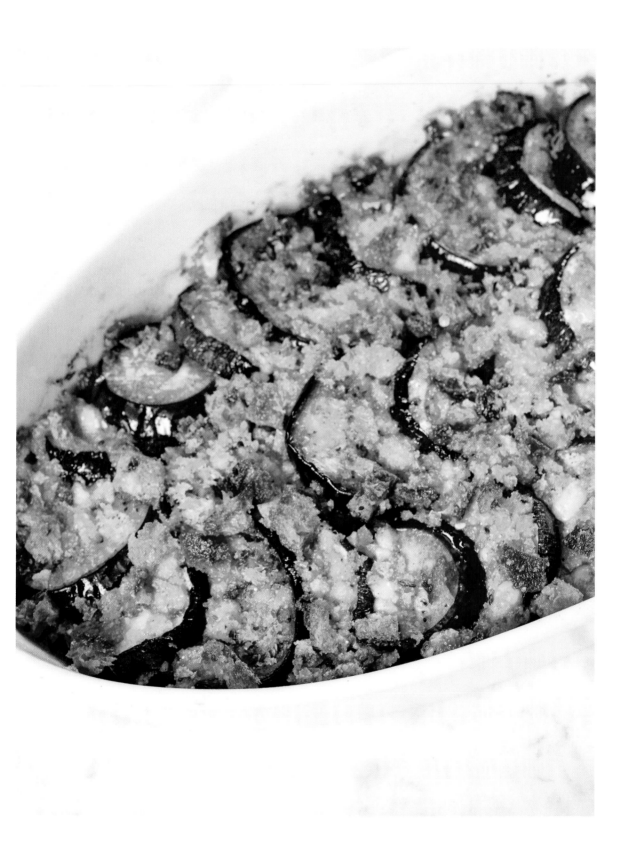

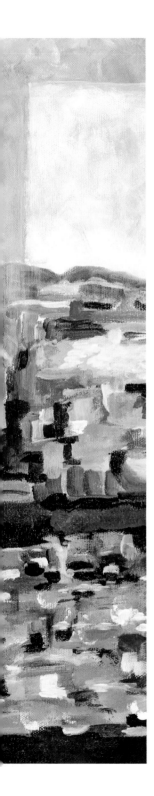

SHELLFISH & FISH

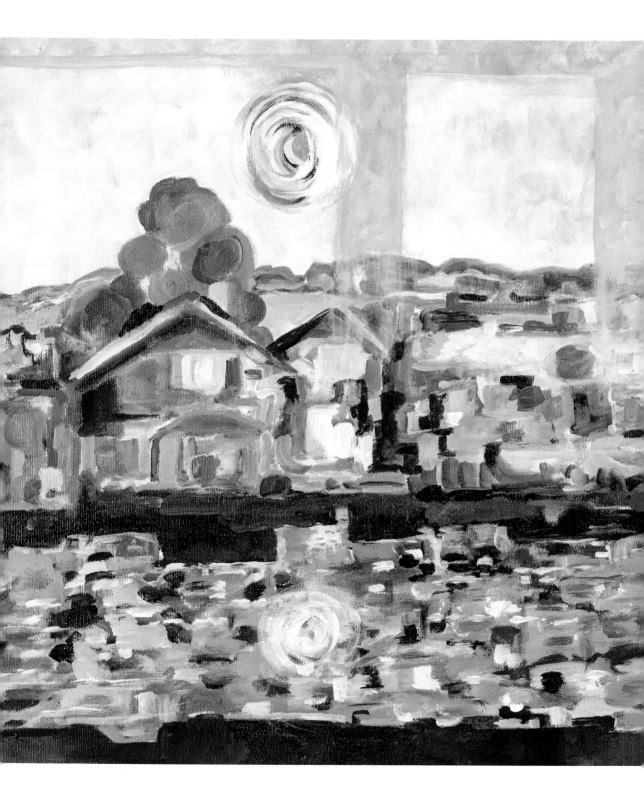

SARDINES IN TOMATO SAUCE

◦ SERVES 4 AS A FIRST COURSE,
2 AS A LUNCH MAIN DISH

About 2 cups salad greens
(such as Boston, red-leaf, or
iceberg lettuce), thoroughly
rinsed and dried

One 16-ounce can sardines
in tomato sauce

1 red onion (about 3 ounces),
peeled and sliced thin

1 tablespoon red wine vinegar

2 tablespoons olive oil

¼ cup flat-leaf parsley leaves

¼ teaspoon freshly ground
black pepper

2 ripe tomatoes (about
10 ounces total)

We often enjoy this as a first course at our house,
especially for lunch. Serve some crusty French bread
alongside.

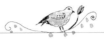

Place the salad greens on a platter and arrange
the sardines, with their sauce, on top. Distribute the
onion slices over the sardines and sprinkle with
the vinegar, olive oil, parsley, and pepper.

Cut the tomatoes lengthwise in half and then into
¼-inch-thick slices. Arrange them attractively around
the edges of the platter and serve.

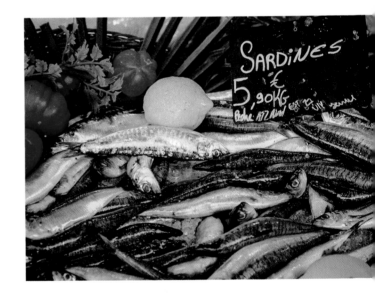

Belgians are great lovers of mussels, and I have a dear friend who often prepares them Belgian-style, garnished with French fries. They are equally good, though, served with sautéed potatoes (see Tip below).

Seasoned primarily with celery and onion, the mussels here are served shells and all in large bowls. If you want to be a bit fancier, remove the empty shells from each one after cooking them and serve them on the half shell, with the cooking juices spooned over them.

The mussels available now are commercially raised and so are much cleaner than they used to be. You don't need to scrape the shells; just wash them thoroughly in cold water. If a shell is open, touch the mussel inside with the point of a knife. If the shell closes, you know the mussel is still alive and will be edible; if it doesn't, discard the mussel.

I do not add any liquid or salt; the mussels release their own juice, which usually has a salty flavor. Add salt if needed after you taste before serving.

Place the mussels in a large bowl of cold water and rub them against one another to clean them. Remove the beards, if any. Check to make certain that all the mussels are alive (see headnote).

Lift the mussels from the water and place them in a saucepan, preferably stainless steel. Add the onions, celery, Tabasco, and olive oil, cover, and bring to a boil over high heat. Stir with a large spoon and cook for 6 to 8 minutes, until all the mussels have opened. Taste for salt and add if needed.

Divide the mussels, vegetables, and broth among four bowls and serve immediately.

MUSSELS A LA BELGE

◦ SERVES 4

3 pounds mussels

2 onions (about 6 ounces total), peeled and cut into ½-inch dice (about 1¼ cups)

1¼ cups sliced celery

1 teaspoon Tabasco sauce

3 tablespoons olive oil

Salt (optional)

▷ **These are good served with sautéed potatoes (see Potatoes Persillade, page 176; Potatoes with Walnuts and Croutons, page 179; and Parsley Potatoes with Butter, page 171).**

MUSSELS IN HOT SAUCE

∘ SERVES 2

2 pounds mussels (about 30), full and heavy

¼ cup dry white wine

2 teaspoons Sriracha or other hot sauce

1 tablespoon olive oil

2 teaspoons toasted sesame oil

1 tablespoon dark soy sauce

1 teaspoon potato starch, dissolved in 2 tablespoons water

⅓ cup coarsely chopped cilantro

I love mussels most when they are plump and full. The season may vary depending on where you live, but usually the shells are really full in late spring. Store-bought mussels are cultivated, usually grown on ropes, and they are quite clean.

I like medium-to-large mussels (about 18 per pound), as heavy as possible, which is an indication of quality. In this recipe, mussels are cooked until they open and then the empty halves of the shells are discarded. The juices are turned into a spicy sauce flavored with cilantro and the mussels served on the half shell with the sauce poured over.

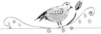

Wash the mussels in a bowl of cold water, rubbing them against one another, and remove the beards, if any. Place the mussels in a deep saucepan along with the wine, hot sauce, oils, and soy sauce. Cover and bring to a boil over high heat, shaking the pan to move the mussels around. Cook for 2 to 3 minutes, until all the mussels have opened. Pull off the empty shells, discarding them, and arrange the mussels on the half shell in two soup plates.

Add the potato starch mixture to the juices in the saucepan. Bring to a boil, stirring, and stir in the cilantro. Pour over the mussels and serve immediately.

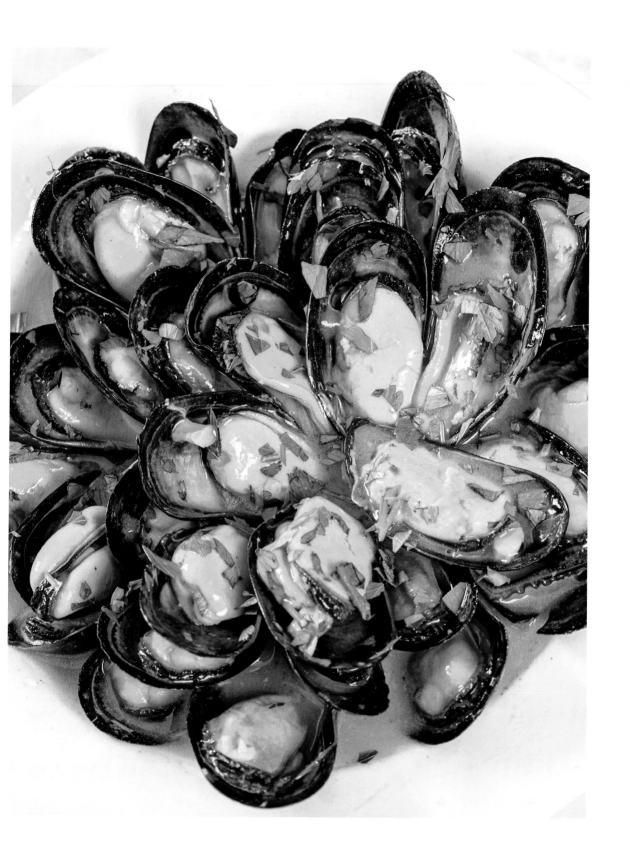

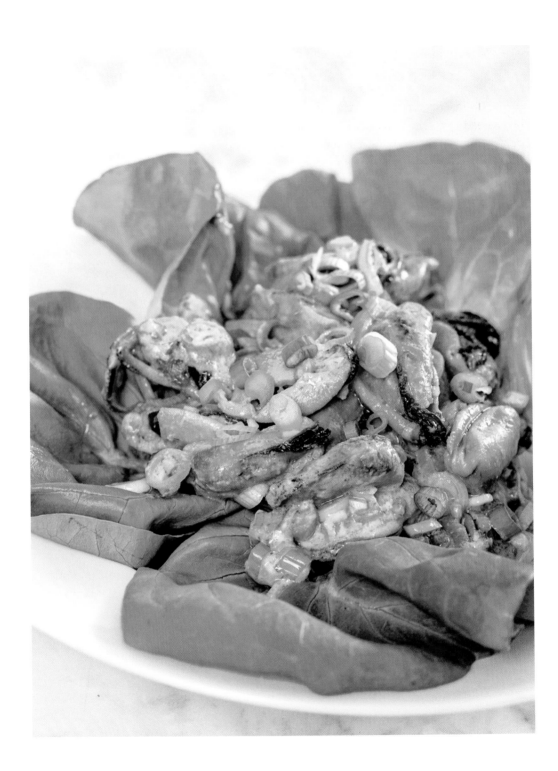

Ravigoter means "to invigorate," which aptly describes the effect the piquant dressing has on the mussels in this dish. There are many reasons to serve mussels: In addition to tasting good, they are inexpensive, usually come already cleaned, and cook in just a few minutes. I don't use the juices from the mussels here; they can be frozen for use in fish soup or fish sauces.

Serve some crusty French bread on the side.

Rinse the mussels in cool water. Don't worry if there is still some incrustation on the outside of the shells, as they will be discarded. Remove any beards.

Place the mussels in a pot, cover, and cook over high heat for 6 to 8 minutes, shaking the pot occasionally, until all the mussels have opened and released their juices. Set aside, covered, to rest for about 5 minutes, then pour into a roasting pan to cool slightly.

When the mussels are cool enough to handle, remove them from their shells and place them in a bowl. Discard the shells. Strain the juices into a plastic container with a tight-fitting lid (you should have about 1½ cups) and freeze for later use in soup, stock, or dishes such as Bllli Bi, page 206.

Add the remaining of the ingredients to the bowl while the mussels are still lukewarm, so they will absorb the seasonings well, and mix well. Serve at room temperature on the lettuce leaves.

MUSSELS RAVIGOTE

∘ SERVES 4

2½ pounds mussels (about 36)

1 tablespoon Dijon-style mustard

3 tablespoons virgin olive oil

2 teaspoons Sriracha or other hot sauce

¼ teaspoon salt

2 scallions, green tops discarded, cleaned and minced fine (about 2 tablespoons)

1 clove garlic, peeled, crushed, and chopped fine (about ½ teaspoon)

4 to 8 Boston lettuce leaves, for serving

▷ **Four reasons to serve mussels: They're good, they're inexpensive, they usually come cleaned, and they cook in a few minutes.**

MUSSELS GRATINEE & BILLI BI

Mussels Gratinée

• SERVES 6 AS A FIRST COURSE

2 pounds mussels (about 36)

1 cup dry white wine

1½ slices white bread

2 tablespoons plus 2 teaspoons olive oil

¼ cup loosely packed flat-leaf parsley

2 cloves garlic, peeled

About 18 hazelnuts

3 tablespoons unsalted butter, softened

½ teaspoon salt

½ teaspoon freshly ground black pepper

These mussels gratinée are seasoned with a garlic-herb butter, just like the classic French *escargots*, or snails. The mussels are first cooked in a little wine until they open and release their juices. Then the empty half shells are removed, leaving the mussels in the half shell, and they are covered with butter and topped with fresh bread crumbs. The mussels are finished under the broiler for a couple of minutes before serving as a first course. They can also be passed around as an hors d'oeuvre, usually six per person.

The juice of the mussels can be frozen for use in fish stew or soup or transformed into the delicious cold soup named Billi Bi; see the recipe on page 206. When I first came to the U.S. in 1959 and worked at Le Pavillon in New York City, we served that soup, which I never saw in any other restaurants. The story is that the soup was created by a cook in Normandy to honor an American GI after the liberation of France in 1945. The GI's name (in the French translation) was Billi Bi. Serve the soup cold, garnished with chives. It is rich and delicious and should be served in small portions.

Place the mussels and wine in a saucepan, cover, and bring to a boil. Stir and cook, covered, for about 2 minutes, until the mussels open. Remove from the heat and let cool for 10 minutes. Separate the shells and discard the empty ones. Strain the cooking liquid, add water if necessary to make 1½ cups, and reserve for the Billi Bi. Arrange the mussels in their half shells on a cookie sheet.

»—>

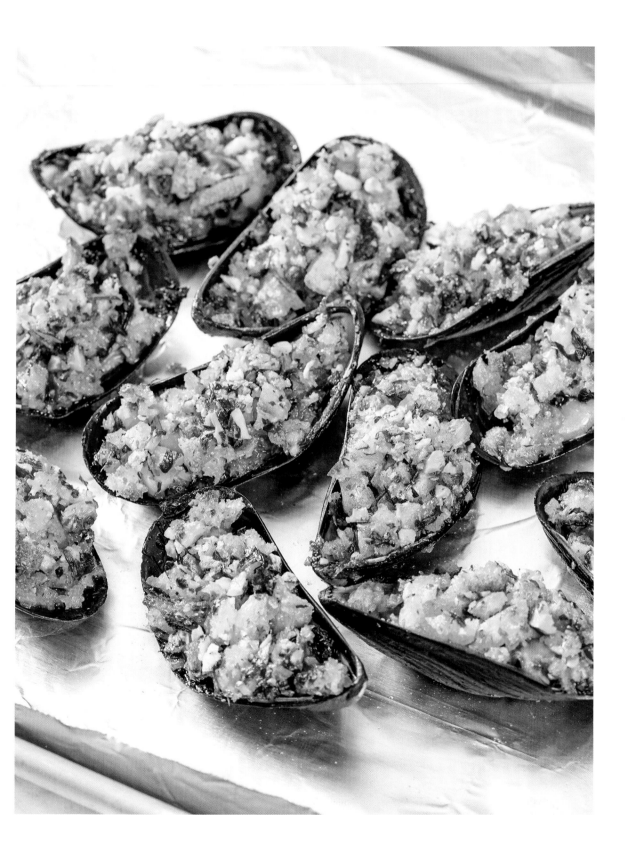

Process the bread in a food processor to make crumbs (you will have about 1 cup). Mix them with 2 teaspoons of the olive oil. Set aside.

Place the parsley, garlic, and hazelnuts in a food processor and process to a fine mixture. Add the butter, the remaining 2 tablespoons oil, the salt, and pepper and process until smooth.

Top each mussel with about a teaspoon of the butter mixture and sprinkle the bread crumbs on top.

At serving time, preheat the broiler. Broil the mussels, about 5 inches below the heat source, for 2 to 3 minutes, until nicely browned. Serve immediately.

Billi Bi

• SERVES 3 AS A FIRST COURSE

1½ cups reserved mussel juices from Mussels Gratinée (see page 204)

1½ teaspoons potato starch, dissolved in 3 tablespoons water

½ cup heavy cream

½ teaspoon Tabasco sauce

½ teaspoon salt, or to taste

1 tablespoon chopped chives, for garnish

Pour the mussel juices into a saucepan, add the dissolved potato starch, and bring to a boil. Stir in the cream, Tabasco, and salt (taste for salt first; you may need less or more than the amount called for, depending on the saltiness of the mussels). Pour the soup into a bowl and let cool, then refrigerate until chilled.

Divide the chilled soup among three small cups and serve with the chives sprinkled on top.

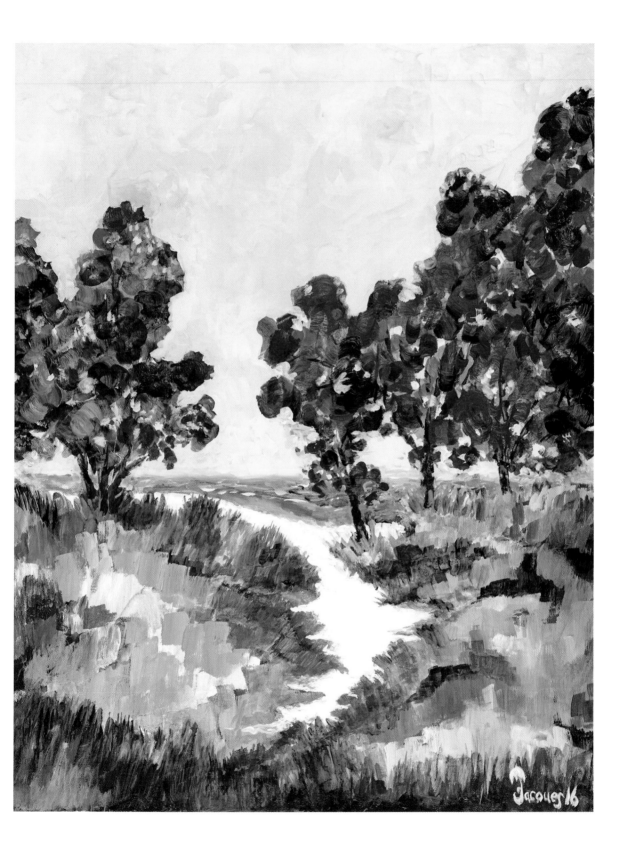

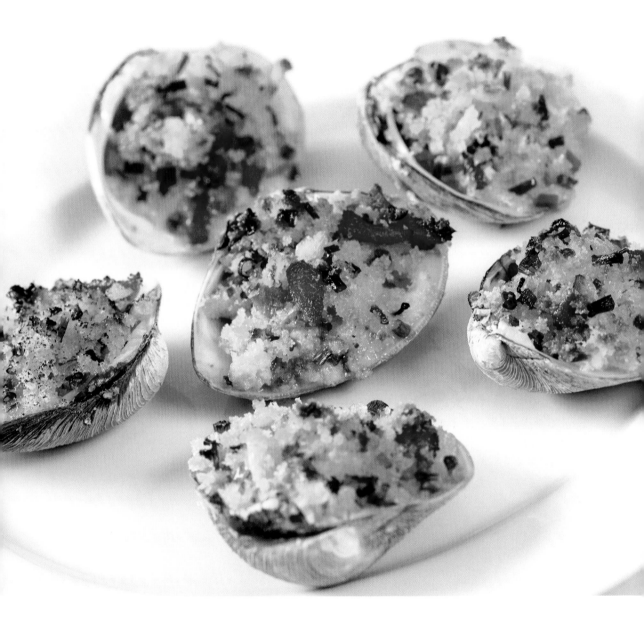

Gloria, my wife, and I love clams on the half shell and we enjoy them throughout the year with a horseradish-ketchup sauce. Occasionally, though, I will cook the clams for linguine and clam sauce or bake them. I like baked clams with a nice crusty topping and the clams just hot, so I cook them under the broiler on the lowest shelf of the oven.

Before shucking the clams, place them in the freezer for 15 minutes to make them easier to open. Then, first cut between the two shells of each clam with a paring knife to sever the adductor muscles. Open the clams, discard the top shells, and cut the clams loose to make them easier to eat, leaving them in their bottom shells. I like the medium-size clams often called top neck.

Open the clams (see headnote), discard the top shells, and cut the clams loose from the bottom shell. Place the clams in their bottom shells on a cookie sheet. Place 1 tablespoon of the olive oil in a medium skillet, add the bacon, and cook over medium heat until the bacon is crisp, about 5 minutes. Add the remaining 2 tablespoons oil, the onion, garlic, and jalapeño and cook for another minute or so, until the vegetables are soft. Transfer the mixture to a bowl and add the bread crumbs. Mix gently to moisten the bread with the oil. Place about 1½ tablespoons of the mixture on top of each clam.

At serving time, place a rack in the lower part of the oven (about 15 inches from the heat source) and preheat the broiler. Broil the clams for 8 to 9 minutes, until the topping is brown and crusty and the clams are hot. Sprinkle with chives and serve.

BAKED CLAMS WITH A BREAD CRUST

∘ SERVES 4 AS A FIRST COURSE

24 medium clams, such as top neck

3 tablespoons olive oil

3 slices bacon, cut into ¼-inch pieces or chopped coarsely

¾ cup chopped onion

2 teaspoons chopped garlic

1 tablespoon coarsely chopped jalapeño pepper

1¾ cups coarse fresh bread crumbs, preferably from a country loaf or baguette

2 tablespoons chopped chives

RAZOR CLAMS IN BUTTER SAUCE

○ SERVES 4 AS A FIRST COURSE

20 razor clams (about 2 pounds)

¼ teaspoon salt

¼ teaspoon freshly ground
black pepper

2 tablespoons olive oil

2 tablespoons grated Parmesan
cheese

Sauce
———
4 tablespoons (½ stick) unsalted
butter, melted

¼ teaspoon salt

2 teaspoons Chinese garlic-chili
sauce or Sriracha or other
hot sauce

1 tablespoon lime juice

2 tablespoons finely chopped
flat-leaf parsley

Of all the clams—littlenecks, cherrystones, quahogs, soft-shell, geoduck—razor clams are one of the most tender, delicious, and underutilized. The East Coast razor clam is slightly curved, about 6 inches long and ¾ inch wide, while the West Coast clam is shorter, straighter, and wider. Razor clam shells are very brittle and sharp, and they are open, exposing the meat. I wash them and then soak them in cold water a couple of times to remove sand before using. Their thick, heavy flesh is very tender and plump, excellent raw or cooked in chowder or baked in the oven, as in this recipe. Five clams per person makes a generous first course.

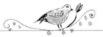

Preheat the oven to 350 degrees. Soak the clams in cold water for 15 minutes. Drain and rinse, then soak them in fresh water for another 15 minutes.

Run a small knife under and along the inside of one shell of each clam to push the meat to the other shell. Run the knife through the hinge to remove the empty shell.

Arrange the clams on their bottom shells on a cookie sheet lined with nonstick aluminum foil. Sprinkle them with the salt, pepper, olive oil, and cheese. Bake for 7 to 8 minutes, until cooked through and hot.

Meanwhile, make the sauce: Mix together all the ingredients in a bowl.

Remove the clams from the oven and arrange 5 clams on each plate. Coat with the sauce and serve immediately.

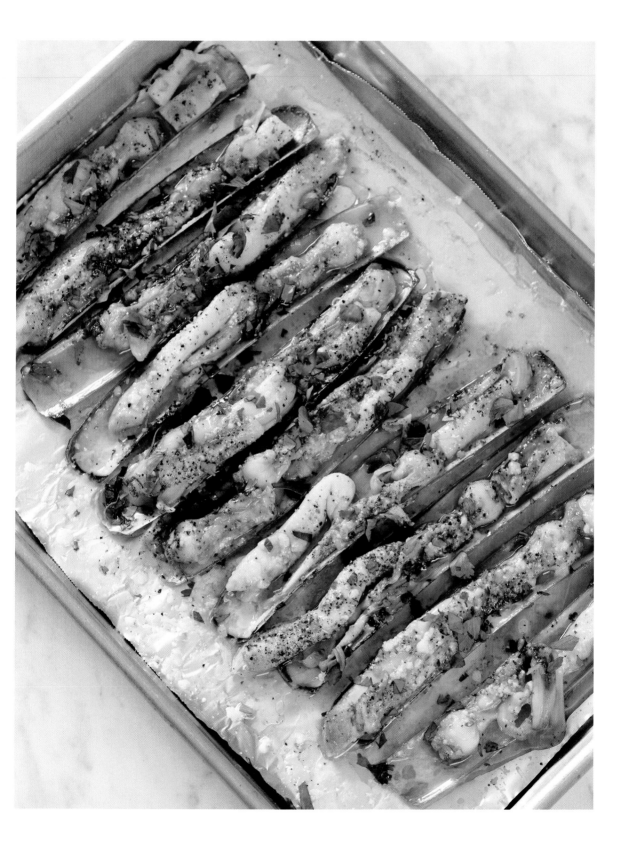

SHRIMP SAUTE PIQUANTE

◦ SERVES 4

1 pound shell-on medium shrimp
(26–30 per pound)

1 teaspoon oregano leaves

½ teaspoon cayenne pepper

¼ teaspoon salt

3 tablespoons virgin olive oil

4 tablespoons water

The secret to preparing this dish is to sauté the shrimp quickly over extremely high heat. This is best done in two skillets, or in two batches with one skillet, so there is only one layer of shrimp to absorb the intense heat. If too many shrimp are cooked at one time, they tend to boil and won't develop the desired taste and texture.

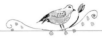

Pat the shrimp dry with paper towels.

Sprinkle the shrimp with the oregano, cayenne, and salt. Heat 2 tablespoons of the olive oil in a large cast-iron skillet. Just when the oil begins to smoke, add half the shrimp in one layer and sauté for about 2 minutes, tossing them in the skillet or turning them with tongs so they cook on both sides. Transfer the shrimp to a bowl and add 2 tablespoons of the water to the pan. Swirl it around to melt any caramelized juices and deglaze the pan. Pour over the shrimp in the bowl.

Repeat this process with the remaining oil and seasoned shrimp and add them to the bowl. Deglaze the pan with the remaining 2 tablespoons water and pour the liquid over the shrimp. Serve immediately.

> **The shrimp can also be served, cooled slightly, as an hors d'oeuvre.**

This was one of my mother-in-law's favorite summer dishes. Since shrimp always taste best when cooked in their shells, we eat this family-style and peel them with our fingers at the table—messy and delicious. Don't forget to suck on the shells to extract the last bit of flavorful juice. Dip the shrimp in melted butter and serve some bread alongside. And since you've already got your sleeves rolled up, serve some hot corn on the cob too!

Place all the ingredients except the shrimp in large saucepan and bring to a boil. Cover and boil for about 1 minute. Add the shrimp, stirring to mix them well with the broth, and bring the mixture barely back to a boil. Cover the pan, remove it from the heat, and set aside; the shrimp will continue to cook in the hot broth.

Serve warm, with melted butter, if desired, or serve cold, with horseradish sauce.

NOTE: These make an excellent shrimp cocktail. Chill the shrimp in the broth, then drain, peel, and serve with horseradish sauce.

SHRIMP IN SPICY BROTH

○ SERVES 4

2 cups water

3 tablespoons cider vinegar

1 onion, peeled and sliced (1 cup)

1 tablespoon herbes de Provence (see Note, page 15)

¾ teaspoon salt

½ teaspoon hot pepper flakes

2 bay leaves

12 sprigs cilantro

1 pound shell-on medium shrimp (26–30 per pound)

Melted butter or Horseradish Sauce (page 13), for serving (optional)

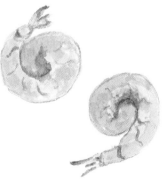

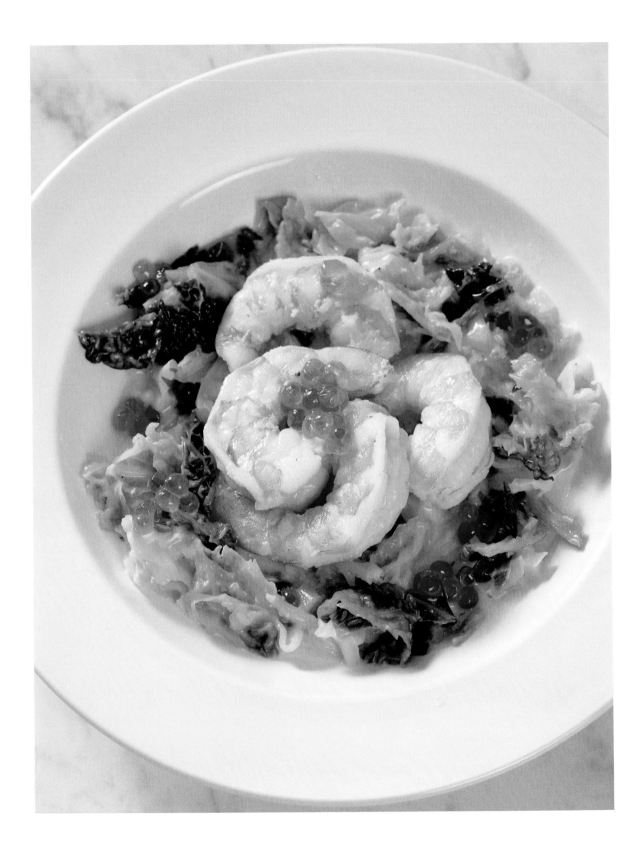

There is an interesting and unusual combination of flavors at play here: The crunchy cabbage is a terrific accompaniment for the just-barely-cooked shrimp, and the saltiness of the salmon caviar, which looks like small pink pearls around the shrimp, complements the dish.

Sprinkle the shrimp with the salt and pepper. Melt the butter in two skillets. When the butter is hot, add the shrimp and sauté over high heat for 60 seconds. Using a slotted spoon, transfer the shrimp to a plate and set aside in a warm place.

Combine the juices from both skillets into one of the skillets, add the cabbage, and sauté for about 2 minutes. Add the cream and water, stir, and bring to a boil over high heat. Boil for about 4 minutes, until the cabbage is soft but still crunchy and the sauce has reduced to a syrupy consistency. Taste and correct the seasonings if necessary.

With a large spoon, transfer the cabbage to a large serving dish or divide it among four individual plates. Arrange the shrimp on top of the cabbage and sprinkle with the caviar. Serve immediately.

SHRIMP WITH CABBAGE AND CAVIAR

○ SERVES 4

16 extra-large shrimp (about 1¼ pounds), peeled and deveined

½ teaspoon salt, plus more if needed

¼ teaspoon freshly ground black pepper, plus more if needed

3 tablespoons unsalted butter

4½ cups shredded savoy cabbage

¾ cup heavy cream

¼ cup water

2 tablespoons red salmon caviar

▷ **This wonderful, distinctly flavored dish makes an easy but elegant first or main course for a special dinner.**

MUSTARD-BROILED SHRIMP

1 pound medium shrimp
(26–30 per pound), defrosted
if frozen, shelled

3 tablespoons honey mustard
(see Note)

2 tablespoons dark soy sauce

¼ teaspoon Sriracha or other
hot sauce

▷ **If you buy shelled shrimp,
this dish will take only
5 minutes to prepare.**

Shelling the shrimp is the hardest part of this recipe—
so buy shelled raw shrimp, usually frozen, at the
market. This is a festive appetizer with a sweet-hot
taste. You can also cool the shrimp and serve them as
an hors d'oeuvre on slices of party rye.

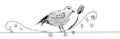

Pat the shrimp dry with paper towels.

Combine the honey mustard, soy sauce, and
hot sauce in a medium bowl. Stir the shrimp into the
sauce to coat them well. Then remove them from
the sauce, reserving what's left, and arrange in a
single layer in a gratin dish or on a cookie sheet
lined with nonstick aluminum foil.

At serving time, preheat the broiler. Broil the shrimp,
about 5 inches from the heat source, for about
2 minutes on the first side, then turn with tongs and
broil on the other side for about 1 minute.

Arrange the shrimp on a serving platter or
individual plates and serve with the reserved sauce.

NOTE: You can create your own honey mustard by mixing
enough honey into whole-grain mustard to achieve a sweet-
hot taste.

Soft-shell crab is ideal as a first course: The crabs are light and small, and cook very fast. They are best at the beginning of the season in the spring, when the delicate crabs have just shed their shells and are very soft.

The crabs can be dusted in flour and sautéed or, as in this recipe, dipped in a tempura batter before sautéing. To cook all four crabs at the same time, you will need two 10-inch nonstick skillets, or cook them two at a time in one skillet.

To prepare the crabs, twist off the skirts, or aprons. Then, using scissors, cut a strip about ½ inch wide from the front of each that includes the eyes and antenna. Remove the soft, tissue-like shells from the tops to expose the insides. This makes the crabs much more tender. Sprinkle with the salt and Tabasco.

Prepare the batter: Mix the flour and baking powder in a bowl. Using a whisk, mix in half the sparkling water until the mixture is smooth. Whisk in the remaining sparkling water to make a thin batter.

Divide the oil between two large skillets and heat it. When the oil is hot, dip the crabs one at a time in the batter, coating them on both sides, and place in the hot oil. Cook for about 3 minutes on each side, until nicely browned and just cooked in the center.

Serve immediately, with wedges of lemon.

SOFT-SHELL CRABS IN TEMPURA BATTER

∘ SERVES 4 AS A FIRST COURSE

4 large soft-shell crabs

¼ teaspoon salt

½ teaspoon Tabasco sauce

Batter

½ cup all-purpose flour

½ teaspoon baking powder

1 cup sparkling water

6 tablespoons peanut oil

1 lemon, cut into 4 wedges, for serving

CRABMEAT CROQUETTES WITH TOMATO RELISH

I prefer to cook these flavorful croquettes at the last moment, but if you have a larger party and want to prepare them ahead, you can; just reheat them under the broiler for a few minutes before serving. You will notice that the crabmeat mixture is soft; it will firm up as it cooks, and the result will be quite delicate. The croquettes are served with a tomato relish.

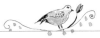

∘ SERVES 4 AS A FIRST COURSE

1 slice white bread

8 ounces cooked crabmeat

2 scallions, cleaned and minced fine (⅓ cup)

1 teaspoon chopped fresh ginger

¼ teaspoon Tabasco sauce

1 large egg, beaten

Relish

1 cup peeled, seeded, and diced (¼-inch) tomatoes

2 tablespoons olive oil

1 tablespoon chopped chives

¼ teaspoon salt

½ teaspoon freshly ground black pepper

2 tablespoons safflower or corn oil

Process the bread to crumbs in a food processor (you should have about ¾ cup).

Place the crabmeat, scallions, ginger, Tabasco, and egg in a bowl and mix gently with a fork to combine. Add the bread crumbs and toss just until incorporated. Using a spoon, divide the mixture into 4 parts and then press each portion together lightly in your hands to form 4 patties, each about 1½ inches thick.

Prepare the relish: Mix all the ingredients together in a bowl.

Heat the safflower oil in a large nonstick skillet. When the oil is hot, add the patties and sauté over medium heat for about 2 minutes on each side, until nicely browned. Transfer them to a plate.

Serve immediately, with the tomato relish, or let cool and then reheat under the broiler for a few minutes before serving.

> The croquettes can be cooked ahead and reheated under the broiler just before serving.

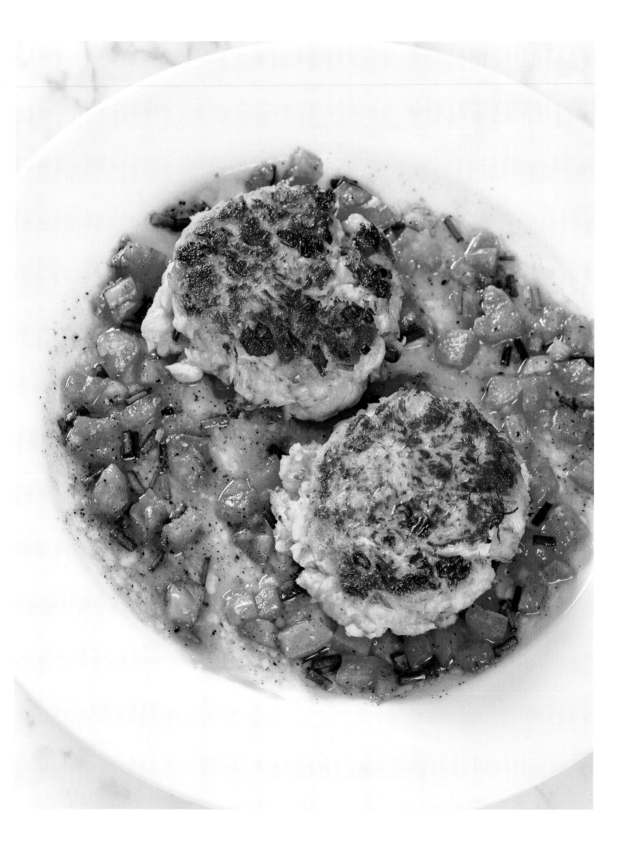

SEAFOOD RISOTTO WITH SQUID INK

◦ SERVES 6

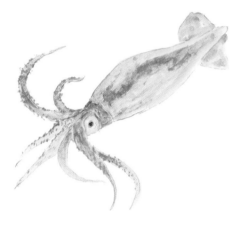

I love to cook with squid ink, which is now available in small jars in specialty markets or can be ordered online. The product is quite adequate, and the little jars will keep for months, if not years, in the refrigerator.

Some cooks prepare risotto from beginning to end in an uncovered saucepan, adding a few tablespoons of liquid (stock or water) every few minutes as the liquid in the pan evaporates. This method requires more liquid for the same amount of rice than partially cooking rice in a pan covered with a lid, as I do, so the liquid does not evaporate. I cook the rice, covered, for 10 to 12 minutes with a precise amount of liquid, which just gets absorbed, and you can do that part ahead to make the recipe easier. Then, during the last 6 to 8 minutes of cooking (risotto cooks in 16 to 18 minutes, depending on your taste), add additional liquid a few tablespoons at a time until the consistency is to my liking. I finish it with a piece of butter and some grated Parmesan cheese, although some cooks object to cheese with seafood. While you can buy clam juice, I've made it a practice to reserve the extra juice when I open oysters or clams and freeze it to use in rice dishes, stews, and chowder.

Place 3 tablespoons of the olive oil in a saucepan set over high heat, add ½ cup of the onion, and cook for about 2 minutes. Add the rice and cook, stirring, for another minute. Add 1½ cups of the clam juice, the water, and ½ teaspoon of the pepper and bring to a boil, then stir well, cover, reduce the heat to low, and cook for 12 minutes. Set aside until serving time or just continue with recipe if you like.

Meanwhile, place the remaining 3 tablespoons oil in another saucepan, add the remaining ½ cup onion and the garlic, and cook for 2 minutes. Add the wine, squid ink, and remaining ½ teaspoon pepper and ½ cup clam juice and bring to a strong boil, then add the seafood, stir, and bring the mixture back to a strong boil. Set aside.

At serving time, reheat the rice and add ½ cup of the juice from the shellfish mixture. Cook, stirring, for a couple of minutes, until the juice has been absorbed. Keep adding the shellfish juice, stirring, until all the juice has been absorbed. Finally, add the shellfish to the rice, along with the cheese and butter, and cook, stirring, until the risotto is silky and creamy.

Serve in hot soup plates, garnished with the parsley.

NOTE: You can make the same recipe without the squid ink for a regular seafood risotto.

6 tablespoons olive oil

1 cup finely chopped onion

1¼ cups Arborio rice

2 cups reserved clam or oyster juice, or a mixture

½ cup water

1 teaspoon freshly ground black pepper

1 tablespoon finely chopped garlic

⅓ cup dry white wine

1 tablespoon squid ink

8 ounces shrimp (about 8), shelled and cut into 2 or 3 pieces each

8 ounces squid, cleaned, bodies cut into 1-inch-wide strips and tentacles left whole

8 ounces scallops, cut into 1-inch pieces

2 tablespoons grated Parmesan cheese

2 tablespoons unsalted butter

Salt (optional, depending on the saltiness of the clam/oyster juice)

1 tablespoon chopped flat-leaf parsley, for garnish

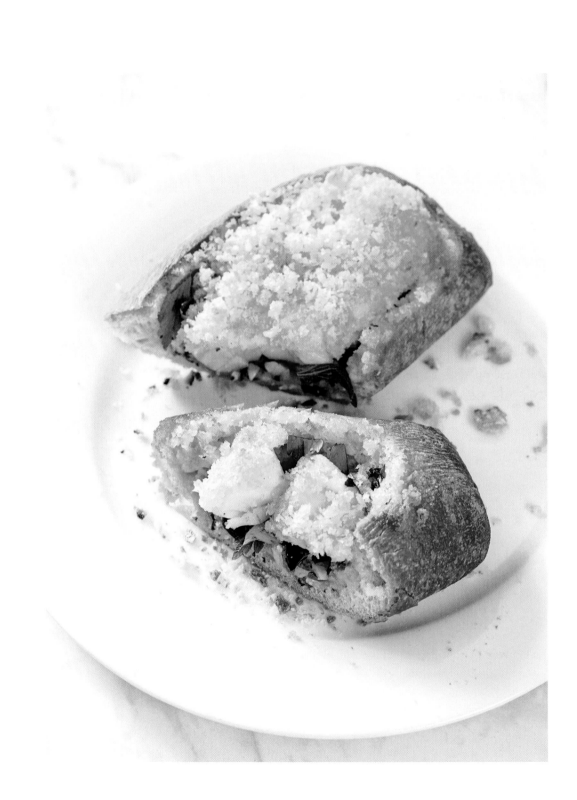

These stuffed rolls, which can be made ahead, become a favorite of everyone who tries them. Although you can use a single large bread loaf and cut it into wedges for serving, I prefer to use hard rolls and serve one per person. Be sure to select rolls that don't have any holes on the sides or bottom, as the butter has a tendency to seep out.

I use medium-size sweet bay scallops or small sea scallops, although any size will work well. If you are not fond of cilantro and ginger, use parsley and either garlic or shallots instead.

Preheat the oven to 375 degrees. Cut off the top of each roll about a third of the way down and, with your fingers, pull out the soft insides. Place the insides and the roll "lids" in a food processor and process to crumbs. Mix 1½ cups of the crumbs (reserving any extra for another use) with the olive oil and set aside.

Rinse the scallops to remove any sand or grit and drain thoroughly.

Combine the butter, garlic, parsley, mushrooms, salt, and pepper in a bowl and mix well. Place about 2 tablespoons of the butter mixture in the bottom of each hollowed-out roll. Arrange the scallops, about 6 per roll, on top of the butter mixture and cover with the remaining mixture. Lightly press the bread crumbs on top, mounding them in the center.

Arrange the rolls on a cookie sheet lined with nonstick aluminum foil and bake for 25 minutes, or until the scallops are cooked through and the tops are nicely browned. Serve.

SCALLOPS IN BREAD SHELLS WITH PARSLEY

○ SERVES 6

6 small round or oval hard rolls (about 3 ounces each)

1 tablespoon virgin olive oil

1 pound bay scallops (about 36)

8 tablespoons (1 stick) unsalted butter, softened

2 cloves garlic, chopped fine (2 teaspoons)

3 tablespoons chopped flat-leaf parsley

½ cup coarsely chopped mushrooms

¼ teaspoon salt

½ teaspoon freshly ground black pepper

> **These stuffed rolls can be prepared a few hours ahead and baked when needed.**

SCALLOPS IN A SKILLET

○ SERVES 4

1 pound large sea scallops
(about 16)

Sauce

1 tablespoon mayonnaise

2 teaspoons lemon juice

1 teaspoon Worcestershire sauce

1 tablespoon peanut oil

1 tablespoon chopped chives

¼ teaspoon Tabasco sauce

2 tablespoons virgin olive oil

½ teaspoon salt

½ teaspoon freshly ground
black pepper

These scallops are cooked quickly in a very hot
cast-iron or aluminum skillet just until their surface is
nicely browned. The lemony sauce is also very good
with other types of shellfish.

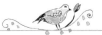

Rinse the scallops well to remove any sand or grit
and dry them thoroughly on paper towels.

Prepare the sauce: Mix all the ingredients together in
a serving bowl and set aside.

Combine the scallops, olive oil, salt, and pepper in
a large bowl and toss well to coat. Place a large
heavy skillet over high heat. When it is very hot,
add the scallops in one layer. Cook for about
1½ minutes on each side, until lightly browned.

Transfer the scallops to individual plates and serve
immediately, with the sauce.

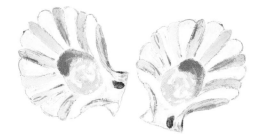

I love scallops cooked just warm, tossed with a vinaigrette, and served as a first course. It is an impressive dish, quite quickly prepared and delicious. It is best done at the last moment, but it takes only a few minutes to prepare. I use medium-size sea scallops.

Place the scallops and 2 tablespoons water in a stainless steel skillet and bring to a boil over medium to high heat. Cook, shaking the pan occasionally, until the scallops are opaque, about 2 minutes. Drain the scallops and set aside on a plate.

Prepare the vinaigrette: Combine all the ingredients in a bowl, adding any moisture that has collected on the plate around the scallops.

Arrange the lettuce leaves on individual plates, divide the scallops among them, sprinkle with the basil, and spoon the vinaigrette over the top. Serve immediately.

▷ **This impressive first-course dish takes only a few minutes to prepare.**

SCALLOPS VINAIGRETTE

○ SERVES 4 AS A FIRST COURSE

1 pound medium sea scallops (about 24), rinsed under cool water to remove sand or grit and patted dry

Vinaigrette

2 teaspoons Dijon-style mustard, preferably "hot"

1 tablespoon red wine vinegar

¼ cup extra-virgin olive oil

¼ teaspoon salt

½ teaspoon freshly ground black pepper

10 to 12 Boston lettuce leaves, for serving

About ⅓ cup minced basil, for garnish

RED LOBSTER STEW

◦ SERVES 4

4 live lobsters (1¼ pounds each)

⅓ cup extra-virgin or virgin olive oil

1½ cups coarsely chopped onion

About 4 cloves garlic, peeled and chopped (1 tablespoon)

One 15-ounce can Italian plum tomatoes, with their juices

1 tablespoon herbes de Provence (see Note, page 15)

1 teaspoon hot pepper flakes

½ cup chopped flat-leaf parsley, basil, and/or chives (a mixture, or one of the three)

Lobster is a favorite at our house, for family meals as well as for company fare. This particular dish is best eaten with family and close friends, since the shells are broken open and the meat extracted with the help of your fingers at the table. Serve it with corn on the cob.

Traditionally raw lobster is cut into equal pieces before it is cooked, but it's a difficult job to perform, so here I divide it into pieces by breaking off the claws and twisting the tail out of the body. (A fishmonger can do this for you if you prefer.) I calculate one lobster per person for a main-course serving, so you will need to cook them in two saucepans to start, then finish the recipe in one of the pans.

Be sure the lobsters you buy are alive and freshly caught. The fresher the lobster, the fuller and firmer the meat will be. Females are the preferred choice.

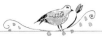

Protecting your hands with a kitchen towel, break off the claws from each lobster. Then twist off the tails, separating them from the bodies.

To make it easier to extract the meat from the claws after cooking, crack the shells: Place each claw on the counter, cover with a clean kitchen towel to prevent splattering, and, using a meat pounder or the bottom of a heavy saucepan, pound on the claw until the shell cracks. Place the tails and cracked claws in a large bowl to capture any juices that they release.

Heat the olive oil in two large saucepans. When the oil is hot, add the lobster claws, tails, and bodies, along with any juices that have accumulated in the bowl. Shaking the pans and stirring occasionally, sauté the lobster pieces, covered, over medium-high heat for about 10 minutes, until the shells are bright red and the meat is almost cooked through.

Transfer the tail and claw pieces to a bowl and combine the drippings and lobster bodies in one of the saucepans. Return the pan to the heat, add the onion, garlic, tomatoes with their juices, and herbes de Provence and bring to a boil, stirring. Boil until the mixture thickens slightly and the taste is concentrated, 6 to 8 minutes. Remove the lobster bodies and discard them.

Return the lobster tail and claw pieces to the sauce and stir in the pepper flakes and herbs. Heat gently for about 5 minutes, until all the lobster is heated through. Arrange on four plates and serve.

NOTE: If you feel inspired, you can remove the meat from the tail and claws before returning them to the sauce for easier enjoyment for your guests.

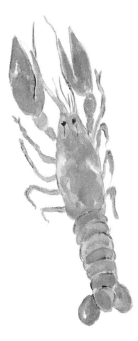

LOBSTER IN PAPRIKA SAUCE ON TOAST

∘ SERVES 4 AS A FIRST COURSE

4 slices firm-textured bread

1 pound cooked lobster meat, cut into 1-inch pieces

1 teaspoon paprika

½ teaspoon salt

¼ teaspoon freshly ground black pepper

2 tablespoons unsalted butter

1 tablespoon Cognac

⅔ cup heavy cream

1 tablespoon chopped chives, for garnish

This is a rich dish, ideal as a first course for a dinner party. Lobster meat is expensive, of course, but in the summer it is more reasonably priced, of the best quality, and available cooked from most fishmongers. All that is involved here is cutting up the meat, combining it with the sauce ingredients, and serving it over toast rounds.

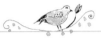

Toast the bread slices in a toaster and trim them to create sticks. Set aside.

Sprinkle the lobster pieces with the paprika, salt, and pepper. Melt the butter in a skillet, and when it is foaming, add the lobster and sauté for about 1 minute, just long enough to heat it through. Add the Cognac and cream, bring to a boil, and simmer gently, uncovered, for about 1 minute to reduce slightly.

Spoon the lobster and sauce on a warm plate and arrange the bread around it. Sprinkle with the chives and serve.

> This couldn't be easier: All you have to do is cut up cooked lobster meat and combine it with a quickly made pan sauce.

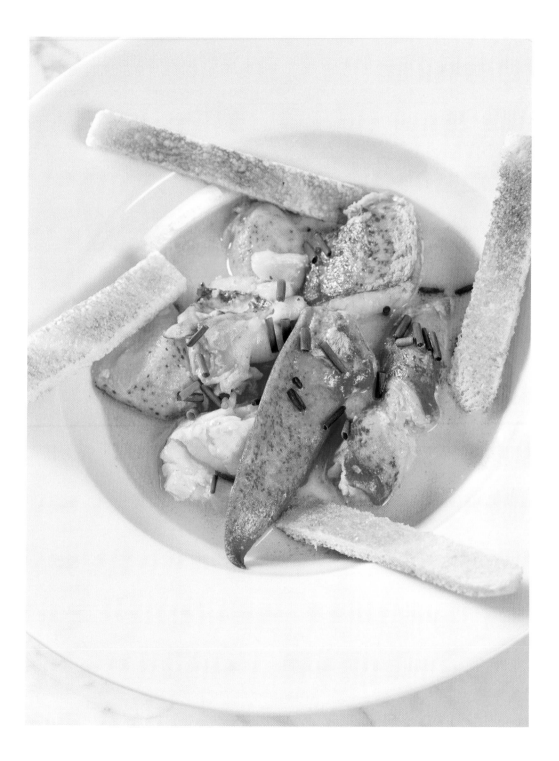

SAUTE OF LOBSTER WITH BASMATI RICE

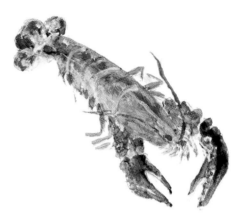

∘ SERVES 4 AS A MAIN COURSE

Rice

2 tablespoons unsalted butter

1 cup chopped onion

1¼ cups basmati rice

1 teaspoon Italian seasoning

½ teaspoon salt

¼ teaspoon freshly ground black pepper

2¼ cups Basic Chicken Stock (page 15) or canned chicken broth

Lobster

About 3 plum tomatoes (8 ounces total), cut into ½-inch dice (about 2 cups), juices and seeds reserved

2 tablespoons unsalted butter

2 tablespoons virgin olive oil

1 cup diced (½-inch pieces) red onion

3 shallots, peeled and cut into ¼-inch dice (about ¼ cup)

3 cloves garlic, peeled, crushed, and chopped coarsely (1 tablespoon)

½ cup dry white wine

½ teaspoon salt

½ teaspoon freshly ground black pepper

1 pound cooked lobster meat, cut into 1-inch pieces

¼ cup minced flat-leaf parsley, for garnish

Cooked lobster meat is available from most fishmongers. Served with basmati rice, which has a distinctive nutty taste, it is perfect as a first course for an elegant dinner or as a main course for a light brunch.

Prepare the rice: Melt the butter in a saucepan with a tight-fitting lid. When the melted butter is hot, add the onion and sauté over medium-high heat for about 1½ minutes. Mix in the rice, Italian seasoning, salt, and pepper, then add the chicken stock and bring to a boil, stirring, over high heat. Cover, reduce the heat to very low, and cook for 20 minutes.

Meanwhile, prepare the lobster: Heat the butter and olive oil in a saucepan. When the mixture is hot, add the onion and shallots and sauté over high heat for 3 minutes. Stir in the garlic and cook for about 10 seconds. Add the tomatoes with their juices and seeds, wine, salt, and pepper and bring to a boil. Cover, reduce the heat to low, and simmer gently for 5 minutes. Add the lobster meat and heat for 1 minute.

Cooked lobster meat from your fishmonger makes this dish easy.

Mound the rice in the center of four plates and spoon the lobster and sauce over each portion. Sprinkle with the parsley and serve immediately.

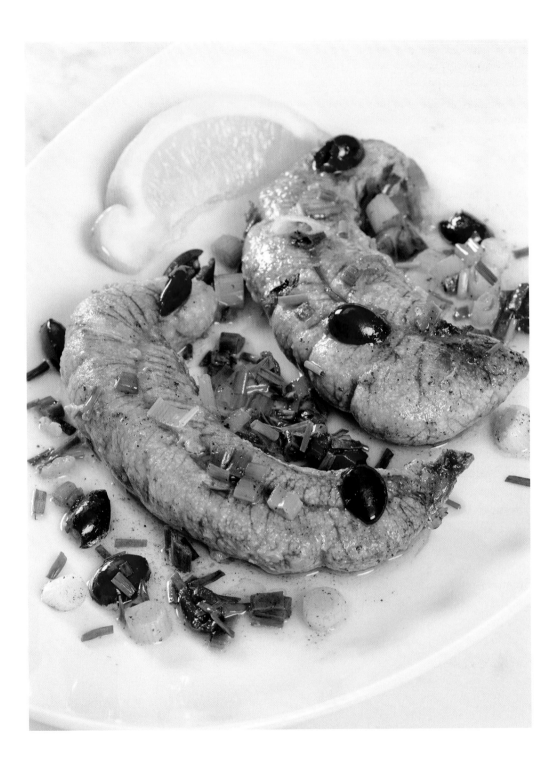

Shad is a river fish, part of the herring family, that is available in spring. The fish is very bony and often sold boneless. The roe is prized and delicious. It is a very special treat in the spring, and my wife, Gloria, always looks forward to it. The delicate roe should not be overcooked—the secret is to sauté it at a low temperature, or it will tend to burst and break open.

For this recipe, I cook two pairs of shad roe lobes, each divided into its two halves, and the individual lobes are the right size for a first course; serve a full pair as a main course. The shad roe will cook in a few minutes and the recipe will take only 10 minutes to prepare. I use small Niçoise olives here, but any olives would work. Serve on hot plates.

Use a knife to separate the lobes of roe in each pair. Sprinkle the roe with the salt and Tabasco. Dust each lobe on both sides with the flour.

Heat the olive oil in a 10-inch nonstick skillet over low heat (high heat will make the roe burst open). Add the roe and cook, partially covered to avoid splattering, for about 3 minutes on the first side. Flip the roe over and cook for about 2 minutes on the other side. Each lobe should be nicely browned but still soft in the middle.

Place a lobe of the roe on each of four warm plates. In the same skillet, melt the butter and when it is hot, add the scallions. Cook over high heat for about 1 minute. Add the olives and chives and cook for about 30 seconds.

Spoon the mixture over the roe and serve with wedges of lemon, if desired.

SHAD ROE WITH NIÇOISE OLIVES AND SCALLIONS

○ SERVES 4 AS A FIRST COURSE

2 large shad roe lobe pairs (8 to 10 ounces each)

½ teaspoon salt

½ teaspoon Tabasco sauce

1 tablespoon all-purpose flour

¼ cup olive oil

4 tablespoons (½ stick) unsalted butter

½ cup sliced scallions

24 small Niçoise olives, pitted

¼ cup chopped chives

1 lemon, cut into 4 wedges, for serving (optional)

NOTE: To pit the olives, crush them with the bottom of a skillet and pry out the pits with your fingers.

INSTANT GRAVLAX WITH OLIVES

○ SERVERS 4 AS A FIRST COURSE

4 pieces salmon fillet (2 ounces each), completely cleaned of sinews, skin, and any bones

1½ teaspoons salt

1½ teaspoons freshly ground black pepper

2 tablespoons finely chopped shallot

2 tablespoons chopped (¼-inch pieces) pitted oil-cured black olives

2 tablespoons extra-virgin olive oil

1 tablespoon coarsely chopped flat-leaf parsley

2 teaspoons lemon juice

6 pieces toast, crusts removed, halved and buttered

Gravlax is cured fish, usually salmon. Traditional Scandinavian gravlax consists of large fillets or sides of salmon cured with sugar, salt, and a great amount of dill. It is often served with a mustard sauce or sweet mustard mayonnaise.

In modern cooking, the gravlax treatment is applied to other types of fish, among them tuna and black sea bass. Often the fish is cut into thin slices and cured with lemon or lime juice.

This instant salmon gravlax could also be called carpaccio, a name that used to be applied only to beef, but can now refer to uncooked meat or fish that is pounded very thin and served with a garnish ranging from mayonnaise to plain olive oil. Most fish markets carry wild salmon, my first choice.

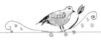

Place the salmon pieces in a single layer, with space between them, on a large square of plastic wrap and cover it with another square of plastic wrap. Using a meat pounder or the bottom of a small heavy saucepan, pound the salmon to flatten it, forming pieces about 7 inches across. The thin pieces should be almost transparent. Remove the top layer of plastic wrap.

Sprinkle half the salt and pepper on four serving plates. Invert a salmon piece onto each plate, peeling off the plastic wrap as you go. Sprinkle the top of the salmon with the remaining salt and pepper. Cover the plates tightly with plastic wrap and refrigerate for at least 1 hour.

Just before serving, place the shallots in a sieve and rinse them under cold water (this removes their harsh, acidic taste); drain thoroughly. Sprinkle the

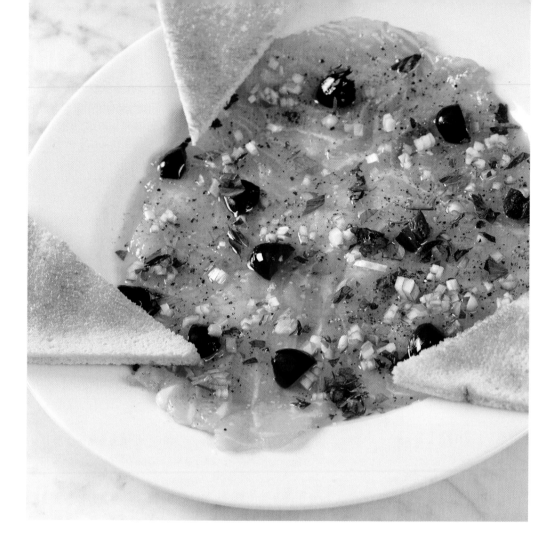

shallots over the salmon, followed by the olives, olive oil, parsley, and lemon juice. Surround with the toasts and serve immediately.

> **This is a great (and relatively inexpensive) do-ahead recipe for a dinner party.**

NOTE: You can keep the gravlax for up to 24 hours in the refrigerator. You can add the shallots, olives, oil, and parsley up to 30 minutes before serving, but don't sprinkle the lemon juice over the fish until the last moment. If the lemon juice is added earlier, it will "cook" the salmon, setting the protein and turning it an opaque white.

MINUTE SALMON STEAKS

4 salmon steaks (5 to 6 ounces each and about 1 inch thick), skin and bones removed

1 teaspoon salt

½ teaspoon freshly ground black pepper

1 tablespoon peanut oil

1 teaspoon chopped tarragon

1 tablespoon chopped flat-leaf parsley

1 clove garlic, peeled, crushed, and chopped fine (½ teaspoon)

¼ cup olive oil

4 teaspoons lemon juice

This is an elegant dish to serve at a special dinner or lunch. Most steamed and buttered vegetables, from potatoes to broccoli, go well with it. Use wild salmon, if you can.

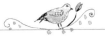

Preheat the broiler. Sprinkle the salmon steaks with the salt, pepper, and oil. Arrange them on a cookie sheet lined with nonstick aluminum foil and set aside.

Mix the tarragon, parsley, garlic, and olive oil together in a bowl.

Place the steaks under the broiler, 5 or 6 inches from the heat source, and cook for 4 to 5 minutes, until just pink inside.

Add the lemon juice to the herb sauce. Transfer the salmon steaks to warmed dinner plates, spoon the sauce over them, and serve immediately.

> **These steaks cook in only a few minutes, and the sauce can be made ahead.**

This dish, which can be prepared at the last minute, makes an excellent lunch or first course at dinner. The croquettes will brown nicely, but be sure to use a nonstick pan and turn them gently, as they are very delicate.

Place the bread in a food processor and process to crumbs (you should have 1 cup crumbs).

Crumble the salmon, with its liquid, into a bowl. Add the scallions, tarragon, bread crumbs, salsa, and mayonnaise and mix gently but thoroughly. Form the mixture into 4 patties.

Heat the olive oil in a large nonstick skillet. When the oil is hot, add the croquettes and cook them over medium to high heat, turning once, until nicely browned on both sides, about 2½ minutes per side—since the croquettes are delicate, turn them carefully with a large flat spatula.

Divide the chopped cucumbers among four plates. Arrange 2 croquettes on each plate and serve immediately.

▷ **Keep a can of red salmon on hand for this quick, easy luncheon dish or first course.**

SALMON CROQUETTES WITH CUCUMBER SALSA

◦ SERVES 4 AS A FIRST COURSE OR LUNCH MAIN COURSE

1½ slices white bread

One 7½-ounce can red salmon in water

3 or 4 scallions, cleaned and minced (½ cup)

1 teaspoon chopped tarragon

1 tablespoon Spicy Red Salsa (page 13) or 2 teaspoons Sriracha or other hot sauce

3 tablespoons mayonnaise

About 2 tablespoons olive oil

½ cup cucumbers from Spicy Cucumber Relish (page 17), drained and coarsely chopped

POTTED SMOKED SALMON

∘ SERVES 4 AS A FIRST COURSE

2 teaspoons chopped chives, plus more for sprinkling

One 4-ounce container soft cream cheese (about 6 tablespoons)

4 large slices smoked salmon (6 ounces), cut crosswise in half

¼ teaspoon freshly ground black pepper

¼ cup very thinly sliced red onion

1 tablespoon small capers, drained

Asparagus

8 medium to large stalks asparagus (about 6 ounces total), trimmed

1 tablespoon peanut oil

1 teaspoon red wine vinegar

⅛ teaspoon salt

⅛ teaspoon freshly ground black pepper

6 slices black bread, buttered, for serving

This dish is impressive to look at and delicious, and it can be prepared up to a day ahead. It is especially elegant accompanied, as it is here, by asparagus in a vinaigrette dressing.

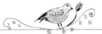

Line each of four ½-cup soufflé molds with a 7-inch square of plastic wrap. Divide the chives evenly among the molds and cover each with 1 good tablespoon of the cream cheese. Press a half-slice of the salmon into the cream cheese to form a flat layer. Sprinkle with half the pepper. Divide the onion among the four molds and then layer on the remaining cream cheese, using about ½ tablespoon for each. Add the capers, distributing them evenly, then top with the remaining salmon and pepper. Press down on the salmon slightly to make the mixture more compact. Cover with plastic wrap and refrigerate for at least 1 hour or as long as overnight.

Prepare the asparagus: Peel the lower third of the asparagus stalks. Cut each stalk into 3 pieces.

To cook the asparagus in a microwave oven, seal it in a plastic bag with 2 tablespoons water and cook for about 2 minutes; drain. To prepare the asparagus on the stovetop, arrange the pieces in one layer in a stainless steel skillet, add ½ cup water, bring to a boil, and cook for 1 to 2 minutes; drain. Slice the lower two-thirds of the asparagus down the middle to make a decorative presentation.

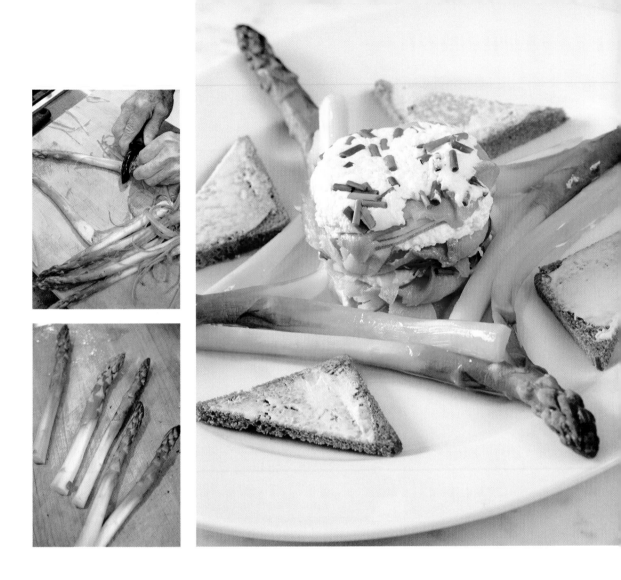

Transfer the asparagus to a medium bowl and toss with the oil, vinegar, salt, and pepper.

At serving time, unmold the potted salmon, lifting it out of the molds using the plastic wrap, and invert onto individual plates. Peel off the plastic wrap. Serve the salmon with the asparagus arranged around it and buttered black bread on the side.

> **Elegant and delicious, the potted salmon can be made up to a day ahead.**

ARCTIC CHAR IN SORREL SAUCE

∘ SERVES 2

Sauce
---

1 cup shredded sorrel (about a handful of leaves, gathered together, rolled, and cut into ½-inch-wide strips)

¼ cup heavy cream

¼ teaspoon salt

¼ teaspoon freshly ground black pepper

2 skinless Arctic char fillets (about 4 ounces each and about ½ inch thick)

1 teaspoon peanut or other oil

¼ teaspoon salt

¼ teaspoon freshly ground black pepper

I have a great deal of sorrel growing in my garden every spring and make a version of a famous dish served in three-star restaurants in France: salmon in sorrel sauce. Sometimes I pick the wild sorrel called sour grass in nearby woods or along the side of the road. Just like the cultivated variety, it is very sour, but it works well with fatty fish like salmon and Arctic char.

In this recipe, thin fillets of Arctic char cook in a nonstick pan in just a couple of minutes, about as long as takes the sorrel to cook, and should, therefore, be cooked just before serving. The dish is finished with cream, and because the cream will thicken as it comes into contact with the sorrel, it is just brought to a boil. This dish is very good with small boiled and peeled potatoes or noodles.

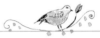

Prepare the sorrel sauce: Place the shredded sorrel in a stainless steel saucepan, add 1 tablespoon water, and bring to a boil; the sorrel will "melt" and change from bright green to a khaki color. Cook for about 30 seconds, then add the cream, salt, and pepper and boil for 10 seconds. Set aside.

At serving time, heat a large nonstick skillet over high heat for 1½ minutes. Rub the fish with the oil and sprinkle with the salt and pepper. Place the fish in the hot skillet and cook, covered, for about 2½ minutes. (No need to turn the fish. Covering it while cooking develops some steam and cook the top of the fish. This gives you fish that is slightly underdone in the center.) Remove from the heat.

Reheat the sorrel sauce and divide among two plates. Place the fish on top of the sauce. Serve immediately.

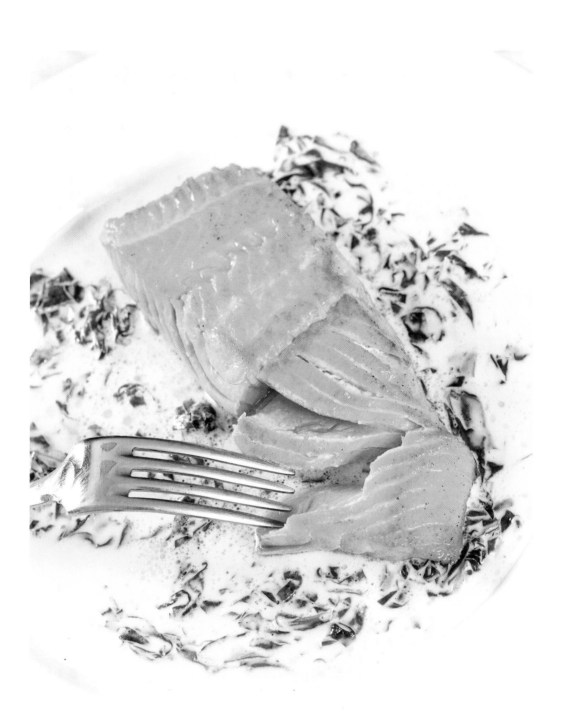

BROILED ARCTIC CHAR WITH LEMON VINAIGRETTE

∘ SERVES 4

4 skin-on fillets Arctic char (about 5 ounces each)

½ teaspoon salt

¼ teaspoon freshly ground black pepper

2 teaspoons olive oil

Vinaigrette
—————

2 tablespoons extra-virgin olive oil

2 teaspoons lemon juice

¼ teaspoon salt

½ teaspoon freshly ground black pepper

1 tablespoon chopped chives, for garnish

Do not remove the skin when you broil this fish—it protects the flesh and browns beautifully. If char is not available, substitute striped bass, black sea bass, or other white-fleshed fish fillets.

Serve these with Parsley Potatoes with Butter (page 171) or Potatoes with Walnuts and Croutons (page 179).

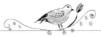

Place the fillets skin side up on a work surface and, using a sharp knife, cut 2 diagonal slits about ¼ inch deep through the skin of each one. (This helps the fish absorb the marinade more readily and cook more evenly.) Place the fillets in a plastic bag, along with the salt, pepper, and olive oil. Seal the bag and toss to mix the ingredients well. Refrigerate for at least 1 hour or up to overnight.

Preheat the broiler. Arrange the fillets skin side up in a single layer on a cookie sheet lined with nonstick aluminum foil or in a gratin dish from which they can be served. Broil, no more than 4 inches from the heat source, for 5 minutes, or until the skin is bubbly, brown, and crusty.

Meanwhile, make the vinaigrette: Combine the olive oil, lemon juice, salt, and pepper in a bowl and blend well.

Transfer the fish to a platter or individual plates. Spoon the vinaigrette over the fish, sprinkle with the chives, and serve immediately.

This attractive, fresh-tasting fish dish makes a perfect first course for an elegant dinner but could also be served as a main course for a special lunch.

When preparing the watercress, remove the bottom 2 inches of the stems, approximately where they are usually bound together with elastic, and reserve for soup.

Heat 2 tablespoons of the olive oil in a large skillet. When the oil is hot, add the garlic and sauté for 5 seconds. Add the watercress, still wet from washing, with ¼ teaspoon each of the salt and pepper. Sauté 1 minute, or until wilted.

Arrange the watercress in a gratin dish large enough to lay the fish in a single layer, creating a bed. Arrange the fish fillets on top. Sprinkle with ¼ teaspoon each salt and pepper.

Place the bread in a food processor and process to crumbs (you should have about 1 cup). Mix the crumbs gently with the remaining 2 tablespoons olive oil and sprinkle on top of the fish. (The dish can be prepared a few hours ahead to this point.)

When you are ready to cook the fish, preheat the broiler. Place the gratin under the broiler, about 10 inches from the heat source, and cook for 10 to 12 minutes, until the fish is just cooked through and the bread crumbs are lightly browned. If you want the crumbs browner yet, move the dish closer to the heat source and cook for another 2 to 3 minutes. Serve immediately.

FISH FILLETS ON WATERCRESS AU GRATIN

∘ SERVES 4

4 tablespoons virgin olive oil

2 cloves garlic, peeled and chopped fine (about 1 teaspoon)

2 bunches watercress, bottom 2 inches of stems removed, washed (about 4 cups)

½ teaspoon salt

½ teaspoon freshly ground black pepper

4 fillets black sea bass, tilefish, red snapper, or cod (about 5 ounces each)

1½ slices white bread

> **Buy your fish already filleted to save yourself time and effort.**

NOTE: You can substitute 4 cups trimmed spinach for the watercress.

FISH PATTIES WITH SPINACH

◦ SERVES 4

It is important to use fresh bread crumbs to coat these fish patties, which are sometimes called croquettes or fish burgers. Two slices of sandwich bread (I like Pepperidge Farm) will give you 1¼ cups fresh bread crumbs. (Dried slices of bread would give you only about ⅓ cup of finer, more powdery crumbs.) Most fish fillets will work well with this simple spinach accompaniment, which I use as a garnish for poultry or meat as well as fish.

Fish Patties

2 slices bread

12 ounces fish fillets, cut into 1- to 2-inch pieces

½ cup chopped (1-inch pieces) onion

1 large egg

3 tablespoons potato starch

¼ cup heavy cream

1 teaspoon salt

1 teaspoon freshly ground black pepper

2 tablespoons peanut oil or other oil

1 tablespoon unsalted butter

3 tablespoons chopped chives

Spinach

2 tablespoons olive oil

1½ teaspoons chopped garlic

One 9-ounce bag baby spinach, cleaned (about 10 cups)

¼ teaspoon salt

¼ teaspoon freshly ground black pepper

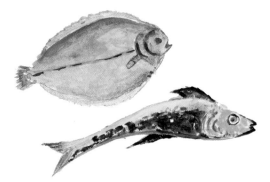

Prepare the fish patties: Place the bread slices in a food processor and process to crumbs. (You will have 1½ cups.) Transfer the crumbs to a bowl.

Add the fish, onion, egg, potato starch, cream, salt, and pepper to the processor bowl and process for 10 seconds. Clean the sides of the bowl and process for another 15 to 20 seconds, until the ingredients are well combined and smooth. Stir in the chives.

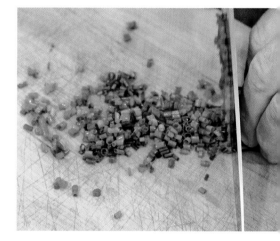

Spread the bread crumbs on a cutting board. Divide the fish mixture into quarters and arrange on top of the bread crumbs. Wet your hands and press on the fish mounds to shape them into patties 3 to 4 inches in diameter and ¾ inch thick. Turn the patties so both sides are well coated with the bread crumbs. Refrigerate the patties until ready to cook.

To cook the fish, heat the peanut oil and butter in a large skillet until hot. Add the 4 patties and cook over high heat for about 3 minutes. Turn the patties over and cook for another 2 minutes on the second side. Transfer to individual plates and sprinkle with chives.

Prepare the spinach: Heat the olive oil in a large skillet for about 1 minute. Add the garlic and cook for 10 to 15 seconds. Pile the spinach in the pan and cover with a lid. Cook, turning the spinach occasionally with tongs, for 2 to 3 minutes, until all the spinach is soft. Add the salt and pepper, mix well, and serve alongside the fish patties.

LEMON SOLE WITH SOUR CREAM AND HORSERADISH SAUCE

◦ SERVES 6

1½ pounds lemon sole fillets

1 cup sour cream

¼ cup water

3 tablespoons grated fresh horseradish, or 5 tablespoons bottled

1 tablespoon small capers, drained

½ teaspoon salt

¼ teaspoon freshly ground black pepper

2 tablespoons chopped cilantro, for garnish

The sole is poached here in a little water, which takes only a few minutes, since the fillets are thin. The sauce, also made very quickly, is an unusual combination of flavors. Because there is a lot of horseradish in it, it tends to be a bit grainy, but this doesn't detract from its taste.

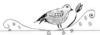

Place the fish fillets in a large stainless steel or nonstick skillet and add ½ cup water. Bring to a boil, immediately turn the fillets over with a spatula, and cook on the other side for about 1 minute. Remove from the heat.

Meanwhile, mix the sour cream, water, horseradish, capers, salt, and pepper together in a saucepan and heat to warm.

Lift the fish fillets from the skillet, dry with paper towels and arrange them on individual plates. Coat with the warm sour cream–horseradish sauce and garnish with the cilantro. Serve immediately.

> The thin sole fillets cook very quickly and the sauce is ready in minutes, so this dish is ideal when you don't have much time.

Several varieties of sole—gray or lemon sole, true Dover sole, or flounder—can be used for this simple but attractive dish. If sole is not available, other white-fleshed fish fillets (small cod or haddock, for example) would be very good prepared this way.

The red pepper sauce can be made ahead. It is also good on pasta or gnocchi.

Prepare the sauce: Cut the bell peppers in half, remove the seeds, and cut into ½-inch pieces. Place the pieces in a blender or a food processor, add the tomato juice, and process until liquefied. (You should have approximately 1½ cups.) Place the mixture in a saucepan (preferably stainless steel), add the butter, olive oil, salt, and black pepper, and bring to a strong boil, mixing with a whisk. Set aside, covered to keep warm.

Sprinkle the fillets with the salt. If they are very thin, fold them in half. Arrange in one layer in a nonstick skillet and add 2 tablespoons water. Bring to a boil, cover, and cook for 1½ to 2 minutes, depending on the thickness of the fillets. Remove them from the pan, pat dry with paper towel, and arrange on individual plates.

Spoon some pepper sauce over each fillet, garnish with the basil, and serve immediately.

▷ **Try the red pepper sauce on pasta or gnocchi.**

FILLETS OF SOLE IN RED PEPPER SAUCE

◦ SERVES 4

Sauce

1 large or 2 medium red bell peppers (about 12 ounces total)

⅓ cup unseasoned tomato juice

1 tablespoon unsalted butter

2 teaspoons extra-virgin olive oil

½ teaspoon salt

½ teaspoon freshly ground black pepper

4 large fillets sole (about 5 ounces each)

¼ teaspoon salt

About 12 basil leaves, shredded coarsely, for garnish

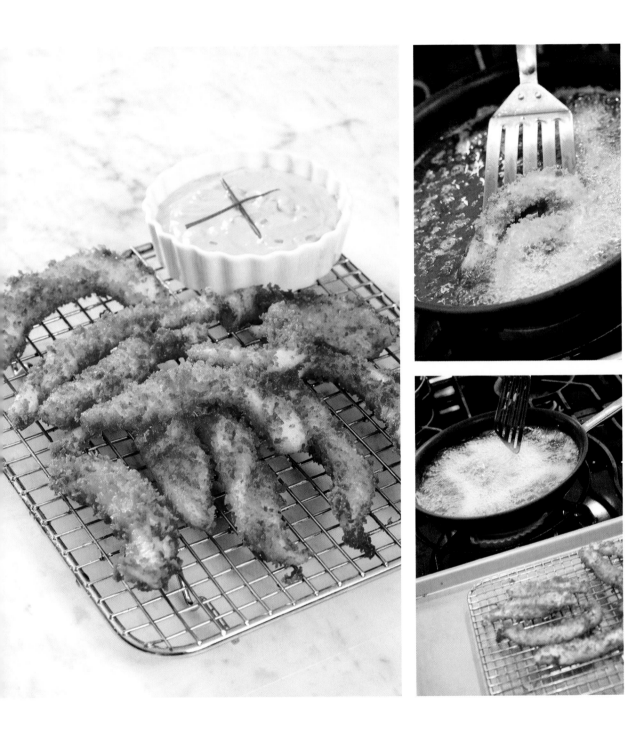

I do not often deep-fry food at home, not only because of the smell, but also because one needs a fairly large amount of oil to deep-fry, and at home, that oil is usually not needed again, as it would be daily in a restaurant. To avoid that problem, I fry the fish in a large pan in a minimal amount of oil. One cup oil gives me a depth of about ½ inch in a large saucepan, so the fish can be fried in one layer in a few minutes. Even if you double the recipe, there is still enough oil to fry a second batch. Then the oil should be discarded, unless you plan to use it again for frying fish in the next few days. Use any sole or flounder, from fluke to lemon, gray, or petrale sole, or any other flatfish. You can make the spicy sauce ahead and refrigerate it until needed.

Prepare the sauce: Mix all the ingredients together in a small bowl. Set aside.

Mix the egg with the Sriracha and salt in a medium bowl. Add the fish, turning to coat. Sprinkle the panko on a plate.

Heat the oil in a large (12-inch) saucepan or skillet to about 350 degrees. Remove the fish strips from the egg mixture, roll them in the panko to coat, and arrange on another plate. Add the strips to the hot oil in one layer. Cook for about 2 minutes and then, using tongs, turn the fish strips over and cook them on the other side for about 2 minutes, or until browned all around. Remove to a serving plate or a wire rack. Serve immediately, with the sauce.

FRIED SOLE FINGERS

○ SERVES 2

Sauce

⅓ cup mayonnaise

2 tablespoons ketchup

1 teaspoon wasabi powder

¼ teaspoon Tabasco sauce

1½ tablespoons chopped chives

1 large egg

1½ teaspoons Sriracha or other hot sauce

⅛ teaspoon salt

2 fillets sole or other flatfish (5 to 6 ounces each), cut into strips ½ to 1 inch wide and about 6 inches long

1 cup panko (Japanese-style bread crumbs)

1 cup peanut or safflower oil

STRIPED BASS GRILLED EN PAPILLOTE

∘ SERVES 4

4 fillets striped bass or sea bass (about 5 ounces each), cleaned

¼ cup extra-virgin olive oil

1 teaspoon salt

1½ cups diced (½-inch pieces) ripe tomato

2 teaspoons freshly ground black pepper

1 teaspoon thyme leaves

2 tablespoons unsalted butter, softened

In the summer, I like to cook fish outside on the grill (see Grilled Red Snapper with Herbs, page 254). One good way of grilling fish—especially when you have fillets—is to cook it *en papillote,* wrapped in parchment paper; in this recipe, I use foil instead of parchment, which is easier to work with. Cooking the fish this way ensures that it will be moist and delicious.

I use striped bass here, but other types of fish fillets—from sole to trout to sea bass—would also be good. You can vary the vegetable too, as long as whatever you select will cook in the 5 minutes allowed.

Rice, steamed potatoes, or pasta makes a good accompaniment.

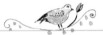

Heat a charcoal or gas grill. Place each fillet in the center of a 12-inch square of aluminum foil. Sprinkle the fish with the olive oil and salt and distribute the tomatoes evenly over and around the fillets. Sprinkle with the pepper and thyme. Fold up each square of foil into a package so that the seam is on top and the contents are securely enclosed.

Place the packages on the hot grill and cook for 5 minutes.

To serve, carefully unwrap the foil packages and transfer the fillets and tomatoes to individual dinner plates. Dot them with the butter and serve. Or place an unopened package on each plate and let your guests open their own packages. Dot the fish with butter and enjoy.

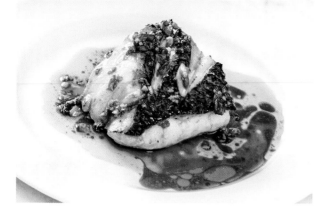

SOY-GARLIC BROILED STRIPED BASS

Once considered a sport fish, striped bass, which has tender white flesh, is now raised commercially. The skin is left on, so the fish should be scaled. Marinate the fish for at least 30 minutes or as long as overnight (refrigerated) to absorb the flavors of the marinade.

Serve the fish with Potatoes with Walnuts and Croutons (page 179), Parsley Potatoes with Butter (page 171), or hash-brown potatoes.

Place the fillets skin side up on a work surface and, using a sharp knife, cut 2 diagonal slits about ¼ inch deep through the skin of each one. (This helps the fish absorb the marinade more readily and cook more evenly.) Place the fillets in a plastic bag, along with the garlic, ginger, scallions, soy sauce, sugar, and oils. Seal the bag and toss to mix the ingredients well. Refrigerate for at least 30 minutes or up to 10 hours.

At cooking time, preheat the broiler. Drain the fillets and arrange them skin side up in a single layer on a cookie sheet lined with nonstick aluminum foil or in a gratin dish from which they can be served. Broil, 4 to 5 inches from the heat source, for 5 to 6 minutes. The skin will brown and bubble and the heat will penetrate the fish through the slits in the skin and cook the flesh. Serve.

○ SERVES 4

4 skin-on fillets striped bass (about 6 ounces each and 1 inch thick)

4 cloves garlic, peeled, crushed, and chopped (about 1 tablespoon)

One 1-inch piece fresh ginger, peeled and chopped (about 1 tablespoon)

4 scallions, cleaned and minced (about ⅔ cup)

2 tablespoons dark soy sauce

2 teaspoons sugar

1 tablespoon peanut oil

1 tablespoon toasted sesame oil

NOTE: This preparation also works well with sea bass or black bass, as well as red snapper and other white-fleshed fish fillets.

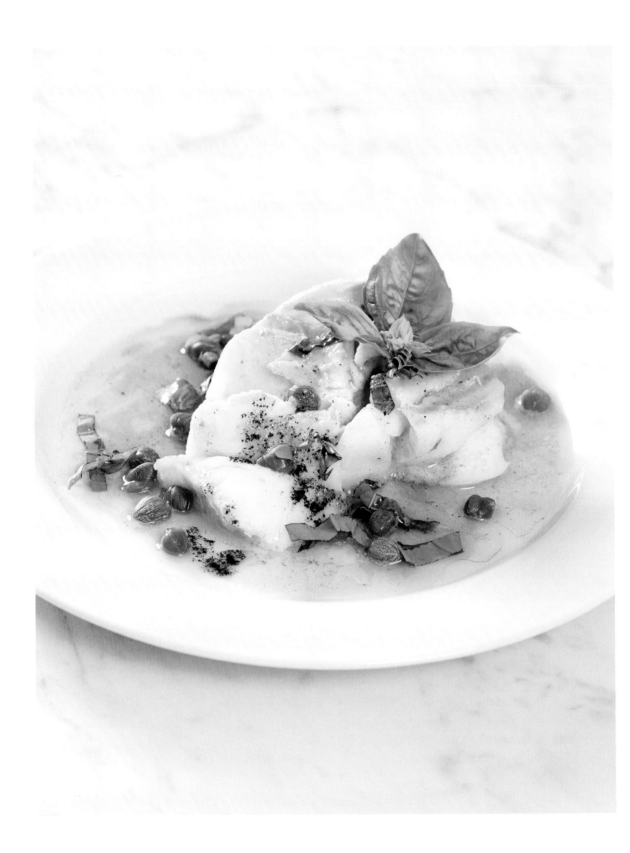

I like white, fleshy fillets—as thick as possible—for this dish so they remain moist in the center. Fresh scrod (a young cod), cod, and haddock are all excellent choices. Black butter, a butter cooked to a dark hazelnut color, has a nutty, rich taste.

Bring about 2 cups water to a boil in a large saucepan. Add the fish and bring the water back to a boil (this will take about 2 minutes). Boil gently for about 2 minutes, until the fillets are tender but still slightly undercooked in the center. Increase the cooking time if the fillets are thicker.

While the fish is cooking, place the butter and olive oil in a skillet and cook over medium to high heat until the mixture turns brown.

Drain the fish, pat dry with paper towels, and arrange the fillets on four plates. Sprinkle with the capers, salt, pepper, and vinegar. Pour the brown butter mixture over the fish, garnish with the basil, and serve.

▷ **It only takes a few minutes to poach the fillets and prepare the sauce for this dish.**

POACHED COD WITH BLACK BUTTER AND CAPERS

∘ SERVES 4

4 thick fillets scrod or cod (about 6 ounces each and 1½ inches thick)

4 tablespoons (½ stick) unsalted butter

1 tablespoon olive oil

2 tablespoons capers, drained

⅛ teaspoon salt

¼ teaspoon freshly ground black pepper

1 tablespoon red wine vinegar

⅓ cup shredded basil leaves, for garnish

GRILLED RED SNAPPER WITH HERBS

∘ SERVES 4

2 red snapper (about 1½ pounds each), scaled and gutted, heads left on

2 tablespoons peanut oil

½ teaspoon salt

8 bay leaves

4 sprigs thyme

2 sprigs mint

2 small jalapeño peppers

2 tablespoons extra-virgin olive oil

When grilling fish, I often use a folding wire grill and "sandwich" the fish between the two racks so that I can manipulate it easily. Before placing the fish inside, heat the wire grill on the hot barbecue for a few minutes so the wires are very hot. And get the fish as close to the heat as possible. The fish will be less likely to stick if the grill is very hot, and the intense heat will give it a nice crusty exterior.

Whole fish is good for a casual family meal. You can use your fingers to separate the flesh from the bones.

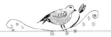

Heat a charcoal or gas grill. Place a folding wire grill on the grill grate to heat for 10 minutes.

Meanwhile, clean the fish well under water, removing any trace of blood from the inside. Dry thoroughly with paper towels. Cut 2 diagonal slits ¼ inch deep and 2 inches apart on both sides of each fish. Sprinkle the fish inside and out with the oil and salt. Place the bay leaves in the cuts, and press a sprig of thyme onto the side of each fish. Place a sprig of mint and a jalapeño inside each fish.

When the wire grill is extremely hot, place the fish inside it, between the two racks. Cook as close to the heat as possible for 5 to 6 minutes on the first side. Then turn the wire grill and cook the fish on the other side for another 5 to 6 minutes.

Remove the fish from the wire grill and place on a large platter. Sprinkle with the olive oil and serve immediately.

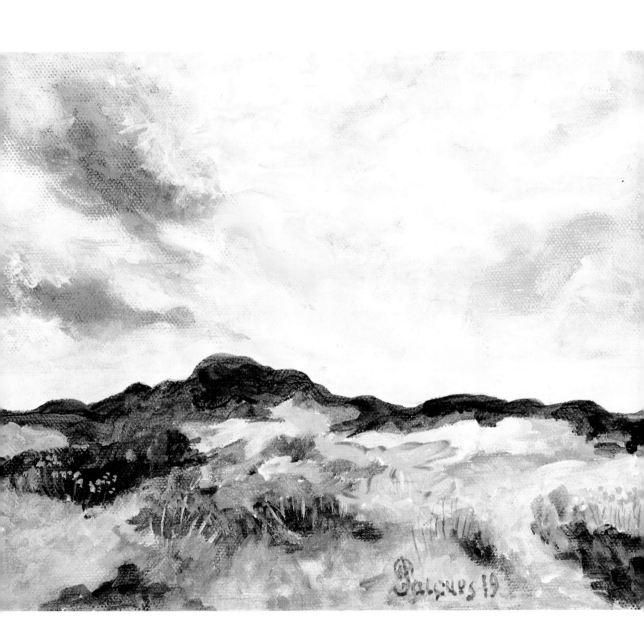

TUNA CARPACCIO

○ SERVES 6 AS A FIRST COURSE

One 1¼-pound tuna steak, cleaned (see Note)

Salt

Freshly ground black pepper

¼ cup finely chopped shallots (about 2 large)

½ cup diced (¼-inch pieces) radishes

½ cup peeled, seeded, and diced (¼-inch pieces) cucumber (about ¼ cucumber)

½ cup diced (¼-inch pieces) mushrooms (about 3 medium)

2 tablespoons finely chopped flat-leaf parsley

1 tablespoon rice vinegar

3 tablespoons extra-virgin olive oil

Classic carpaccio is paper-thin slices of raw beef covered with a flavorful mayonnaise. In this recipe, I use tuna instead of beef and a dressing of oil and vinegar with a garnish of diced vegetables. This is particularly good as a first course for an elegant dinner party, because it can be prepared a few hours ahead—then all you have to do at serving time is to add the garnish.

Be sure to buy the freshest-possible fish. If you are not absolutely certain about its freshness, purchase it frozen, then defrost it slowly in the refrigerator.

Serve this with black bread or crunchy French bread.

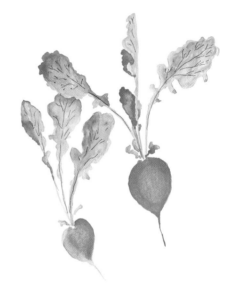

Cut the tuna into 6 equal pieces. Place a piece of tuna on a sheet of plastic wrap and lay another piece of plastic wrap on top. Pound the tuna with a meat pounder or a small heavy saucepan until it has flattened out into a thin piece 5 to 6 inches across. Remove the top layer of plastic wrap and sprinkle salt and pepper on the fish. Using the bottom layer of plastic wrap, invert the tuna onto a serving plate; peel off the plastic. Sprinkle the fish with more salt and pepper. Re-cover the fish with the plastic wrap. Repeat this procedure with the remaining pieces of tuna. Refrigerate while you prepare the garnishes or for up to 24 hours.

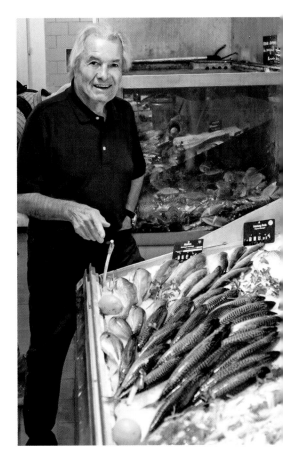

About 1 hour before serving, prepare the garnishes: Place the shallots in a sieve and rinse under cool water. (Rinsing removes the sulfuric acid, which tends to make chopped shallots and onions discolor and stings the eyes.) Drain, dry on a paper towel to remove the moisture, and place in a bowl.

At serving time, remove the plastic wrap from the tuna. Sprinkle the shallots, radishes, cucumber, mushrooms, and parsley evenly on top, then sprinkle each portion with approximately ½ teaspoon of the vinegar and 2 teaspoons of the olive oil. Serve immediately.

NOTE: If you will have to remove skin, sinew, and/or bone from the tuna, buy about 1½ pounds of tuna.

TUNA STEAK AU POIVRE WITH CUCUMBER SAUCE

◦ SERVES 6

Sauce
———

1 cucumber (about 10 ounces)

⅓ cup water

⅓ cup olive oil

¼ cup cider vinegar

2 teaspoons soy sauce

½ teaspoon Tabasco sauce

2 teaspoons sugar

¾ teaspoon salt

3 tablespoons coarsely chopped cilantro

1 tablespoon black peppercorns (see Note)

6 tuna steaks (about 6 ounces each 1 inch thick)

½ teaspoon salt

3 tablespoons olive oil

Classic steak au poivre is traditionally made with beef. Tuna steaks make an excellent variation; they are meaty but lean, filling, and juicy. This is an easy and fast dish, and the sauce can be made ahead and stored in the refrigerator.

Prepare the sauce: Peel the cucumber, cut it lengthwise in half, and remove the seeds by scraping them out with a spoon. Cut the cucumber halves into 1-inch pieces and place them in a food processor. Add the remaining sauce ingredients except the cilantro and process for a few seconds, until the mixture is chopped fine but still grainy. Add the cilantro and pulse to blend. Transfer the sauce to a serving bowl and set aside.

Spread the peppercorns on a work surface and, using a rolling pin or the bottom of a heavy saucepan, coarsely crush them. Spread the crushed pepper on both sides of the tuna steaks. Sprinkle with the salt.

Heat one large or two medium skillets until very hot. Add the olive oil, tilting the pan(s) to quickly coat the bottom, and add the steaks. Cook for 1 minute on each side. Turn off the heat, cover the skillet(s), and let the tuna steam for 4 to 5 minutes (the interior of the steaks should be medium-rare).

Serve immediately, with the cucumber sauce.

NOTE: Instead of all black peppercorns, try a mixture of black, white, pink, green, and, if you like, Szechuan peppercorns with some allspice berries.

> This preparation also works well with swordfish steaks. The sauce can be used with other fish dishes, cold meats, and grilled meat or poultry.

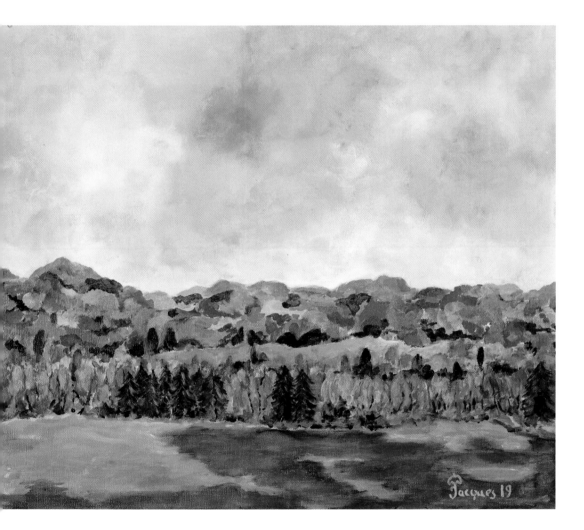

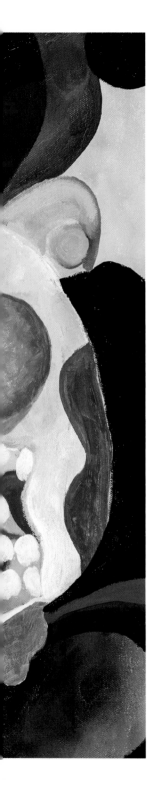

EGGS, POULTRY & MEAT

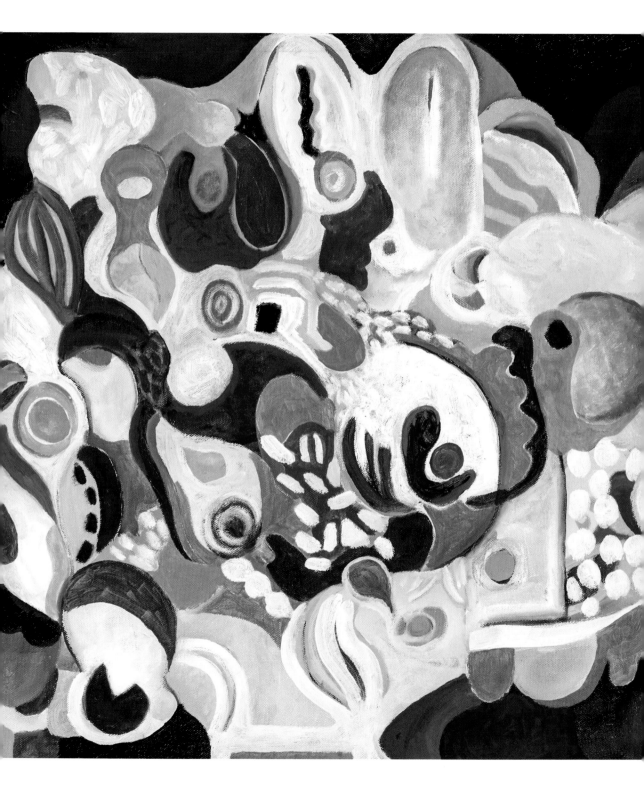

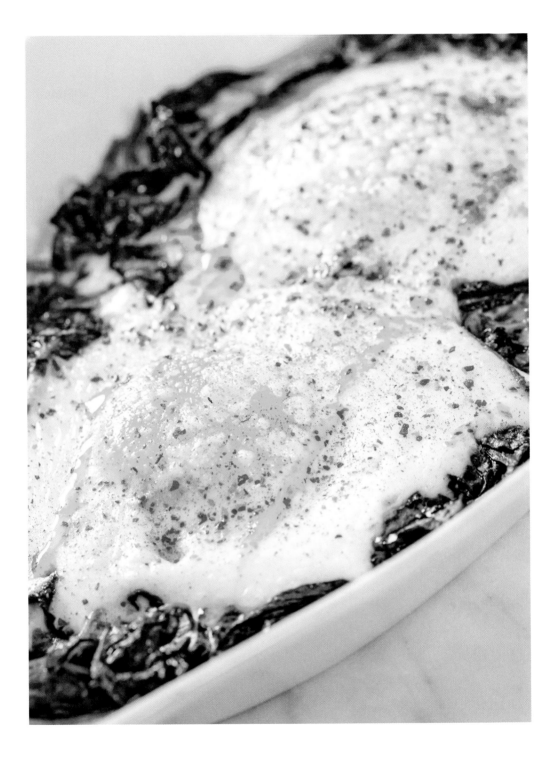

This makes a terrific main dish for brunch or first course for dinner, typical of the way eggs are often served in France.

If you like, you can cook the spinach ahead and reheat it in the oven before adding the eggs to finish the dish.

Preheat the oven to 400 degrees. Pile the spinach into an oval gratin dish about 14 inches long and 8 inches wide. Place the dish on a cookie sheet and bake for about 12 minutes, until the spinach has wilted considerably and is beginning to "melt" down into the dish.

Remove the dish from the oven and press on the spinach with a fork to gather it together. Sprinkle with the salt, pepper, and olive oil, stir to mix well, and press again into one compact layer in the dish.

If you are serving the dish immediately, make 4 "nests" in the spinach with a spoon. Break an egg into each nest, sprinkle the eggs with the cheese and paprika, and bake for 7 to 10 minutes, until the egg whites are set but the yolks are still soft and runny. (Cook longer if you like your egg yolks hard.) Spoon the cream over the entire surface of the dish and serve immediately.

If you will be serving it later, allow the spinach to cool. When you are ready to complete the recipe, return the dish to a 400-degree oven for 5 minutes to reheat the spinach, then proceed as described above.

EGGS IN A SPINACH NEST

° SERVES 4 AS A FIRST COURSE OR BRUNCH MAIN COURSE

One 12-ounce package prewashed baby spinach

¼ teaspoon salt

¼ teaspoon freshly ground black pepper

¼ cup extra-virgin olive oil

4 large eggs, preferably organic

1 tablespoon grated Parmesan cheese

Dash of paprika

¼ cup heavy cream

GRATIN OF EGGS WITH MUSHROOMS AND HAM

◦ SERVES 6 TO 8

8 large eggs, preferably organic

1 tablespoon unsalted butter

1 tablespoon olive oil

4 ounces oyster mushrooms, washed and cut into 1-inch pieces (2 cups)

3 tablespoons all-purpose flour

2½ cups milk

¾ teaspoon salt

¾ teaspoon freshly ground black pepper

4 ounces boiled ham, cut into ½-inch pieces (1 cup)

3 tablespoons chopped chives

½ cup grated sharp cheddar cheese

There is something very elegant about egg dishes, which are versatile and can be served for breakfast, brunch, lunch, or dinner. When I was a kid, we ate a gratin of eggs in one form or another at least once a week. The important thing is to cook the hard-cooked eggs the right way. Use organic eggs, and make a hole in the rounder end of each egg with a pushpin, penetrating the air chamber. This will relieve the air pressure when the eggs are placed in boiling water and prevent them from cracking.

Cook the eggs at a low boil to prevent the whites from toughening. As soon as the eggs are cooked, pour out the hot water and shake the pan to crack the shells, which will make the eggs easier to peel. Add cold water and ice to the pan and set aside until the eggs are thoroughly cooled. (This quick method of cooking the eggs releases the sulfur in them and prevents the yolks from having that green color and sulfur smell.) Shell the eggs under cool running water.

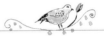

Bring a large saucepan of water to a boil. With a pushpin, punch a hole in the rounder end of each egg and lower them into the boiling water. When the water comes back to a boil, reduce the heat so the eggs cook at a gentle boil. After 10 minutes, pour out the water and shake the eggs in the pan to crack their shells. Add cold water and ice to the pan and let the eggs cool.

Drain the eggs and shell them under cool running water, then quarter them lengthwise and arrange them in a 6-cup gratin dish.

Preheat the broiler. Heat the butter and olive oil in a medium saucepan and add the mushrooms. Cook until the moisture is released from the mushrooms and they are sizzling in the butter, about 5 minutes. Sprinkle the flour on top and mix it in. Add the milk, salt, and pepper and bring to a boil, stirring with a whisk until the mixture thickens. Remove from the heat.

Sprinkle the ham, chives, and half the cheese over the eggs. Pour the sauce on top and sprinkle on the rest of the cheese.

Place the dish under the broiler, not too close to the heat source, and broil for about 10 minutes, until the surface is brown and bubbling. Serve.

NOTE: To prepare the gratin ahead (even the night before), assemble the dish and refrigerate, covered. When ready to serve, preheat the oven to 400 degrees. Bake the gratin for about 30 minutes, until it is brown, bubbling, and hot.

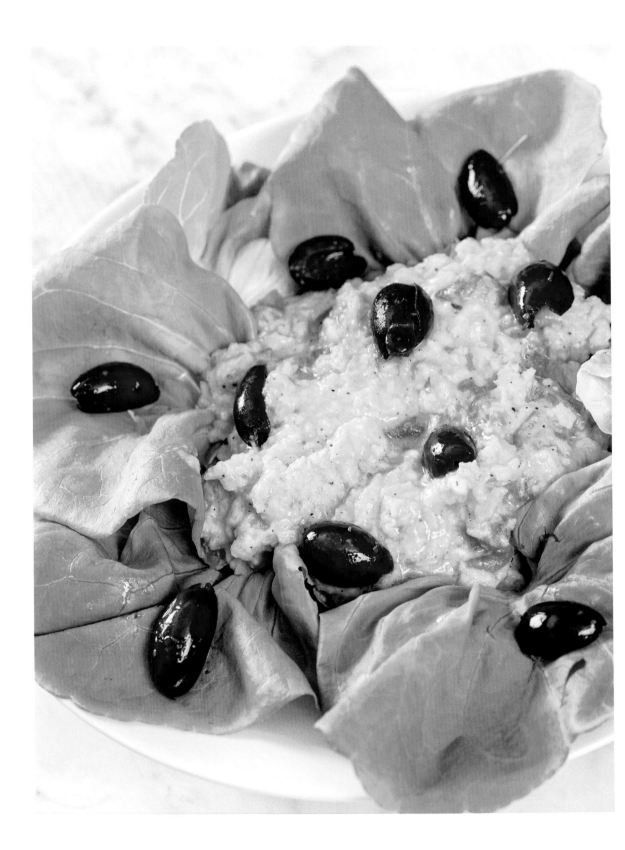

A *brouillade* is a mixture of scrambled eggs combined with tomato (as in my recipe), a mushroom, or herbs or other vegetable, like zucchini, eggplant, etc. I serve it in lettuce cups—Boston lettuce is best for this—as a first course for a dinner or as a brunch or lunch main course. The tomatoes can be prepared ahead and then combined with the eggs at serving time.

Heat the olive oil and butter in a saucepan. When the mixture is hot, add the onion and cook for about 45 seconds. Add the tomato, salt, and pepper and cook over low heat, stirring occasionally, for about 5 minutes, until the tomato is soft. Set aside.

At serving time, crack the eggs into a bowl. Add the chives and beat with a fork until well combined.

Heat the tomato mixture, add the eggs to the saucepan, and cook over medium to high heat, moving and stirring the mixture with a rubber spatula, until the eggs form large curds and are well combined with the tomatoes, about 2 minutes. Do not overcook; the mixture should still be moist. Stir in the olives.

To serve, place a lettuce leaf on each plate and form it into a cup. Spoon the egg mixture into the lettuce cups and serve immediately.

TOMATO BROUILLADE WITH OLIVES

○ SERVES 4 AS A FIRST COURSE OR BRUNCH OR LUNCH MAIN COURSE

2 tablespoons olive oil

2 tablespoons unsalted butter

½ cup chopped onion

1 large ripe tomato (10 to 12 ounces), cut into ½-inch pieces (about 2 cups)

¾ teaspoon salt

¾ teaspoon freshly ground black pepper

6 large eggs, preferably organic

3 tablespoons chopped chives

20 oil-cured black olives, pitted and halved

6 large Boston lettuce leaves, for serving

COCOTTE EGGS WITH SHRIMP

∘ SERVES 4 AS A FIRST COURSE
OR LUNCH MAIN COURSE

7 or 8 shrimp (frozen shrimp
can be used), shelled and cut into
½-inch pieces (about ⅔ cup)

½ cup heavy cream

½ teaspoon salt

½ teaspoon freshly ground
black pepper

4 large eggs, preferably organic

1 tablespoon finely chopped
chives, for garnish

Oeufs en cocotte are eggs cooked in small soufflé
molds, cups, or bowls with a ½- to ¾-cup capacity.
The molds are placed in a saucepan with water
around them; the pan is then covered and the water
brought to a boil on the stovetop. The saucepan
should be deep enough so there is some space
between the eggs and the lid so the steam generated
by the boiling water will cook the eggs. They will have
the consistency of poached eggs. An elegant way of
serving eggs, this makes a wonderful first course for
dinner or main course for lunch.

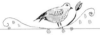

Place the shrimp pieces, cream, and half the salt
and pepper in a saucepan and bring just to a
boil. Immediately remove from the heat and divide
among four ½- to ¾-cup cocotte or soufflé molds.

At serving time, break an egg on top of the shrimp
mixture in each cup and sprinkle the eggs with the
remaining salt and pepper. Arrange the filled molds
in a large saucepan with 1 cup water around them,
cover, and bring to a boil. Cook, covered, for about
5 minutes, until the eggs whites are cooked but the
yolks are still runny. Sprinkle with the chives and
serve immediately. Eat with a spoon.

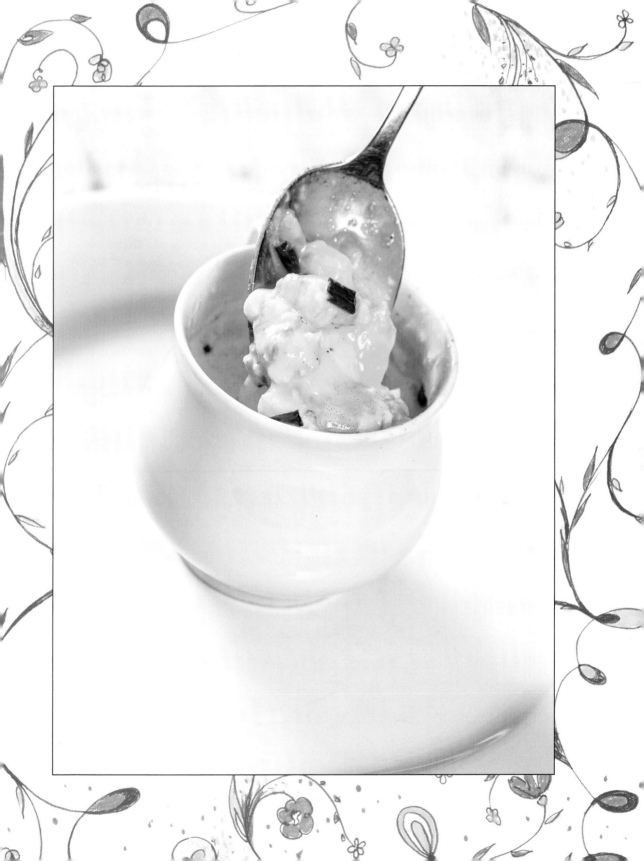

SUPREMES OF CHICKEN WITH PAPRIKA

◦ SERVES 4

4 tablespoons (½ stick) unsalted butter

4 skinless, boneless chicken breasts (about 6 ounces each)

1 teaspoon smoked paprika

½ teaspoon salt

½ teaspoon freshly ground black pepper

1 tablespoon lime juice

A supreme of chicken is simply a boneless, skinless chicken breast. Available at any supermarket, these are virtually fat-free and cook in a few minutes. The trick is to avoid overcooking them. The best way I've found to do this is to sauté the breasts until they are about three-quarters done, then set them aside to finish cooking in their residual heat. The result is very tender meat.

You can use these in a salad, like the Chicken and Spinach Salad (opposite), or serve them with White Bean Puree (page 146), sautéed potatoes, peas, or almost any vegetable dish in this book.

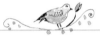

Melt the butter in a large skillet. Sprinkle the chicken breasts with the paprika, salt, and pepper, place them in the foaming butter, and cook for approximately 2½ minutes on each side. Then remove from the heat, cover the pan, and set aside for 8 to 10 minutes to let the chicken finish cooking.

Arrange the chicken breasts, whole or sliced, on individual plates. Add the lime juice to the drippings in the pan, bring the mixture to a boil, and pour over the chicken. Serve immediately.

▷ **Skinless, boneless chicken breasts make a quick and nutritious meal.**

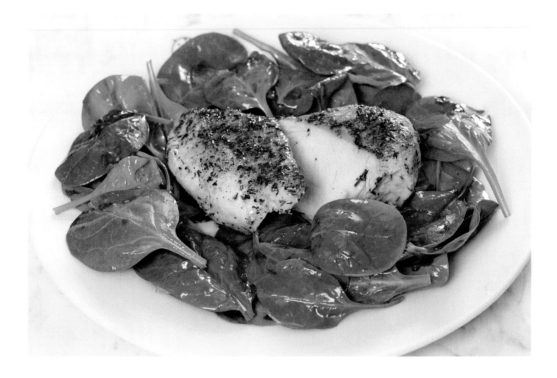

Toss the spinach with the vinaigrette in a large bowl and divide it among four plates. Slice the chicken breasts, arrange them in the center of the salads, and sprinkle with the cooking juices. Serve immediately.

Chicken and Spinach Salad

• SERVES 4

4 cups baby spinach, usually pre-washed

¼ cup Mustard Vinaigrette (page 12)

Supremes of Chicken with Paprika (opposite), cooled to room temperature in the covered pan

GRILLED CHICKEN BREASTS WITH SUNFLOWER-CILANTRO SAUCE

◦ SERVES 6

If you cannot cook the chicken on a grill (which gives it a distinctive taste), cook the breasts in a cast-iron skillet over very high heat for approximately the same length of time.

The recipe yields about 2 cups Sunflower-Cilantro Sauce, so you will have leftovers. It can be made ahead and stored in the refrigerator for up to 1 week. It is spicy and invigorating and goes well not only with the chicken breasts, but also with leftover beef, veal, pork, or lamb roasts; fish (poached, steamed, or grilled); and grilled scallops or shrimp.

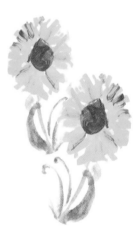

6 skinless, boneless chicken breasts (about 6 ounces each)

¾ teaspoon salt

¾ teaspoon freshly ground black pepper

1 teaspoon dried oregano

1 tablespoon virgin olive oil

Sauce
———

1 jalapeño pepper

1 cup lightly packed flat-leaf parsley leaves

1 cup lightly packed cilantro leaves

6 cloves garlic, peeled

⅓ cup sunflower seeds

1 teaspoon salt

¼ cup virgin olive oil

¾ cup water

3 ripe tomatoes (about 1 pound total), thinly sliced

Sprinkle the chicken breasts with the salt, pepper, and oregano, then coat with the olive oil. Cover with plastic wrap, and refrigerate for at least 1 hour or as long as 8 hours.

Meanwhile, prepare the sauce: Halve the jalapeño, remove the seeds, and cut the pepper into a few pieces. Place the jalapeño pieces, parsley, cilantro, garlic, sunflower seeds, salt, olive oil, and water in a blender and blend until pureed to a smooth green liquid. Transfer to a bowl.

> **You can prepare the sauce and season the chicken ahead of time, with the grilling done at the last minute.**

At serving time, heat a charcoal or gas grill until very hot. Remove the chicken breasts from the refrigerator and place them on the hot grill. Cover and cook for about 2½ minutes on each side, until the chicken is well marked. Move it to a cooler place on the grill, or transfer it to a baking dish and keep warm in a 150-degree oven.

Arrange a few spoonfuls of the sauce on each of six plates and top with the grilled chicken breasts. Garnish with tomato slices arranged attractively around the border and serve.

CHICKEN NIÇOISE IN PUFF PASTRY

∘ SERVES 4

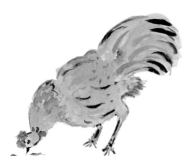

Frozen puff pastry shells are available in many supermarkets. They go directly from the freezer to the oven and can accommodate a variety of fillings, including shrimp, scallops, vegetables, and scrambled eggs. In this recipe, I fill them with chicken in a delicious sauce containing diced black olives— definitely "dressy" enough for company.

To make the pastry shells taste richer, rub them with butter before baking. Then, after the shells are baked, you remove the "lids" with the point of a sharp knife. Inside you will find a soft dough that is cooked but not crisp. Fill the shell as needed. The chicken filling can also be served by itself.

4 frozen puff pastry shells

1 tablespoon unsalted butter, softened

Filling

2 tablespoons unsalted butter

2 tablespoons olive oil

3 skinless, boneless chicken breasts (about 6 ounces each), cut into ½-inch-wide strips

¾ teaspoon salt

½ teaspoon freshly ground black pepper

2 large shallots, peeled and chopped (about ¼ cup)

2 cloves garlic, peeled, crushed, and chopped very fine (about 1 teaspoon)

2 tablespoons balsamic vinegar

1 teaspoon bottled steak sauce

¼ cup water

1½ cups halved, seeded, drained, and cut into ½-inch dice ripe tomatoes

2 tablespoons ketchup

½ cup oil-cured black olives (about 20), pitted

1 teaspoon chopped tarragon

Preheat the oven to 400 degrees. Rub the tops and bottoms of the frozen puff pastry shells with the butter. Place them on a cookie sheet lined with nonstick aluminum foil and bake for 30 minutes, or until well puffed and quite brown. Turn the oven off, prop the door slightly open, and allow the shells to cool in the warm oven (this allows them to cool slowly and helps keep them from collapsing).

When the pastry shells have cooled enough to handle, remove them from the oven and lift off the lids with the point of a sharp knife. Then return the shells to the warm oven until serving time.

Meanwhile, prepare the filling: Heat the butter and olive oil in a large skillet until the mixture is very hot. Sprinkle the chicken strips with the salt and pepper and place them in the hot skillet. Sauté over high heat for about 1½ minutes, stirring to separate the pieces. Using a slotted spoon, transfer the chicken to a plate. Add the shallots and garlic to the drippings in the skillet and cook for about 30 seconds. Add the vinegar and cook until the mixture begins to sizzle. Add the steak sauce, water, and tomatoes and bring the mixture to a boil. Boil for about 1 minute, then stir in the ketchup and olives. Return the chicken to the pan, heat through, and sprinkle with the tarragon.

NOTE: To prepare this dish ahead, sauté the chicken and prepare the sauce, but do not combine them until just before serving. If you don't have frozen pastry shells on hand, you can serve the chicken mixture on its own or on toast.

Place the pastry shells on individual plates and spoon the chicken mixture into and around them. Serve immediately.

CRUSTY CHICKEN LEGS

◦ SERVES 4

4 chicken legs (2½ pounds total)

¾ teaspoon salt, plus more to taste

½ teaspoon freshly ground black pepper, plus more to taste

1 onion, peeled and chopped fine (about ¾ cup)

2 cloves garlic, peeled and chopped fine (1 teaspoon)

1 tablespoon red wine vinegar

1 tablespoon balsamic vinegar

2 teaspoons bottled steak sauce

½ cup water

1 tablespoon finely chopped flat-leaf parsley, for garnish

I do this sauté using chicken legs rather than breasts—the legs stay moister. Notice that the chicken is cooked mostly skin side down for quite a long time: 30 minutes. This technique constitutes a recipe in itself—you can serve the chicken as is right out of the skillet, with a salad alongside. Or, if you want to make it a little fancier, discard some of the fat from the skillet, add a little water to melt the solidified juices, and pour this mixture over the chicken. Here I take the basic idea a step further, creating a sauce with the chicken drippings (after first removing the chicken so its skin stays crisp).

Using a good sturdy skillet, preferably heavy nonstick aluminum, is important to ensure that the chicken becomes crusty and brown but doesn't burn.

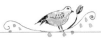

With a sharp heavy knife, cut off the tips of the chicken drumsticks and discard them. Cut halfway through the leg between the thigh and drumstick (this helps with the cooking). Sprinkle the legs with the salt and pepper.

Heat a large heavy nonstick skillet for 1 minute, then add the chicken legs, skin side down, in one layer. Cook over medium to high heat for about 5 minutes on each side, until the legs have begun to brown. Turn the legs skin side down, cover, reduce the heat to medium-low, and cook for about another 20 minutes, until the chicken is well browned and cooked through. Remove the chicken legs from the skillet, arrange them skin side up on an ovenproof plate, and place in a warm oven.

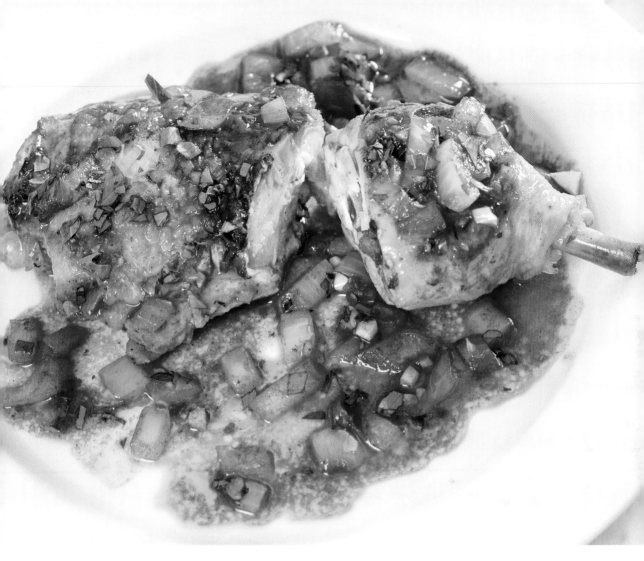

Discard all but 1 to 2 tablespoons of the fat from the skillet. Add the onion and garlic to the skillet and cook for about 1 minute. Then stir in both vinegars and the steak sauce and cook, stirring, for a minute or so, until most of the liquid has evaporated. Add the water and salt and pepper to taste and cook, stirring to melt and mix in the solidified juices, for about 2 minutes. Pour the sauce over the chicken, garnish with the parsley, and serve immediately.

BAKED CHICKEN LEGS WITH MUSTARD CRUMBS

∘ SERVES 4

4 skinless chicken legs (about 10 ounces each)

½ teaspoon salt

½ teaspoon freshly ground black pepper

3½ tablespoons olive oil

2 slices white bread

2 tablespoons Dijon-style mustard

▷ **The chicken legs can be prepared ahead through the initial cooking, then finished in the oven just before serving.**

I prefer the dark meat of chicken and find the legs remain nicely moist when prepared this way. The initial cooking can be done ahead, then return the legs to the oven just before serving to finish cooking.

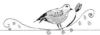

Preheat the oven to 425 degrees. Using a sharp heavy knife, cut halfway through the joint between the drumstick and thigh of each leg to help the cooking process. Cut off and discard the tips of the drumsticks. Sprinkle the meat with the salt, pepper, and 2 tablespoons of the olive oil and arrange the legs on a cookie sheet lined with nonstick aluminum foil. Bake for 15 minutes; the chicken will be only partially cooked.

Meanwhile, place the bread in a food processor and process to crumbs (you will have about 1½ cups crumbs). Gently mix the bread crumbs with the remaining 1½ tablespoons oil to moisten them.

Remove the chicken from the oven, brush the surface with the mustard, and pile the bread crumbs on top, pressing lightly to make them adhere. (You can prepare the chicken ahead to this point.)

Return the chicken to the oven and bake for 20 to 25 minutes, until the bread crumbs are brown and the meat is tender.

Transfer the legs to individual plates and serve immediately, spooning any spilled crumbs alongside the meat.

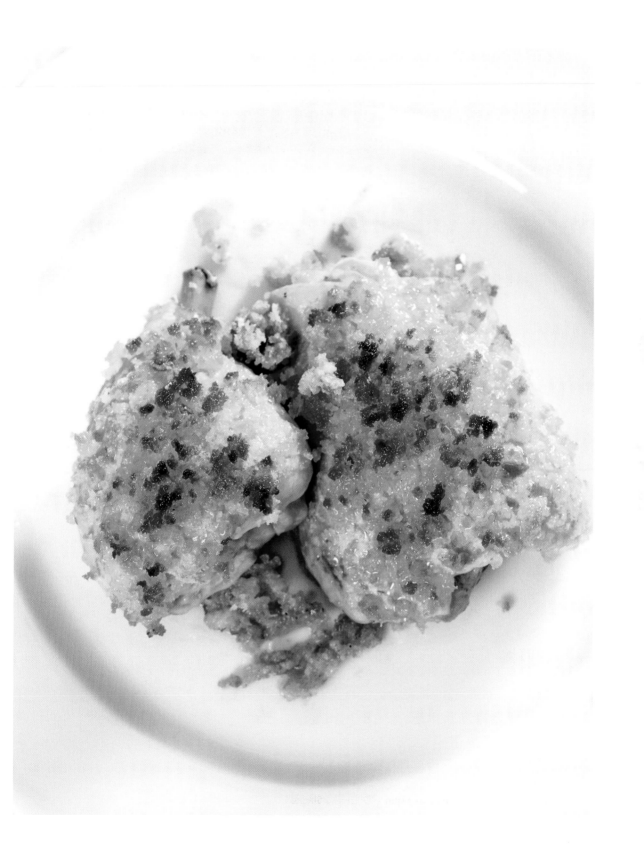

SAUTÉED CHICKEN WINGS WITH HOT SAUCE

◦ SERVES 4

About 1¾ pounds chicken wings
(12 wings)

½ teaspoon salt

Sauce
———
1 tablespoon Sriracha or other
hot sauce

1 tablespoon hoisin sauce

1 tablespoon dark soy sauce

2 teaspoons balsamic vinegar

2 teaspoons toasted sesame oil

▷ **This dish requires
practically no prep.**

You have to eat chicken wings with your fingers, so these are best prepared for informal family dinners or friendly reunions. I always have the ingredients for the sauce in my refrigerator, but it can be changed based on your taste and what you have on hand, such as balsamic vinegar, ketchup, honey, etc. Use a large (12-inch) skillet for this recipe. The wings are arranged in one layer in the cold pan (with no oil) and are cooked over high heat for about 25 minutes.

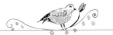

Arrange the chicken wings in one layer in a 12-inch nonstick skillet. (Use two skillets if necessary.) Sprinkle the wings with the salt. Cook over high heat, uncovered, for 10 minutes, shaking the pan occasionally so the wings don't stick.

Meanwhile, prepare the sauce: Mix all the ingredients together in a bowl.

Turn the chicken wings. They should be nicely browned on the first side. Cover the skillet, reduce the heat to medium-low, and cook the wings for another 12 minutes, or until they are browned on the second side and tender. Using the lid to hold the wings in the pan, pour out the accumulated fat. Pour the sauce over the wings and cook over high heat, tossing the wings in the sauce, until the sauce has reduced enough that it coats the wings like a glaze, 2 to 3 minutes.

Serve immediately.

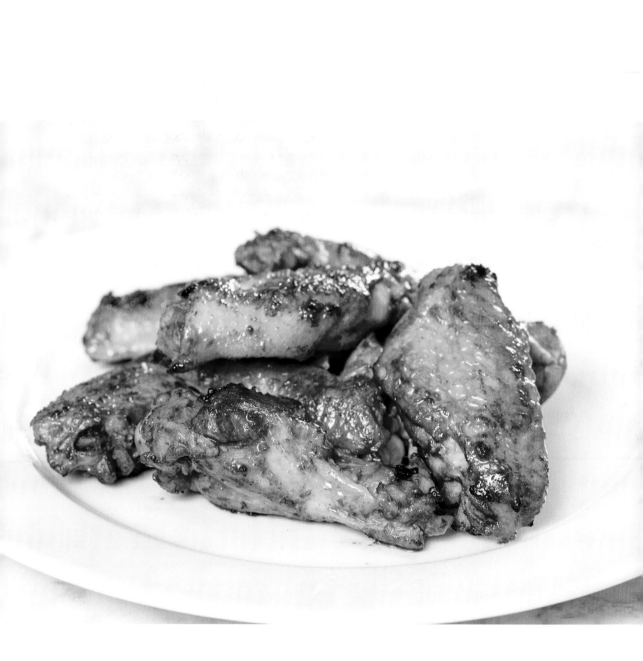

CHICKEN IN VINEGAR WITH GARLIC AND TOMATO SAUCE

◦ SERVES 4

4 chicken thighs (about 2 pounds)

¾ teaspoon salt

1 teaspoon freshly ground black pepper, or to taste

3 garlic cloves, peeled, crushed, and chopped finely (1 tablespoon)

⅓ cup best-quality red wine vinegar

⅓ cup water

1½ cups chopped peeled tomatoes (fresh or canned)

½ teaspoon Tabasco sauce, or to taste

2 teaspoons chopped chives, for garnish

Chicken in vinegar with garlic is a bistro specialty in Lyon. The spicy, piquant sauce of vinegar, garlic, and tomatoes has an assertive flavor that complements the bird well. The chicken thighs are cooked only on the skin side, covered, so the skin is crispy and the flesh is cooked by the steam. The cooked chicken could be served with a salad. In this recipe, the chicken is removed from the skillet and a sauce is made in just a couple of minutes, then spooned over the chicken and served.

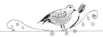

Place the chicken thighs skin side down on your cutting board. Make a ½-inch-deep cut along both sides of the bone of each thigh. Sprinkle the thighs with half the salt and pepper.

Place the chicken pieces skin side down in a large nonstick skillet and cook over high heat for a couple of minutes, until sizzling. Turn the heat to medium-low, cover tightly, and cook for 18 to 20 minutes. Remove the chicken to a serving platter and keep warm.

Add the garlic to the skillet and sauté for 30 seconds. Add the vinegar and water and bring to a boil, stirring to melt all the solidified juices. Boil for 1 minute, until the liquid has almost completely reduced. Add the tomatoes, the remaining salt and pepper, and the Tabasco. Simmer for 2 to 3 minutes to thicken the sauce. (If the sauce separates, whisk in 2 tablespoons warm water.)

Pour the sauce around the chicken, sprinkle with the chives, and serve.

This quick dish should be prepared at the last moment and served immediately. It makes a nice appetizer for dinner, and it can also be served with a salad as a main course for a brunch or light lunch.

Chicken livers are readily available and inexpensive. For best results, cook them over very high heat to seal in their juices, and cook them only briefly—they should still be slightly pink inside. For this recipe, the livers are sautéed, mixed with garlic and parsley (a mixture called *persillade*), and served on toasted bread.

Separate each liver into its two halves, discarding any connecting sinews. Pat dry with paper towels and sprinkle with the salt and pepper. Heat the butter and oil in a nonstick pan at least 9 inches in diameter. When the mixture is a hazelnut color, add the livers in one layer and cook over high heat for 1 minute. Turn and cook on the other side for 1 minute, taking care to avoid splatters. Add the garlic and parsley, immediately remove the pan from the heat, and mix well.

Place a slice of toast on each plate, top with the liver, and serve immediately.

> For best results, select pale, plump
> chicken livers and cook them for only
> a couple of minutes.

CHICKEN LIVERS PERSILLADE

∘ SERVES 4 AS A FIRST COURSE OR BRUNCH OR LUNCH MAIN COURSE

12 ounces chicken livers (about 14), preferably plump and pale in color

¼ teaspoon salt

¼ teaspoon freshly ground black pepper

3 tablespoons unsalted butter

1 tablespoon peanut oil

4 cloves garlic, peeled and chopped fine (2 teaspoons)

3 tablespoons coarsely chopped flat-leaf parsley

4 slices from a large country loaf (½ inch thick and about 5 inches in diameter), toasted

DUCK LEGS WITH SHALLOTS AND POTATOES

∘ SERVES 2

2 duck legs (about
12 ounces each)

½ teaspoon salt

½ teaspoon freshly ground
black pepper

4 large shallots (about 6 ounces),
peeled

6 large cloves garlic, peeled

6 small golden potatoes (about
8 ounces total), peeled

¼ cup cold water

2 teaspoons chopped chives,
for garnish

Duck legs are usually available in my market and I often make this recipe for dinner. The legs are started skin side down in a nonstick saucepan and cooked, covered, for a whole hour; the garnishes are added to the pan after about 35 minutes. Although it does take some time, this is an easy dish.

Serve the duck leg crusty skin side up with the garnishes around it. Reserve the rendered fat for sautéing potatoes or browning meat. For a quick extra bonus, you make a sauce by adding water to the drippings, boiling it, and mixing the glaze and water together. A salad completes the meal.

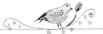

Season the duck legs with half the salt and pepper. Place the legs skin side down in a saucepan, place over high heat, and cook for 3 minutes. Reduce the heat to very low, cover, and cook for 30 minutes.

Arrange the shallots, garlic, and potatoes around the duck legs, cover, and cook for about another 15 minutes. Add the remaining salt and pepper, turn the vegetables over so they brown on both sides, and cook for another 10 to 15 minutes.

Place the duck legs crusty side up on two warm plates and arrange the vegetables around them.

Pour the fat from the saucepan (about ⅓ cup) into a container and reserve for another use. Add the cold water to the saucepan and bring to a boil. Stir to melt the solidified juices and cook for 1 minute.

Spoon the pan sauce over and around the duck and serve, sprinkled with the chives.

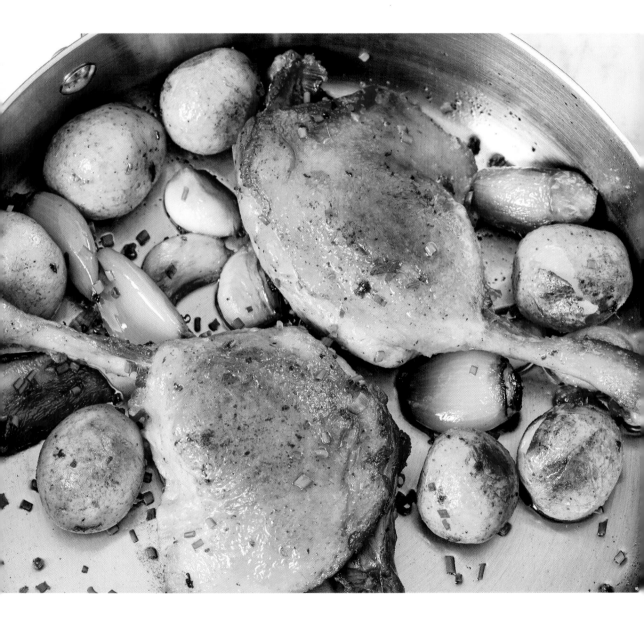

BROILED QUAIL WITH SPICY MARINADE

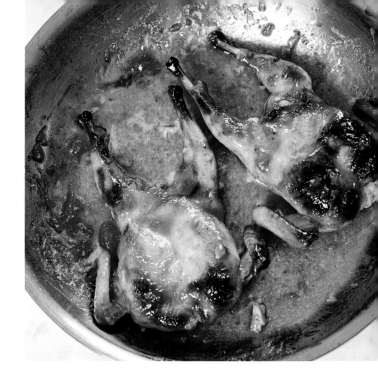

∘ SERVES 2

Marinade

1 tablespoon Worcestershire sauce

1 tablespoon ketchup

1 tablespoon honey

½ teaspoon Tabasco sauce

½ teaspoon ground coriander

¼ teaspoon salt

2 quail (4½ to 5 ounces each), semi-boned and butterflied

> **Combine the marinade ingredients directly in the plastic bag so you won't have to wash a mixing bowl.**

This recipe will work well with either fresh or frozen semi-boned quail that are butterflied.

Serve with Cornmeal Mush with Cheese (page 139), rice, or pasta and a vegetable dish.

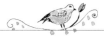

Prepare the marinade: Combine all the ingredients in a large plastic bag and shake to mix well. Add the quail and toss to coat with the marinade. Seal the bag and refrigerate for at least 2 hours.

When ready to cook, preheat the broiler. Remove the quail from the marinade and arrange them skin side up in a skillet. Broil, about 5 inches from the heat source, for 3 to 4 minutes. Turn and broil for about 2 minutes on the other side.

Arrange the quail skin side up on individual plates and serve drizzled with any juices from the skillet.

I enjoy turkey at all times of the year, but especially over the holidays, when fresh organic turkeys are available in most markets.

I prefer small turkeys—about 12 pounds—because they cook quickly and remain moist, and you won't have to worry about leftovers. In this recipe, I cook the turkey mostly upside down. I start it breast side up to brown the skin, then turn it over—the juices naturally flow through the breast meat if the bird is cooked in this position, and the turkey comes out moist without any basting.

I cook the dressing separately from the turkey. The turkey cooks faster this way, because the heat can circulate through the cavity. Serve with a salad alongside.

Preheat the oven to 425 degrees. Remove the neck, gizzard, and heart from the turkey and place them in a saucepan. (I usually sauté the liver and enjoy it with a glass of wine.) Add the water and bring to a boil. Cover, reduce the heat to low, and cook for about 1 hour. Drain, reserving the liquid and the solids separately (you should have about 1½ cups liquid—add water if needed to make 1½ cups).

Meanwhile, pat the turkey dry with paper towels. Make an incision about 1 inch deep at the fold between the thighs and drumsticks; this helps decrease the cooking time. Cut the 3 largest garlic cloves into slivers (about 12 total). Making small incisions here and there around the breasts and legs, insert the garlic slivers under the skin of the

»—>

GARLICKY ROAST TURKEY

◦ SERVES 8 TO 10

1 small turkey (12 pounds)

2 cups water

8 cloves garlic, peeled

½ teaspoon salt

½ teaspoon freshly ground black pepper

3 onions (about 12 ounces total), peeled and cut into 1-inch dice

3 carrots (8 ounces total), peeled and cut into ½-inch dice

1 teaspoon potato starch, dissolved in 1 tablespoon water

1 tablespoon soy sauce

Cornbread and Ham Dressing (recipe follows)

turkey and into the flesh. Sprinkle the turkey with the salt and pepper, inside and out.

Place the turkey breast side up in a large roasting pan and roast for about 30 minutes, until nicely browned.

Using pot holders, turn the turkey so it is breast side down. Arrange the onions, carrots, and remaining garlic cloves around it. Reduce the oven temperature to 325 degrees and roast for 1¼ hours.

Add the 1½ cups reserved cooking liquid to the roasting pan and cook for another 30 minutes. Turn the oven off and let the turkey rest in the warm oven while you complete the rest of the preparations.

Pull the meat from the turkey neck and cut the neck meat, gizzard, and heart into ¼-inch dice. Set aside.

Transfer the turkey breast side up to an ovenproof platter and return it to the warm oven. Pour the vegetables and cooking juices from the roasting pan into a saucepan. Let the sauce rest for 4 to 5 minutes, until most of the fat has risen to the top, then skim off as much fat as possible (at least 1 cup). You should have approximately 2 cups of defatted juices remaining. Add the chopped neck meat, gizzard, and heart and simmer the mixture for 10 minutes to reduce it slightly. Stir in the dissolved potato starch and the soy sauce until smooth.

Carve the turkey and serve it with the gravy and dressing.

NOTE: Use any leftover turkey instead of chicken in salads (see page 47), and reserve the bones for chicken stock (see Basic Chicken Stock, page 15).

This is good with goose and pork as well as turkey. Spoon it onto individual plates, place slices of the turkey or other poultry or meat over it, and ladle on some gravy or sauce.

You can make your own cornbread for this recipe, but I often use packaged cornbread; if you can't find cornbread, buy corn muffins, selecting those with the least amount of sugar. I add ham and scallions to the crumbled cornbread, with just enough stock to moisten the mixture; it should be crumbly, not gooey. The dressing can be prepared ahead.

Preheat the oven to 350 degrees. Melt the butter in a large skillet. When the melted butter is hot, add the onion, celery, and scallions and sauté over medium-high heat for about 3 minutes.

Transfer the vegetables to a bowl and add the crumbled cornbread, corn kernels, ham, herbes de Provence, pepper, parsley, and chicken stock. Toss lightly and place in a 6-cup (8½ by 4½-inch) loaf pan.

Bake the dressing for about 30 minutes, until nicely browned on top and hot inside.

> **You can make your own cornbread for this recipe, but packaged cornbread or corn muffins from the supermarket work well, too.**

Cornbread and Ham Dressing

• SERVES 8 TO 10

4 tablespoons (½ stick) unsalted butter

1 onion, peeled and coarsely chopped (1 cup)

2 ribs celery, rinsed and cut into ¼-inch dice (¾ cup)

5 scallions, cleaned and minced (about ¾ cup)

12 ounces cornbread or corn muffins, crumbled

1 cup fresh or frozen corn kernels

1 thick slice cooked ham (3 ounces), cut into ½-inch pieces

1 teaspoon herbes de Provence (see Note, page 15) or Italian seasoning

½ teaspoon freshly ground black pepper

3 tablespoons chopped flat-leaf parsley

¼ cup Basic Chicken Stock (page 15) or canned chicken broth

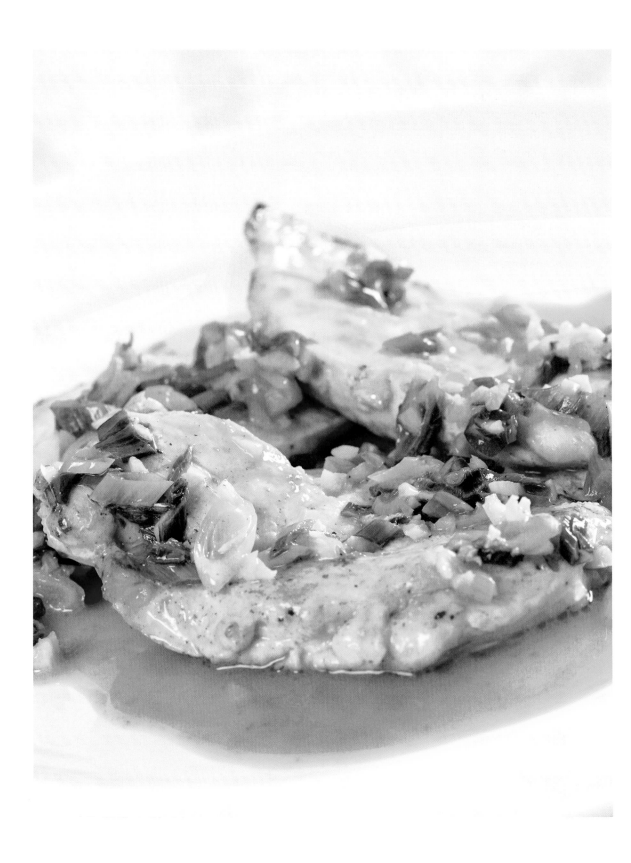

Veal scaloppini are expensive, so I sometimes substitute turkey, either cutting a whole fresh turkey breast into thin slices or buying it already sliced. The most common mistake you can make when preparing scaloppini—either veal and turkey—is to overcook them. These thin pieces of meat will remain moist, tender, and delicious if cooked for only 1½ minutes or so per side, depending on thickness.

Veal scaloppini can be prepared in exactly the same manner.

Heat the olive oil and butter in a large (12-inch) skillet preferably nonstick). Meanwhile, season the scaloppini with the salt and pepper. When the butter-oil mixture is hot, add the scaloppini and sauté over medium to high heat for about 1½ minutes on each side. Remove the scaloppini from the pan, arrange them on a serving platter, and set aside in a warm place or a low oven (140 degrees).

Add the scallions and garlic to the drippings in the pan and sauté for about 10 seconds. Add the chicken stock and cook, stirring to loosen and dissolve the solidified juices, for about 45 seconds.

Pour the mixture over the scaloppini and serve immediately.

SCALOPPINI OF TURKEY WITH SCALLIONS

∘ SERVES 4

1 tablespoon virgin olive oil

1 tablespoon unsalted butter

1 pound turkey scaloppini, ½ inch thick (4 slices)

½ teaspoon salt

¾ teaspoon freshly ground black pepper

6 scallions, greens removed, cleaned and minced (about 1 cup)

2 cloves garlic, peeled and chopped fine (about 1 teaspoon)

½ cup Basic Chicken Stock (page 15) or canned chicken broth

CASSOULET WITH SAUSAGES

○ SERVES 4

1 tablespoon olive oil

¼ cup water

4 sweet Italian-style sausages (12 ounces)

8 ounces pancetta, cut into ½-inch pieces

1 onion, peeled and sliced thin (about 1 cup)

5 scallions, cleaned and cut into ½-inch pieces (about ¾ cup)

2 cloves garlic, peeled and sliced (about 2 teaspoons)

Two 16-ounce cans white kidney (cannellini) beans

8 ounces kielbasa, peeled if the casing is tough, cut into 4 pieces

1 teaspoon Tabasco sauce

1 teaspoon herbes de Provence (see Note, page 15) or Italian seasoning

2 slices country bread

2 tablespoons peanut oil

Cassoulet is a famous dish from southwestern France. It always contains white beans and usually duck or goose—as well as roast pork and sausages. This satisfying simplified version is easily made with sausages and canned white kidney (cannellini) beans. I prepare it in large ovenproof soup bowls, but you could also serve it into individual bowls without browning it in the oven.

A simple stew of sausage and beans, the ingredients can be assembled in the individual bowls and refrigerated, ready to cook, the night before serving. The cassoulet will then take slightly longer to cook, since the ingredients will be cold.

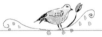

Place the olive oil and water in a large saucepan and add the Italian sausages and pancetta. Cook over medium-to-high heat for about 10 minutes, shaking the pan occasionally so the sausages roll over and cook on all sides.

When most of the moisture has evaporated and the sausages are browning, add the onion, scallions, and garlic and sauté for about 30 seconds. Add the beans, with their liquid, and the kielbasa, Tabasco, and herbes de Provence. Cover, bring to a boil, and cook for 10 minutes. Set aside.

Meanwhile, preheat the oven to 400 degrees. Place the bread in a food processor and process to crumbs (you should have 1½ cups crumbs). Lightly toss the bread crumbs with the peanut oil.

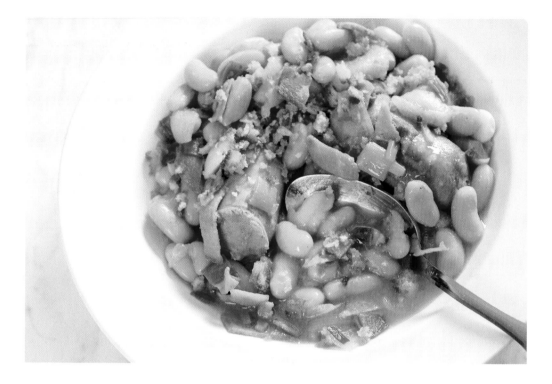

Spoon the sausage mixture into four 2½-cup ovenproof soup bowls, filling the bowls to within ¾ inch of the top. Sprinkle the bread crumbs over the top and arrange the bowls on a cookie sheet lined with aluminum foil. Bake for about 30 minutes, until the mixture is bubbling and very hot and brown. If you want the crumbs a little browner, turn on the broiler and place the bowls under the broiler for a few minutes. Serve hot.

> **To avoid last-minute work, place the ingredients in the bowls the night before and refrigerate, then finish in the oven the next day.**

NOTES: The cassoulet can be made ahead and refrigerated. Bake it for approximately 40 minutes and then finish under the broiler, if desired. Leftover roast pork, veal, or lamb can be used in place of the sausages.

LENTIL AND SAUSAGE STEW

∘ SERVES 8 TO 10

1½ pounds hot Italian-style sausages or sausage patties

5½ cups water

1 pound dried lentils, preferably French Le Puy lentils

3 large cloves garlic, peeled and chopped (1 tablespoon)

1 large onion (6 ounces), peeled and cut into 8 pieces

2 carrots (about 6 ounces total), peeled and cut into ½-inch pieces

1 teaspoon Italian seasoning

1 jalapeño pepper, minced (optional)

½ cup dry white wine

1 tablespoon organic roasted chicken base

Dijon-style mustard, for serving

A great deal can be done with sausages from the supermarket, whether it be Polish-style kielbasa, link sausages, patties of seasoned freshly ground pork, or Italian-style pork sausages. I especially like hot Italian sausages, sometimes grilled, sometimes cooked in a stew or used in soup.

This recipe makes enough to serve eight or more. Any leftover stew will keep for up to a week in the refrigerator and for weeks in the freezer. The best way to reheat the stew is in a microwave oven, although it can be reheated over low heat on the stovetop— just add a little water to keep it from sticking to the bottom of the pan.

Serve the stew with some Dijon mustard on the side. A green salad is all you need as an accompaniment.

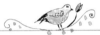

Cut the sausages or separate the patties into 1½-inch pieces and place them in a large deep saucepan or Dutch oven. Add ½ cup of the water and bring to a boil over high heat. Cover and cook for 5 minutes, by which time the meat will have released some fat. Uncover the pan and cook until all the moisture has evaporated and the meat is frying in its own fat.

Meanwhile, rinse the lentils under cold water. Add them to the pan, along with the remaining 5 cups water and all the other ingredients except the mustard. Mix well and bring to a boil. Cover the pan, reduce the heat to very low, and boil very gently for 40 to 45 minutes, until most of the liquid has been absorbed and the lentils are cooked.

Serve with Dijon mustard.

CREAM OF LENTIL SOUP

Puree leftover Lentil and Sausage Stew in a food processor, adding chicken stock or water to thin it to the consistency of a soup. Season with salt and pepper to taste. Ladle into soup bowls, sprinkle with grated Swiss cheese, and serve with crusty French bread.

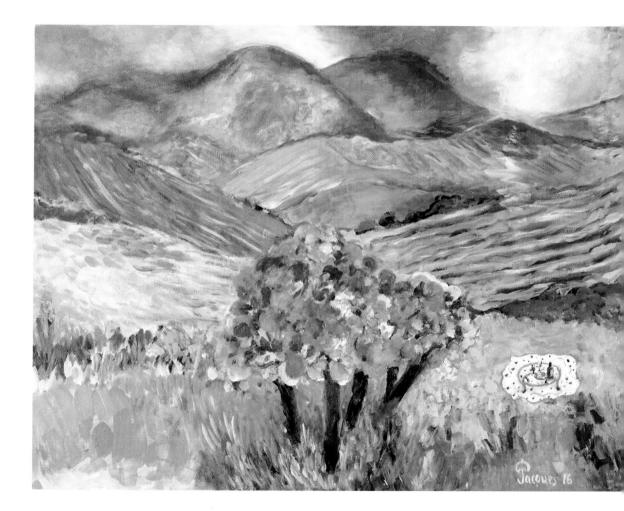

SAUSAGE WITH BROCCOLI RABE

○ SERVES 4 AS A FIRST COURSE
OR SIDE DISH

2 pounds broccoli rabe

1 pound sweet Italian-style
sausage meat

4 cloves garlic, peeled and sliced
(about 1½ tablespoons)

¼ teaspoon hot pepper flakes

½ teaspoon anise seeds

¼ teaspoon salt

2 tablespoons olive oil, plus
more for serving

▷ Make this versatile dish
ahead of time and serve it
at room temperature as a
first course or side dish.

Broccoli rabe, a leafy broccoli with thin stems and small yellow flowers, is available almost year-round at most supermarkets. Its slightly bitter and nutty taste goes particularly well with sausage. For this recipe, use sweet Italian-style sausage meat.

This is good as a first course or as a side dish with pasta, served at room temperature. If it has been refrigerated, warm it to room temperature in a microwave oven for about 20 seconds.

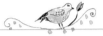

If the broccoli stems are tough and fibrous, peel the outer layer by pulling it off the stems. (This takes some time, but it is well worth the effort, since the stems will be much more tender.) Cut the broccoli into 2- to 3-inch chunks and rinse it thoroughly in a sieve under cold water.

Form the sausage meat into 1-ounce balls, each the size of a jumbo olive, and arrange them in one layer in a large saucepan. Cover and cook over low to medium heat for 10 to 12 minutes. (Liquid will emerge from the sausage balls and they will begin frying after 6 or 7 minutes.) Stir in the garlic, pepper flakes, anise seeds, salt, and olive oil.

Add the broccoli to the sausage mixture a handful at a time, then cover and lower the heat. Cook, covered, for 6 to 8 minutes. Serve with a drizzle of olive oil on top.

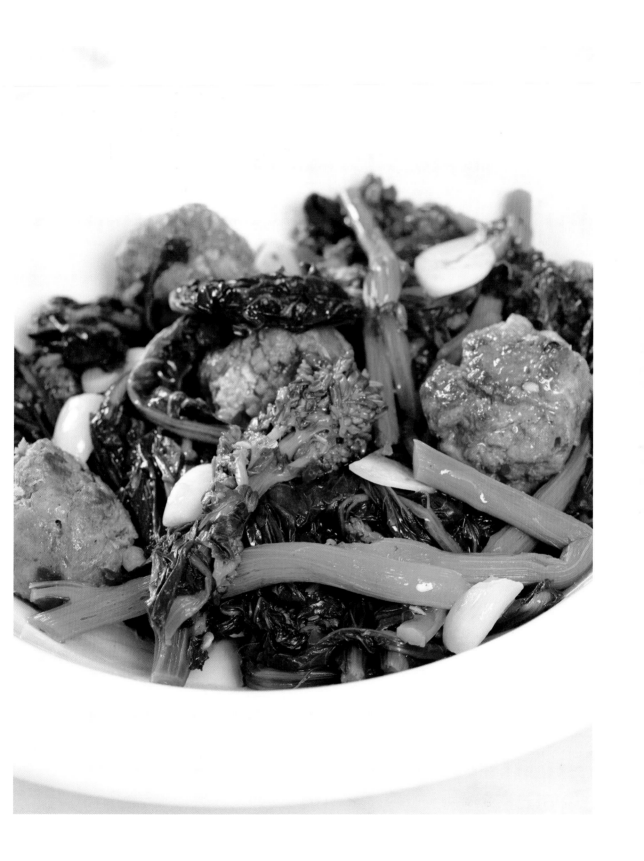

SAUSAGE STEW WITH MUSTARD GREENS AND BEANS

∘ SERVES 6

1¼ pounds Italian-style sausage meat

2 onions (about 8 ounces total), peeled and quartered

12 ounces mustard greens, cut into 2-inch pieces

Two 16-ounce cans red kidney beans

1 small jalapeño or serrano pepper, minced (optional)

1 teaspoon ground cumin

This one-dish meal is a familiar feature on our table. It is easy to make, using canned beans, mustard greens, and Italian sausage meat from the supermarket. You could substitute spinach, broccoli rabe, bok choy, or Swiss chard for the mustard greens, if you prefer. The stew is good reheated—most easily done in a microwave oven—and it can also be frozen.

Serve with a salad and crunchy French bread.

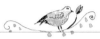

Separate the sausage meat into pieces. Dampen your hands and form the meat into balls, each about 1½ ounces.

Heat a large cast-iron Dutch oven or large heavy saucepan over low to medium heat and place the meatballs in the pot. Cook, covered, for 10 to 12 minutes, turning them every 3 to 4 minutes. The sausage will release its juices during the first 10 minutes of cooking and then, after another 10 minutes, will begin to brown.

Add the onions and mustard greens and cook for 10 minutes. Add the beans with their liquid, the jalapeño, if using, and the cumin. Bring to a boil, cover, and boil gently for about 5 minutes. Serve.

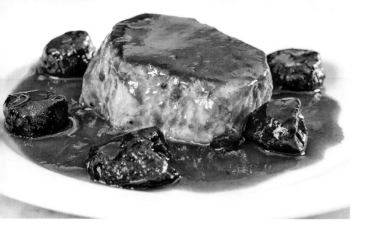

PORK LOIN WITH PORT AND PRUNES

° SERVES 4

Boneless pork loin steaks can be sautéed quickly for a delightful entrée. Pork is rich and so is complemented quite well by the prunes and sweet port wine in this sauce.

16 large pitted prunes (about 6 ounces)

½ cup water

1½ tablespoons unsalted butter

4 boneless pork loin steaks (5 ounces each and 1 inch thick), trimmed of all fat

⅓ cup port

1 teaspoon bottled steak sauce

1½ teaspoons ketchup

¼ teaspoon salt

½ teaspoon freshly ground black pepper

Combine the prunes and water in a bowl and heat in a microwave oven for about 2½ minutes (or combine in a saucepan and boil, covered, for 5 minutes, or until reduced by half). Set aside.

Melt the butter in a large skillet. When the butter is hot, add the pork and sauté over medium to high heat for about 2½ minutes on each side; it should still be slightly pink in center. Remove to a platter and set aside.

Add the port to the drippings in the pan and boil for about 1 minute. Add the steak sauce, ketchup, and the prunes with their soaking liquid and bring to a boil. Add the salt and pepper and simmer for about 2 minutes to reduce the sauce until it coats the back of the spoon.

Arrange the pork on plates, coat with the sauce, and serve.

> This elegant but easy entrée can be prepared in about 20 minutes.

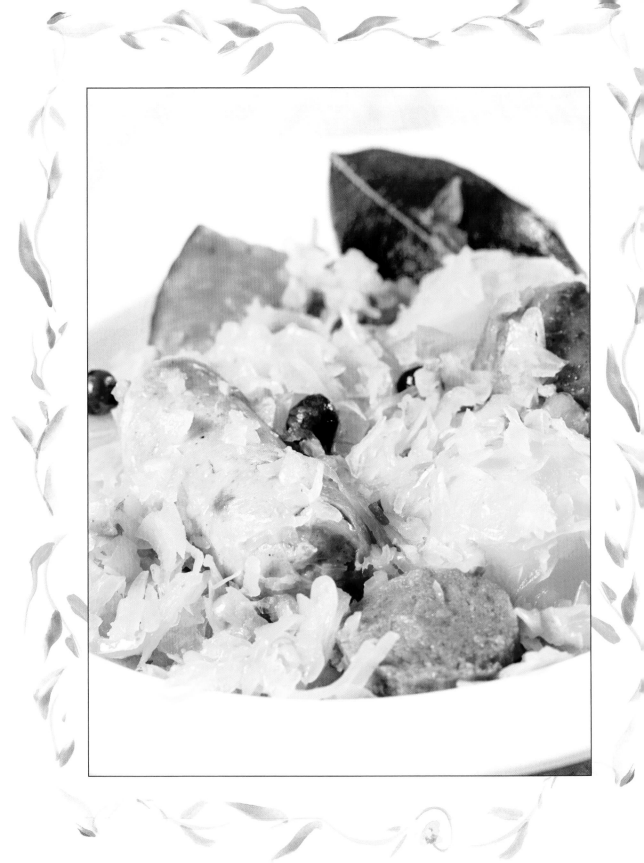

Choucroute, which means "sauerkraut" in French, is a stew with sausages, ham, and potatoes, and is a specialty of Alsace, in northeastern France. Unlike the very crunchy sauerkraut often served with hot dogs, the sauerkraut in this dish is cooked for a long time, giving it a mild, nutty taste. Flavored with juniper berries and white wine, the sauerkraut is usually cooked first and the garnishes added near the end of cooking. It is particularly good served with hot mustard, black or rye bread, and a cold white wine from Alsace, such as a Pinot Blanc, Traminer, or Sylvaner.

Place the pancetta in a Dutch oven or other heavy pot large enough to hold the sauerkraut, potatoes, and meat and cook over medium to high heat for 2 to 3 minutes, until it is lightly browned and some of its fat is rendered. Add the onion and sauté for 5 minutes.

Meanwhile, drain the sauerkraut in a sieve. Press it lightly between your palms to extract more liquid.

Add the sauerkraut, chicken stock, juniper berries, bay leaves, pepper, and wine to the pot. Bring to a boil, cover, reduce the heat to very low, and boil gently for 45 minutes. (The recipe can be prepared to this point up to a day ahead; cool, cover, and refrigerate. Reheat before continuing.)

Add the drained potatoes and the ham and cook over medium heat, covered, for 20 minutes.

Add the bratwurst and knockwurst and cook for 15 minutes longer. Serve directly from the pot.

CHOUCROUTE

∘ SERVES 4

4 ounces pancetta, cut into ½-inch pieces

1 onion, peeled and sliced thin (1 cup)

One 2-pound bag sauerkraut in brine

2 cups Basic Chicken Stock (page 15) or canned chicken broth

12 juniper berries

3 bay leaves

¼ teaspoon freshly ground black pepper

½ cup dry white wine

1 pound potatoes, peeled and held in water to cover (1 potato per person)

1 pound cooked ham, cut into 4 or 5 pieces

4 bratwurst

4 knockwurst or other sausages

▷ **Since this can be partially prepared ahead, it is an ideal party dish.**

GRILLED ROSEMARY PORK CHOPS

○ SERVES 4

4 pork loin chops (about 8 ounces each and 1 to 1¼ inches thick)

2 teaspoons chopped rosemary

¼ teaspoon salt

½ teaspoon freshly ground black pepper

4 teaspoons olive oil

In the summer, when it's hot inside the house, I like to cook food outside on the grill. Pork chops are as good grilled as they are sautéed, providing they are not overcooked. Buy thick loin chops and grill them over high heat until they are just nicely crusted and brown on both sides. Then let them finish cooking in their own residual heat—that way, the meat will relax and become more tender. The center should still be slightly pink and the meat juicy.

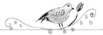

Heat a charcoal or gas grill (the grill grate should be very clean).

Sprinkle the pork chops with the rosemary, salt, and pepper. Pour the olive oil onto a plate and dip the chops into the oil, turning them to moisten both sides. (If you will not be cooking them immediately, cover the chops with plastic wrap and set aside for up to 2 hours.)

Place the chops on the grill, cover with the grill lid, and cook for about 4 minutes. Turn the chops and cook, covered, for another 4 minutes on the other side. Transfer them to the far side of the grill, or transfer to a platter and place in a 150-degree oven. Let rest for 10 to 15 minutes before serving.

▷ **For tender, juicy pork chops, after grilling, let them rest in a warm place to finish cooking in their own residual heat.**

Seasoned with five-spice powder, available in most supermarkets, this stew has a pronounced taste. You can make your own five-spice powder by combining ground star anise, cinnamon, cloves, Szechuan peppercorns, and anise seeds. Here honey adds sweetness to the dish.

Cook this stew in a Dutch oven or other attractive cast-iron pot so the stew can go directly from the stove to the table.

Heat the oil in a large Dutch oven or other heavy pot. When the oil is hot, add the pork cubes in one layer, cover, and brown over high heat, turning the meat occasionally, for about 15 minutes. (The meat will not brown immediately; it will release moisture and steam for about 7 minutes, at which point the moisture will have evaporated and the meat will begin to brown.)

Add the onions and garlic and stir well. Add the flour and five-spice powder and stir well. Mix in the soy sauce, honey, Worcestershire sauce, chicken stock, salt, and pepper and bring to a boil, then reduce the heat to very low and cook, covered, for 1 hour.

Stir in the bamboo shoots and mushrooms and simmer for 5 minutes. Serve sprinkled with the chives.

NOTE: This stew freezes well. Wait to add the bamboo shoots and straw mushrooms (and chives) until just before serving. The best way to reheat the stew is portion by portion in a microwave oven.

PORK STEW A LA SAIGON

∘ SERVES 6

2 tablespoons peanut oil

3 pounds boneless pork shoulder or shoulder blade, cut into 2-inch cubes (about 18 cubes)

2 onions (about 8 ounces total), peeled and chopped coarsely (about 2 cups)

3 large cloves garlic, peeled, crushed, and chopped (about 1 tablespoon)

2 teaspoons all-purpose flour

2 teaspoons five-spice powder

2 tablespoons dark soy sauce

2 tablespoons honey

1 tablespoon Worcestershire sauce

1 cup Basic Chicken Stock (page 15) or canned chicken broth

½ teaspoon salt

½ teaspoon freshly ground black pepper

One 10-ounce can sliced bamboo shoots, drained

One 16-ounce can straw mushrooms, drained

2 tablespoons chopped chives, for garnish

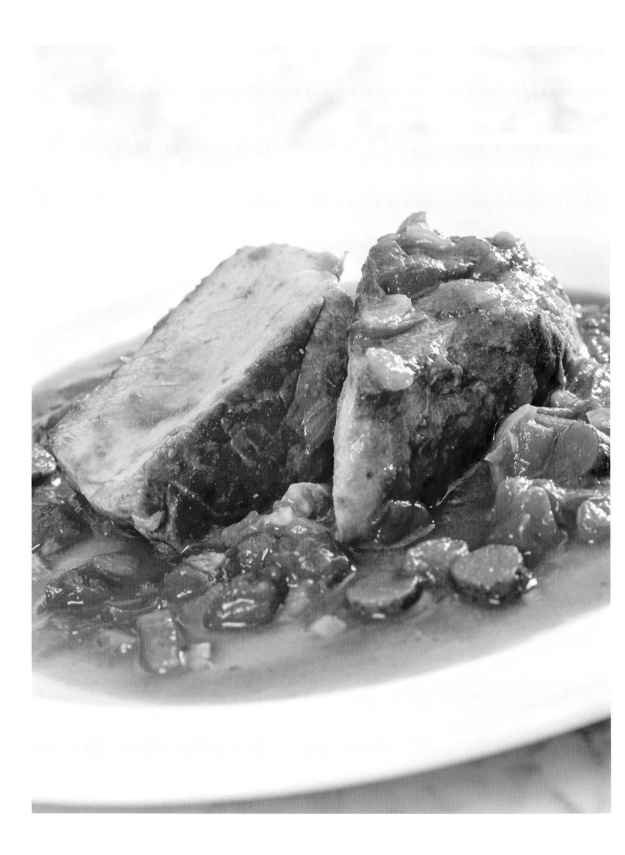

These pork fillets are served with a spicy sauce that contains cornichons, sour French gherkins. The pork is not cooked for very long; the amount of fat in the meat is minimal, so it cooks quickly and should still be pink inside when sliced.

Cut the tenderloin into 4 equal pieces and pound each one to about 1½ inch thick. Sprinkle the pork with the salt and pepper.

Melt the butter in a large skillet, and when it is hot, add the fillets. Cover and sauté over high heat for about 2½ minutes on each side. Transfer the meat to a plate and keep warm in a 150-degree oven while you make the sauce.

Add the onion to the drippings in the skillet and cook for 30 seconds. Add the garlic and cook for 10 seconds. Add the vinegar and boil until most of it has evaporated. Stir in the tomato, ketchup, Worcestershire sauce, and water, bring to a boil, and boil for 30 seconds. Add the cornichons and Tabasco and remove from the heat. Serve the pork coated with the sauce.

NOTE: You can cook the meat and sauce ahead of time. Reheat the pork briefly in the sauce before serving.

> **There's not much fat in these pork fillets, so they cook quickly.**

FILLET OF PORK WITH SAUCE CHARCUTIERE

◦ SERVES 4

1 large pork tenderloin (about 1¼ pounds), cleaned of any surrounding fat

¼ teaspoon salt

¼ teaspoon freshly ground black pepper

2 tablespoons unsalted butter

1 onion (6 ounces), peeled and chopped (1 cup)

4 cloves garlic, peeled and chopped (1 tablespoon)

3 tablespoons red wine vinegar

1 ripe medium tomato, cut into ¼-inch pieces (about 1 cup)

¼ cup ketchup

1 tablespoon Worcestershire sauce

½ cup water

2 tablespoons thinly sliced French sour gherkins (cornichons)

½ teaspoon Tabasco sauce

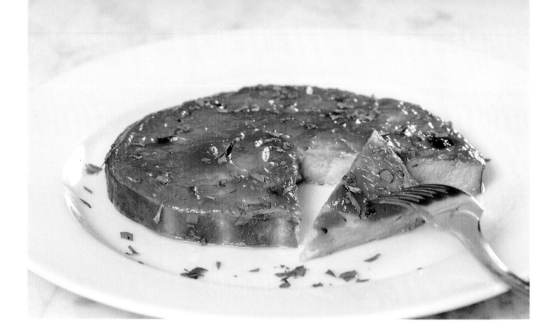

BROILED HAM STEAKS

∘ SERVES 4

4 small ham steaks (about
4 ounces each and ½ inch thick),
cut from precooked boneless ham

2 tablespoons ketchup

4 teaspoons brown sugar

¼ teaspoon Tabasco sauce

1 teaspoon dry mustard

> **These flavorful ham steaks cook in a few minutes under the broiler.**

I often buy ham shoulders, precooked boneless hams that are available at the supermarket. The meat is good in sandwiches or cooked with peas or lentils (see pages 142 and 166), and it can also be sliced into steaks. These cook in a few minutes under the broiler and are quite flavorful. They are especially good served with Steamed Cauliflower with Lemon Butter (page 148) or Zucchini Flan (page 193), along with potatoes.

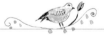

Preheat the broiler. Arrange the ham steaks on a cookie sheet lined with nonstick aluminum foil. Mix together the ketchup, brown sugar, Tabasco sauce, and mustard in a small bowl and spread evenly over the steaks.

Broil the steaks, about 5 inches from the heat source, for about 10 minutes, until nicely browned. Serve.

I use a young, tender rabbit about three months old for this recipe. The rabbit is butterflied first and then seasoned with Chinese chili-garlic sauce (hot sauce like Sriracha will work too), roasted in a hot oven, and finished with a bread topping. Rabbit is available in most supermarkets nowadays. The lean, mild, tender meat is good roasted or in stews.

Preheat the oven to 400 degrees. Place the rabbit breast side up on your cutting board and, using kitchen shears, cut through the center of the rib cage to split it open. Turn the rabbit breast side down and press down on it firmly to flatten it to a thickness of about 2 inches so it cooks uniformly.

Rub the rabbit on both sides with the salt, pepper, and chili-garlic sauce and place it breast side down on a cookie sheet lined with nonstick aluminum foil. Sprinkle with 2 tablespoons of the olive oil and roast for 20 minutes.

Meanwhile, break the bread into pieces, place in a food processor with the parsley, and process until finely chopped. (You should have about 1½ cups.) Mix with the remaining 3 tablespoons olive oil to moisten the bread so it browns nicely instead of burning.

Spread the crumb mixture over the rabbit and roast for 20 minutes longer. Let the rabbit rest for 15 minutes, then cut it into pieces with kitchen shears or a knife and serve.

ROASTED RABBIT WITH SPICY CRUST

∘ SERVES 4

1 cleaned rabbit (2½ to 3 pounds)

1½ teaspoons salt

½ teaspoon freshly ground black pepper

2 tablespoons Chinese chili-garlic sauce, Sriracha, or other hot sauce

5 tablespoons olive oil

2 slices bread

3 tablespoons coarsely chopped flat-leaf parsley

ROAST LEG OF LAMB WITH GARLIC

○ SERVES 6

1 boneless lamb roast from the leg, trimmed and tied (2½ pounds)

2 to 3 large cloves garlic, peeled and cut diagonally into wedges (about 12 total)

½ teaspoon salt

½ teaspoon freshly ground black pepper

1 tablespoon olive oil

⅓ cup Basic Chicken Stock (page 15) or canned chicken broth

My supermarket sells small boned and tied roasts of lamb from the leg, and that is what I use in this recipe. Weighing about 2½ pounds—more than enough for 6 people—the roast should be well trimmed.

Try to get a roast that is plump and round so it will yield slices of equal size. The ones I usually use are about 6 inches long and 5 inches in diameter, and the roasting time given below produces medium-rare meat. If your roast is of slightly different dimensions, or if you prefer your lamb cooked more or less, adjust the cooking time accordingly—keeping in mind that the amount of time you let the meat rest after cooking is important too. A roast like this one needs to rest for at least 15 minutes to be appealingly pink throughout. If need be, it can be kept for as long as 45 minutes to 1 hour in a 140-degree oven before serving.

This dish is particularly good with Mashed Potatoes with Garlic (page 173), roasted potatoes, or noodles.

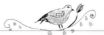

Preheat the oven to 425 degrees. Place the roast in a heavy baking pan. With the point of a knife, puncture the lamb in about 12 places, making ¾-inch-deep slits, and push the garlic into them. Sprinkle the meat with the salt, pepper, and olive oil.

Roast the lamb for 30 minutes, then turn the meat and roast for another 30 minutes, or until the internal temperature of the meat is about 120 degrees.

Pour out most of the fat from the pan, leaving about 1 tablespoon in the bottom of the pan. Stir the chicken stock into the fat and drippings left in the pan and return the meat to the oven for 5 minutes to

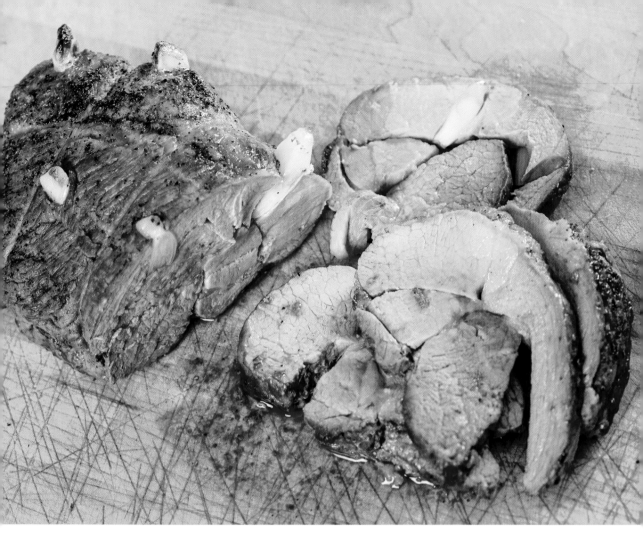

cook the sauce. Remove the pan from the oven and allow the meat to rest for 15 to 20 minutes before serving. (If you are not going to serve the meat right away, place a piece of aluminum foil loosely over the top and set the roast aside in a warm place.)

At serving time, slice the meat and serve it with the sauce.

> **After cooking, the roast will remain moist and flavorful for up to an hour in a 140-degree oven.**

BROILED MARINATED LAMB CHOPS

○ SERVES 4

Marinade

6 scallions, cleaned and chopped fine (1 cup)

3 cloves garlic, peeled, crushed, and chopped fine (2 teaspoons)

1 tablespoon grated lemon peel

1 tablespoon Sriracha or other hot sauce

2 tablespoons dark soy sauce

4 lamb shoulder chops (7 to 8 ounces each) or 8 center-cut loin chops

Large shoulder lamb chops, which are very flavorful and much less expensive than the small center-cut chops from the loin, are very good prepared this way. Although the chops can be coated with the marinade at the last minute and then broiled, it's best if you marinate the meat for at least a couple of hours.

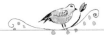

Prepare the marinade: Place all the ingredients in a plastic bag and shake the bag to combine them. Add the lamb chops, seal the bag, and allow them to marinate for 2 to 3 hours at room temperature.

When you are ready to cook the chops, preheat the broiler. Line a cookie sheet with nonstick aluminum foil. Remove the chops from the marinade (reserve the marinade) and place them on the foil-lined sheet. Broil, about 5 inches from the heat source, for about 3 minutes, then turn and cook on the other side for about 3 minutes. Remove from the oven, pour the reserved marinade over the chops, and let the meat rest for 5 minutes before serving.

▷ **Mix the marinade ingredients right in the plastic bag in which you will marinate the chops.**

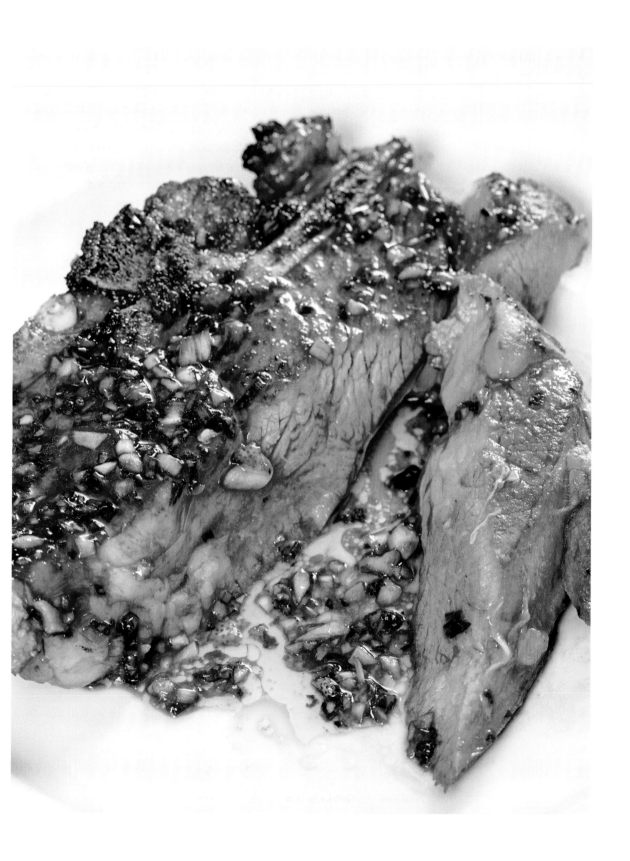

LAMB SHANKS WITH SPLIT PEA PUREE

◦ SERVES 4

4 lamb shanks (about
1 pound each)

One 16-ounce package split peas

About 2 onions (8 ounces total),
peeled and cut into 2-inch pieces
(about 2 cups)

2 carrots (4 ounces total), peeled
and cut into ½-inch pieces (about
¾ cup)

4 cloves garlic, peeled and sliced
thin (about 2 tablespoons)

2 bay leaves

1 sprig thyme

3 cups water

½ cup dry white wine

1½ teaspoons salt

½ teaspoon freshly ground
black pepper

This hearty stew can be prepared in a little over an hour in a pressure cooker.

Lamb shanks, which are available in most supermarkets, are at least 50 percent bone. Be sure to remove most of the fat, but leave the silver skin intact. The shanks are browned in the uncovered pressure cooker until crusty on all sides, which imparts a lot of flavor to the dish, before they are cooked with split peas.

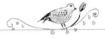

Trim the shanks to remove most of the surrounding fat and place them in a pressure cooker. Cook, covered (not under pressure), over low to medium heat for about 20 minutes, turning every 5 or 10 minutes, until browned on all sides.

Place the split peas in a sieve and rinse them under cool water. Drain the fat from the pressure cooker and add the peas and the remaining ingredients. Bring the mixture to a boil, stir, and lock on the lid. Bring the cooker to the appropriate pressure, following the manufacturer's guidelines, and cook for about 45 minutes.

Depressurize the cooker (again, according to the manufacturer's instructions) and serve.

NOTE: Leftovers reheat well in a microwave oven, or they can be transformed into soup; see opposite.

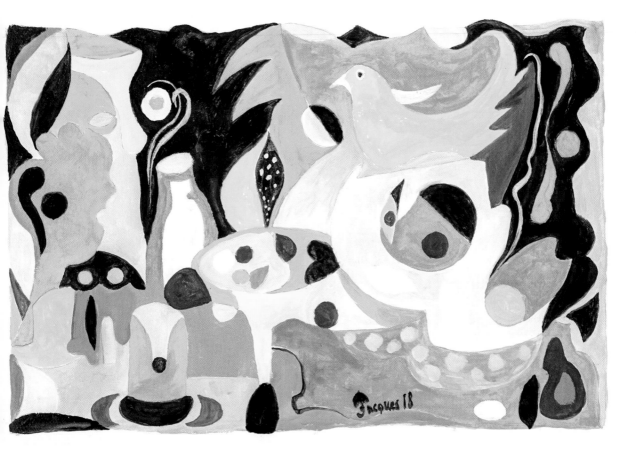

Split Pea Soup with Croutons

Cut or tear the leftover meat into smaller pieces and discard the bones. Combine the meat and leftover split peas in a saucepan. Add enough water or chicken stock to thin the mixture to the desired consistency and bring to a boil. Season with additional salt and pepper, and a dash of Tabasco sauce, if desired, and serve with croutons (see page 40).

> **Cover the pot when you brown the shanks to prevent splatters.**

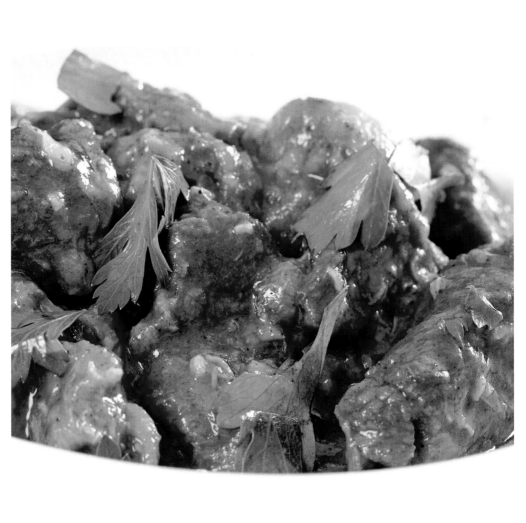
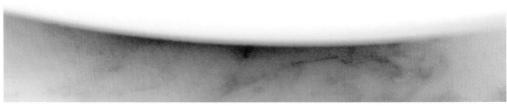

This lamb curry is made in a pressure cooker. After the pressure has built up, it takes just 30 minutes to cook, compared to over an hour in a Dutch oven on the stovetop. You can also make the curry ahead and either refrigerate or freeze it, then reheat. (Alternatively, though, you can cook the curry in a saucepan for about 1½ hours, adding the apple and banana in the last 30 minutes of cooking.)

I have flavored this curry in the conventional way with onion, garlic, and ginger, but I also like to add a banana and an apple, with great results. I use a soft white-fleshed apple, like a McIntosh or Rome Beauty, and I leave the skin on to lend some texture. Apple cider intensifies the flavor.

Serve this over rice, plain noodles, or potatoes.

Melt the butter in a pressure cooker. When the melted butter is hot, add the meat and cook over high heat for 15 minutes, stirring every 2 minutes, until the meat is seared and lightly browned on all sides.

Sprinkle the flour, curry powder, and cumin over the meat and mix well. Add the remaining ingredients, mix well, and bring to a boil, stirring. Lock on the lid and bring up to the correct pressure following the manufacturer's instructions. Reduce the heat to very low and cook for 30 minutes.

Depressurize the cooker (again according to the manufacturer's instructions) and serve.

PIQUANT LAMB CURRY

◦ SERVES 4

2 tablespoons unsalted butter

2 pounds boneless lean lamb, cut into 2-inch cubes

1 tablespoon all-purpose flour

1½ tablespoons curry powder

1 teaspoon ground cumin

2 onions (6 ounces total), peeled and cut into 1-inch pieces (1½ cups)

4 cloves garlic, peeled and chopped (1 tablespoon)

1 tablespoon chopped fresh ginger

1 banana, peeled and sliced

1 large apple (about 8 ounces), cored and cut into 1-inch pieces

1½ cups apple cider

1½ teaspoons salt

SAUTEED LAMB CHOPS WITH SPINACH

∘ SERVES 4

2 tablespoons unsalted butter

4 lamb shoulder chops (about 6 ounces each and ½ inch thick)

¾ teaspoon salt

¾ teaspoon freshly ground black pepper

¼ cup chopped onion

One 16-ounce bag baby spinach

¼ teaspoon ground nutmeg

Lamb shoulder chops are large, flavorful, and less expensive than loin chops. For a more elegant dinner, make this recipe with small loin chops, two per person.

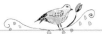

Melt the butter in a large skillet. Sprinkle the chops with ¼ teaspoon each of the salt and pepper. When the melted butter is hot, add the chops and sauté over medium heat for about 3 minutes a side, until medium-rare. Transfer them to a platter and keep warm in a 140-degree oven.

Add the onion to the drippings in the skillet and sauté for 1 minute. Add the spinach to the skillet, piling it up high, and sprinkle with the remaining ½ teaspoon each salt and pepper and the nutmeg. Sauté for 2 to 3 minutes, pushing the spinach down as it wilts. Cook until most of the water from the spinach has evaporated and the spinach it is tender.

Arrange the spinach on individual plates, place the lamb chops on top, and serve immediately.

When cooking meat or fish on an outdoor grill, always be certain that the grill rack is very clean, which will help prevent the food from sticking. My grill has a lid, which makes it work like an oven and helps in the cooking.

The most common mistake made in preparing veal chops is overcooking them—they take only a few minutes. When grilled, they should be well browned on the outside but still juicy and pink inside. The cooking time will be determined, of course, by the thickness of the chops.

This dish goes well with many vegetables, from Buttery Peas and Lettuce (page 168) to most potato dishes.

Heat a charcoal or gas grill with the grill grate positioned 3 to 4 inches above the heat. Spread the olive oil on a large plate. Sprinkle the veal chops on both sides with the thyme, paprika, salt, and pepper and then dip both sides in the olive oil.

Place the chops on the hot grill, cover with the lid, and cook for about 2½ minutes per side. The chops should be brown on the outside but still pink on the inside. Transfer the chops to a plate and let rest, uncovered, either in the grill (away from the heat) or in a 140-degree oven, for 5 to 30 minutes. The meat will relax and continue to cook slightly in its own residual heat.

Serve.

GRILLED THYME VEAL CHOPS

∘ SERVES 4

2 tablespoons virgin olive oil

4 veal chops (about 8 ounces each and ¾ inch thick)

2 teaspoons fresh thyme leaves, or 1 teaspoon dried

1 teaspoon paprika

¼ teaspoon salt

½ teaspoon freshly ground black pepper

VEAL CHOPS IN COGNAC AND MUSHROOM SAUCE

◦ SERVES 4

4 center-cut veal chops
(10 to 12 ounces each and
about 1¼ inches thick)

½ teaspoon salt

½ teaspoon freshly ground
black pepper

2 tablespoons unsalted butter

3 or 4 shallots, peeled and
chopped (½ cup)

8 ounces mushrooms, washed
and sliced (about 3½ cups)

1 tablespoon Cognac

⅔ cup heavy cream

2 tablespoons chopped chives,
for garnish

This dish of veal loin chops in a rich sauce of cream and mushrooms is ideal for a special-occasion dinner. The meat should still be pink inside.

Sprinkle the chops with ¼ teaspoon each of the salt and pepper. Melt the butter in a large heavy skillet or saucepan, and when it is hot, add the chops. Sauté, uncovered, over medium to high heat for about 4 minutes, until nicely browned. Turn, cover, reduce the heat to low, and cook for another 4 minutes on the other side. (At this point, the chops should be medium-rare.) Place the chops on a serving platter and set aside in a warm place while you make the sauce.

Add the shallots to the drippings in the pan and sauté for about 30 seconds. Add the mushrooms and Cognac and sauté for about 2 minutes. Add the cream and simmer for about 1 minute to reduce and thicken the sauce slightly. Stir in the remaining ¼ teaspoon each salt and pepper.

Pour the sauce over the chops, sprinkle with the chives, and serve immediately.

> **If it's more convenient, you can cook the chops ahead and just rewarm them at serving time.**

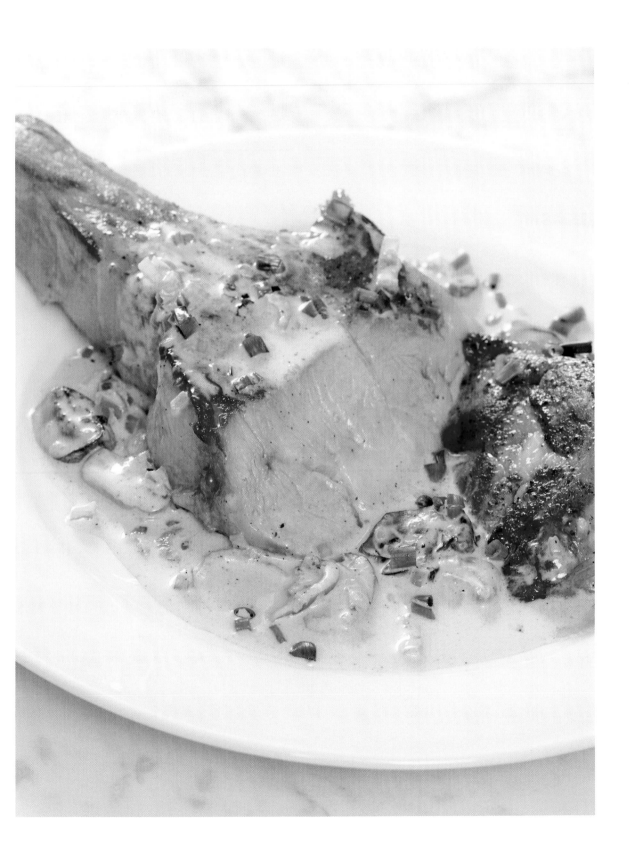

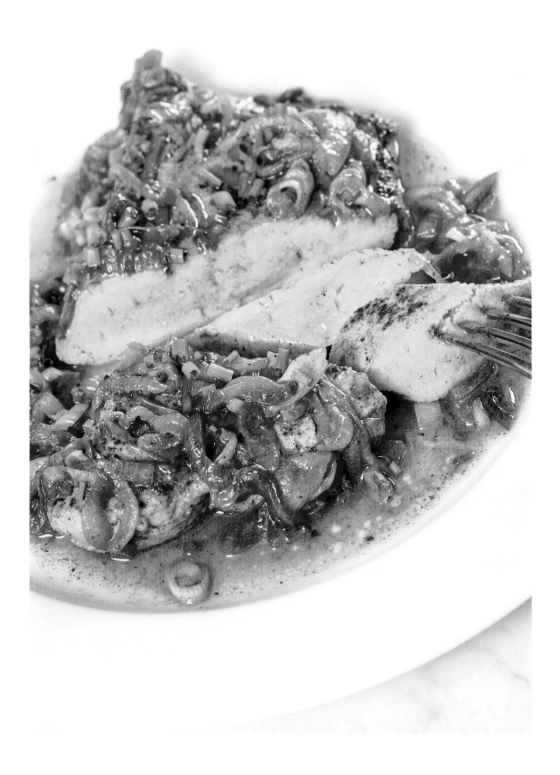

I like calf's liver cooked medium-rare; if you like yours cooked more or less, adjust the cooking time accordingly. When a dish is termed "Lyonnaise," it means it contains sautéed onions. Here I add vinegar, which lends an acidity that works well with liver. Potatoes, pasta, or a rice dish would go well with the liver.

Place the onions in a skillet, add 1 cup water, bring to a boil, and cook, covered, for 7 to 8 minutes, until most of the water is gone and the onions are soft. Set aside.

Divide the butter and olive oil between two large skillets and place the skillets over medium to high heat. Sprinkle the liver with ½ teaspoon of the salt and ¼ teaspoon of the pepper. When the butter and oil are hot, place the liver in the skillets and sauté for about 1 minute on each side. Transfer the liver to a platter and keep warm in a 140-degree oven.

Combine the drippings from both skillets in one of the skillets. Add the onions to the skillet, stir thoroughly, and sauté for 30 seconds. Mix in the vinegar, water, and the remaining ½ teaspoon salt and ¼ teaspoon pepper. Cover and cook over high heat for 1 minute.

Arrange the liver on warm plates, spoon the onion mixture around, sprinkle with the chives, and serve.

CALF'S LIVER LYONNAISE

○ SERVES 4

2 large onions (about 12 ounces total), peeled and sliced thin (about 4 cups)

2 tablespoons unsalted butter

2 tablespoons olive oil

4 slices calf's liver (6 ounces each and about ½ inch thick)

1 teaspoon salt

½ teaspoon freshly ground black pepper

2 tablespoons red wine vinegar

2 tablespoons water

1 tablespoon chopped chives, for garnish

▷ **You can make the liver at the last minute, since it takes only about 2 minutes to cook.**

FIVE-SPICE STEAK

○ SERVES 4

4 sirloin tip or New York strip
steaks (7 to 8 ounces each and
½ to ¾ inch thick), cleaned of all
fat and sinew

1 teaspoon five-spice powder

2 tablespoons unsalted butter

2 tablespoons oyster sauce

2 teaspoons Chinese chili-garlic
sauce

2 teaspoons toasted sesame oil

2 teaspoons dark soy sauce

⅓ cup water

8 scallions, green tops removed,
cleaned, and minced fine (about
1 cup)

▷ **The ingredients for this
tasty sauce should be in
your pantry.**

The sauce for this dish is an interesting mixture of
Asian spices and sauces—five-spice powder, oyster
sauce, chili-garlic sauce, sesame oil, and soy sauce—
all of which I have on my pantry shelf.

You can use either sirloin tip steak or New York
strip, but be sure the meat is completely cleaned of
fat and sinew. If your steaks are a different weight
and thickness than suggested, adjust the cooking time
accordingly to get the same result.

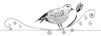

Sprinkle the steaks on both sides with the five-spice
powder. Melt the butter in a large heavy saucepan
or skillet, and when it is foaming, add the steaks in
one layer. Cook for about 2 minutes on each side
for medium-rare.

Meanwhile, combine the oyster sauce, chili-garlic
sauce, sesame oil, soy sauce, and water in a bowl.

When the steaks are cooked, remove them to a
platter and let rest in a 140-degree oven. Add the
scallions to the drippings in the pan and cook,
stirring, for about 30 seconds. Add the oyster sauce
mixture, bring to a boil, and stir to dissolve all the
solidified juices. Cook for 45 seconds to 1 minute.

Pour the sauce over the steaks and serve
immediately.

Beef tenderloin steaks are available in any supermarket. Prepared as here—with shallots, garlic, and parsley—the meat is flavorful, very lean, and cooks in a few minutes. Very tender, beef fillet goes well with most vegetables, from carrots to green vegetables to potatoes, as well as with noodles or rice.

Melt the butter in a heavy saucepan. Sprinkle both sides of the steaks with the salt and pepper. When the melted butter is hot, sauté the steaks for about 3 minutes on each side for medium-rare (or cook them less or more, depending on how you like your steaks). Transfer the steaks to a serving platter. Add the shallots and garlic to the drippings in the pan and sauté for about 1 minute.

Add the water and cook for another minute or so, until most of the moisture has evaporated and the solidified juices in the skillet have dissolved.

Pour the sauce over the steaks, garnish with the parsley, and serve immediately.

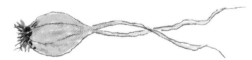

BEEF FILLET STEAKS WITH SHALLOTS

◦ SERVES 4

2 tablespoons unsalted butter

4 beef tenderloin steaks (6 ounces each and 1¼ inch thick), trimmed of any fat or sinew

½ teaspoon salt

½ teaspoon freshly ground black pepper

6 ounces shallots, peeled and sliced thin (about 1½ cups)

2 cloves garlic, peeled and chopped (1 teaspoon)

¼ cup water

2 tablespoons chopped flat-leaf parsley, for garnish

STEAK MARCHAND DE VIN

◦ SERVES 4

3 tablespoons unsalted butter

4 chuck-eye or New York strip steaks (about 6 ounces each and about ¾ inch thick), trimmed of all fat

½ teaspoon salt

½ teaspoon freshly ground black pepper

3 cloves garlic, peeled and chopped fine (about 1½ teaspoons)

1 teaspoon chopped oregano

½ cup dry red wine, such as Beaujolais

⅓ cup spicy V8 juice

⅓ cup water

2 teaspoons Dijon-style mustard

As the name *marchand de vin* (wine merchant) indicates, this steak is served with a red wine sauce. Traditionally a brown stock, or demi-glace, is used in the sauce; here I use a mixture of V8 juice and red wine instead, and thicken it with mustard to create a very satisfying, rich sauce.

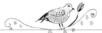

Melt the butter in a large heavy skillet. Sprinkle the steaks on both sides with the salt and pepper and sauté in the hot butter over medium to high heat for about 2 minutes on each side for medium-rare. Remove the steaks to a platter and set aside in a warm place while you make the sauce.

Add the garlic and oregano to the drippings in the skillet and cook for about 30 seconds. Add the wine and cook until the liquid in the pan has almost completely evaporated, then stir in the V8 juice and water. Bring to a boil and cook for about 30 seconds. Mix in the mustard and just heat through.

Arrange the steaks on individual plates, coat with the sauce, and serve immediately.

> **A wonderfully rich-tasting sauce is created easily here with wine, V8 juice, and mustard.**

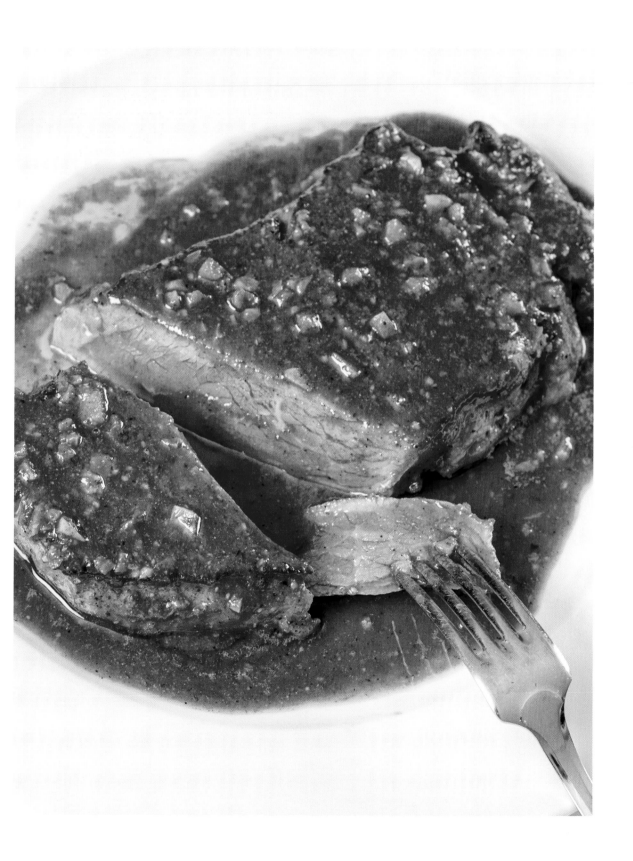

BRAISED SHORT RIBS IN RED WINE SAUCE

◦ SERVES 4

4 well-trimmed short ribs (about 2¼ pounds total), as lean as possible

2 onions (12 ounces total), peeled and cut into 1-inch pieces

4 or 5 carrots (12 ounces total), peeled and cut into 1-inch pieces

12 cloves garlic (from about 1 head), peeled

1 tablespoon all-purpose flour

1 sprig thyme

1 teaspoon salt

½ teaspoon freshly ground black pepper

1 pound small Yukon Gold potatoes (10 to 12), peeled

1 cup dry robust red wine, such as Merlot or Cabernet Sauvignon

1 tablespoon chopped flat-leaf parsley, for garnish

This beef dish is easy to make in a pressure cooker. Very little liquid—only a cup of red wine—is needed, because the meat releases a lot of its juices in the pressure cooker.

I use short ribs because they are so tender and flavorful. Choose ribs that are as lean, thick, and meaty as possible for a stew with an intense flavor and rich color. With the vegetables cooked alongside the meat, this makes a complete, generous meal.

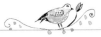

Arrange the short ribs in a single layer in the bottom of a pressure cooker and brown, partially covered, over medium heat for about 20 minutes, turning occasionally, until nicely browned on all sides. (No additional fat is needed since enough fat will emerge from the meat for it to brown well.)

Remove all but 1 tablespoon fat from the pressure cooker and add the onions, carrots, and garlic. Mix well and cook for about 5 minutes, until the vegetables are lightly softened. Sprinkle the flour on top, stirring it in, then stir in the thyme, salt, pepper, potatoes, and wine and bring to a boil. Lock on the lid and bring the cooker up to correct pressure according to the manufacturer's instructions. Reduce the heat to very low and cook for 40 to 45 minutes. Release the pressure following the manufacturer's instructions.

Sprinkle the short ribs with the parsley and serve.

▷ **For a family dinner, this dish can be served directly from the cooker.**

Beef tripe (cow's stomach) is available in most supermarkets. It looks like a honeycomb, and so is often called honeycomb tripe. It is a favorite of my daughter, Claudine, who likes it sautéed with onions and vinegar, as well as in stews or soups. No matter how tripe is prepared, it requires long cooking to become tender, tasty, and digestible. Cooking it in a pressure cooker, as I've done here, reduces the time by more than half and helps seal in the flavor. Because the tripe still takes a while to cook, however, I always prepare extra and freeze it in small containers for later use. Unfrozen, it will keep in the refrigerator for up to a week.

Serve the ragoût with Basic Boiled Potatoes (page 170).

Rinse the tripe thoroughly under cool water and cut it into 2- to 3-inch pieces. Place the tripe and all the remaining ingredients in a pressure cooker and bring to a boil over high heat. Lock on the lid and bring up to the correct pressure according to the manufacturer's instructions. Reduce the heat to very low and cook for 1¼ hours.

Release the pressure according to the manufacturer's instructions. Remove the pig's feet, remove the meat from the bones, and cut the meat into 1-inch pieces. Return the meat to the pot, reheat, and serve.

NOTE: To make the ragoût in a regular pot, place all the ingredients in a large Dutch oven or other heavy pot and bring to a boil, then reduce the heat to very low and cook very gently, covered, for 3 hours. Then proceed as directed.

TRIPE RAGOUT

○ SERVES 6

4 pounds honeycomb beef tripe

2 pig's feet (about 1¼ pounds total)

3 or 4 onions (1 pound total), peeled and cut into 1-inch pieces

3 or 4 carrots (8 ounces total), peeled and cut into ½-inch dice (about 1½ cups)

1 leek, trimmed, washed, and cut into 1-inch slices

1 rib celery, rinsed and cut into ¼-inch dice

6 cloves garlic, crushed, peeled, and chopped coarsely (about 1½ tablespoons)

¼ cup tomato paste

2 bay leaves

2 sprigs thyme

1 medium jalapeño pepper

1½ cups dry white wine

1½ cups Basic Chicken Stock (page 15) or canned chicken broth

2 teaspoons salt

½ teaspoon freshly ground black pepper

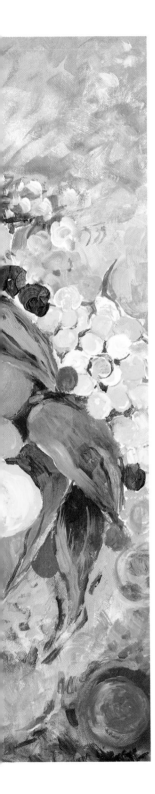
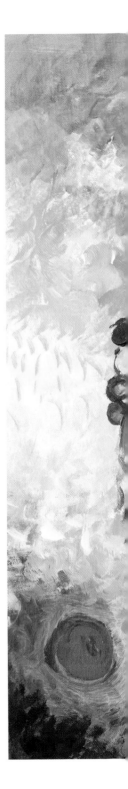

DESERTS

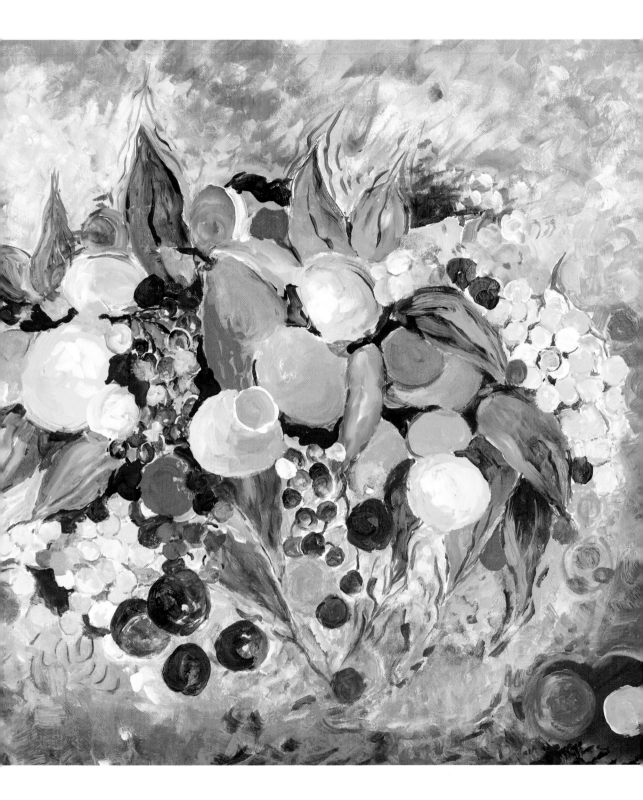

APPLE AND GRAPE GRATIN

◦ SERVES 6

4 medium Russet or Golden Delicious apples (about 1¼ pounds total)

2 cups seedless white grapes (12 ounces)

⅓ cup apricot jam or preserves

⅓ cup maple syrup

4 tablespoons (½ stick) unsalted butter

1 cup sour cream, for serving (optional)

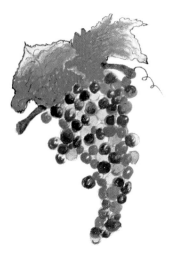

This tarty dessert is made with unpeeled apples—the skin gives it a chewy texture. I use white grapes, but red grapes would be good too. The dish should be served at room temperature.

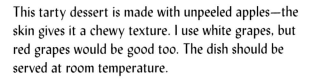

Preheat the oven to 375 degrees. Cut the apples lengthwise in half, remove the cores, and cut each half into 4 wedges. Place them in a bowl and stir in the grapes, apricot jam, and maple syrup. Arrange the mixture in a gratin dish and dot with the butter.

Place the gratin dish on a cookie sheet lined with nonstick aluminum foil and bake for 1 hour, checking after 30 minutes to see if the liquid in the dish is caramelizing. If it is, add 2 to 3 tablespoons water and continue baking.

Serve warm, with sour cream, if desired.

> **Don't peel the apples—the skins give the dessert a wonderfully chewy quality.**

This dessert tastes great and is easy to make. I like to use soft flavorful apples like McIntosh, Rome Beauty, or Macoun, but any other variety to your liking would be good too. Notice that I don't peel the apples; the skin adds texture to the dish.

I like to cook the brown Betty in a 6-cup gratin dish, because the shallow dish allows a lot of the mixture to be exposed to the heat of the oven. The surface will caramelize, producing a great intensity of taste. Instead of the bread, you can also use leftover croissants, Danish, pound cake, cake, and the like.

Preheat the oven to 400 degrees. Mix together all the ingredients except the sour cream in a bowl. Pack the mixture into a 6-cup oval gratin dish.

Set the gratin dish on a cookie sheet and bake for about 45 minutes, until nicely browned and caramelized on top. Cool until lukewarm, and serve as is or with sour cream.

▷ **To eliminate last-minute work, make this dessert ahead and rewarm it at serving time.**

APPLE BROWN BETTY

◦ SERVES 6

6 McIntosh or other apples (about 1½ pounds total), halved, cored, and each half cut into 3 wedges

5 slices firm-textured white bread (about 5 ounces total), broken into 2-inch pieces

8 tablespoons (1 stick) unsalted butter, melted

½ cup apricot preserves

2 teaspoons ground cinnamon

½ cup apple cider

¼ cup sugar

⅓ cup raisins

1 cup sour cream, for serving (optional)

BANANA BREAD

○ MAKES 1 LOAF

1 tablespoon peanut oil

2 cups all-purpose flour

1 tablespoon double-acting baking powder

4 tablespoons (½ stick) unsalted butter

½ cup sugar

2 very ripe bananas

2 large eggs

¼ cup milk

½ cup sunflower seeds

▷ **It takes less than a minute to make this batter in a food processor.**

There is practically no work involved in this recipe—the ingredients can be combined in a food processor in three stages and take less than a minute to put together. Use ripe bananas: Those with some dark, spotted skin have the intense flavor that makes this bread so special.

This is excellent for breakfast and makes a nice addition to a bread basket. Well wrapped, it will keep for a few days at room temperature or for weeks in the freezer.

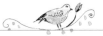

Preheat the oven to 350 degrees. Grease a 9 by 5-inch loaf pan with the oil. Place the flour, baking powder, butter, and sugar in a food processor and process for 10 to 15 seconds, until the ingredients are well combined.

Peel the bananas, break them into pieces, and add them to the processor. Process for 5 to 10 seconds, until the bananas are incorporated. Add the eggs, milk, and sunflower seeds and process for a few seconds, just until the ingredients are well combined.

Pour the batter into the greased loaf pan and place the pan on a cookie sheet. Bake for about 60 minutes, until well set and nicely browned on top. Cool for a few minutes in the pan on a wire rack before unmolding.

These sautéed bananas can also be eaten cold with sour cream and a slice of pound cake, but here they are served warm, with ice cream on top. I prefer vanilla ice cream with the bananas, but almost any flavor you like will be good.

Peel the bananas and slice them crosswise.

Heat the butter and sugar in a skillet until the butter melts, then cook over medium heat, stirring occasionally, for about 1 minute, until the sugar starts to brown lightly and the mixture begins to caramelize. Add the bananas and sauté, stirring, for about 1 minute. Stir in the water, rum, and lemon juice. Cover and cook for about 1 minute, until a sauce has formed.

Spoon the mixture onto dessert plates or into individual glass bowls or wine goblets, top each with a scoop of ice cream, and serve immediately.

NOTE: Use bananas that have some black spots on their skin to ensure they are well ripened.

BANANAS FOSTER WITH ICE CREAM

○ SERVES 4

4 ripe bananas

2 tablespoons unsalted butter

¼ cup sugar

¼ cup water

¼ cup dark rum

2 tablespoons lemon juice

1 pint best-quality vanilla ice cream

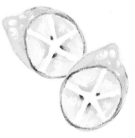

BLUEBERRY TART

◦ SERVES 6

¾ cup pecan pieces

¾ cup sugar

3 tablespoons all-purpose flour

One 1-pound bag frozen unsweetened blueberries (preferably small wild berries)

One 9-inch frozen pie shell

1 cup sour cream, for garnish

You can make your own pie shell for this tart, but if you have a packaged frozen pie shell in your freezer, you can assemble this dessert in a few minutes. Bake it ahead—it is best served at room temperature, with a garnish of sour cream.

Fresh blueberries would be good here, but packaged IQF (Individually Quick Frozen) berries, which are unsweetened, work very well.

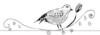

Preheat the oven to 400 degrees. Place the pecan pieces, sugar, and flour in a food processor and process to a powder. Combine with the frozen berries in a bowl and pour into the frozen pie shell.

Place the tart on a cookie sheet and bake for 50 to 60 minutes, until the dough is well cooked and the filling is lightly browned on top. Cool for at least 1 hour before serving.

To serve, cut the tart into wedges and garnish with the sour cream.

▷ **You can assemble this tart and put it in the oven while the berries and the pie shell are still frozen.**

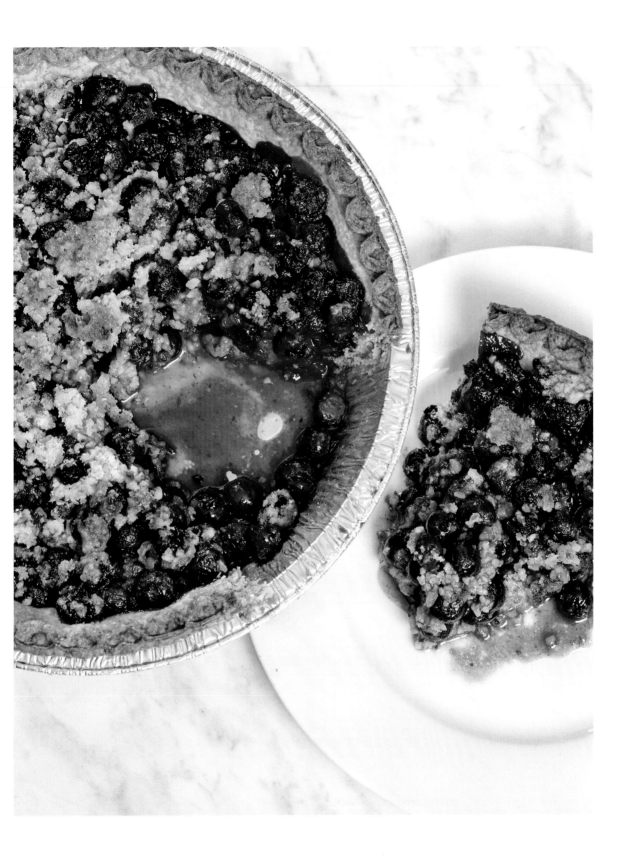

BLUEBERRY CRISP

∘ SERVES 6

Filling

⅓ cup sugar

1 tablespoon cornstarch

About 5 cups fresh or frozen
blueberries (1½ pounds)

Dough

1 cup all-purpose flour

⅓ cup sugar

½ cup walnut pieces

8 tablespoons (1 stick) unsalted
butter, cut into pieces

¼ cup half-and-half

1 cup lightly whipped heavy
cream or sour cream, for serving

You don't need to wait for blueberry season to enjoy
this dessert. Often frozen blueberries cannot replace
fresh—in a soufflé or in a fruit mixture, for example—
because they will "bleed." But cooked as they are
here, with a crumbly dough topping, they work
perfectly well.

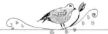

Preheat the oven to 400 degrees.

Prepare the filling: Stir the sugar and cornstarch
together in a bowl. Add the blueberries and toss
gently to mix. Pour into a 6-cup gratin dish (the
mixture should be about 1 inch deep).

Prepare the dough: Place the flour, sugar, and nuts in
a food processor and process for 15 to 20 seconds.
Add the butter and process for 5 seconds. Add the
half-and-half and process for another 5 seconds, or
just until the mixture holds together.

Crumble the dough evenly over the berries. Bake
for 45 minutes, or until the crisp is nicely browned
on top. Serve warm, with whipped cream or sour
cream.

▷ **The dough topping for this crisp is quickly
made in a food processor.**

At the end of the summer, Damson plums—the oval variety sometimes called prune plums or Italian plums—are available at my market. They are excellent poached and make an elegant dessert. Prepared ahead, the poached plums will keep in the refrigerator for about a week. I like to serve them garnished with a spoonful of sour cream and a slice of pound cake. Black currant syrup, *cassis* in French, is the classic syrup of Burgundy to make kir, the white wine drink. If it is unavailable, grenadine can be substituted.

Place the plums, preserves, and syrup in a stainless steel saucepan, stir gently, and bring to a boil. Cover, lower the heat, and boil gently until the plums are tender, 7 to 8 minutes, depending on the ripeness of the fruit. Set aside, covered, to cool in the poaching liquid.

When you are ready to serve, trim the pound cake, cut it into ½-inch-thick slices, and cut each slice in half to form 2 triangles. Arrange about 6 plums, with some of the poaching liquid, in each dessert dish and top with a large spoonful of sour cream. Serve garnished with the pound cake triangles.

▷ **Refrigerated in their poaching liquid, these plums will keep for about a week.**

DAMSON PLUMS IN BLACK CURRANT SYRUP

∘ SERVES 4

1½ pounds damson plums (about 24)

One 12-ounce jar cherry preserves

½ cup black currant syrup (cassis)

1 store-bought pound cake (8 to 10 ounces)

1 cup sour cream

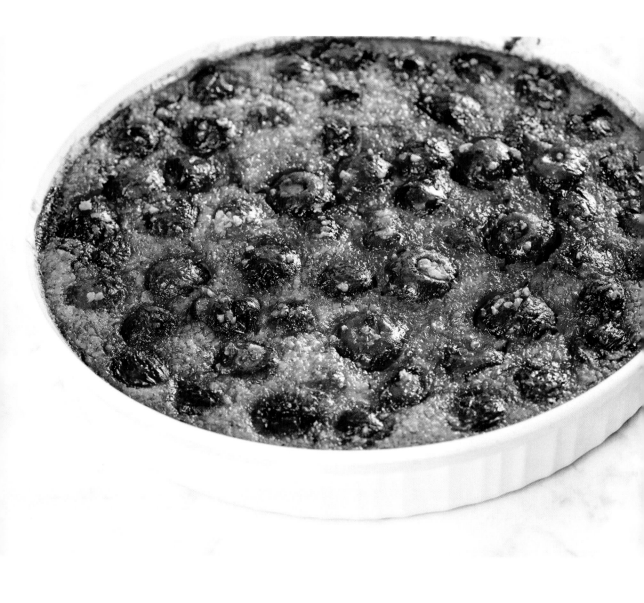

A clafoutis is a French country dessert in which cherries are cooked in a batter of milk, eggs, and flour. In this version, I add almonds and rum for a nice flavor combination. A scoop of vanilla or coffee ice cream is good with this. A frangipane is a mixture often made with almond paste, butter, and eggs. In my recipe I use almonds and sugar to replace the almond paste.

Preheat the oven to 375 degrees. Place the cherries in a gratin dish or porcelain pie dish (suitable for serving) that is about 1½ inches deep and 10 inches in diameter. Add the preserves, mix, and set aside.

Prepare the frangipane: Place the almonds, granulated sugar, and cornstarch in a food processor and process to a powder. Add the melted butter, eggs, and rum and process for a few seconds, until well mixed.

Pour the frangipane mixture over the cherries and mix gently. Set the dish on a cookie sheet and bake for 40 minutes, or until the top is browned and the custard is cooked through. Allow the clafoutis to cool to lukewarm.

Dust with confectioners' sugar if desired, and serve.

NOTE: Either sweet or tart cherries can be used in this classic French dessert.

CLAFOUTIS OF CHERRIES AMANDINE

◦ SERVES 6 TO 8

One 20-ounce bag frozen pitted cherries, or about 1½ pounds fresh cherries, pitted (see Note)

⅔ cup cherry preserves

Frangipane

1 cup unskinned almonds

½ cup granulated sugar

1 tablespoon cornstarch

2 tablespoons unsalted butter, melted

2 large eggs

2 tablespoons dark rum

Confectioners' sugar, for dusting (optional)

GATEAU CLAUDINE

∘ SERVES 6

1 cup heavy cream

One 3½-ounce package instant vanilla pudding

1 cup milk

1 round sponge cake (8 ounces), about 7 inches in diameter and 1½ inches thick

¼ cup apricot preserves (warm to make spreadable)

This is a cake I've made many times for my daughter, Claudine. Even though I often make fancy multilayered cakes and decorate them elaborately with rich buttercream frostings, Claudine likes this one, which is frosted with a mixture of instant vanilla pudding and whipped cream.

The cake can be one you make yourself or a store-bought sponge cake. Decorate it as elaborately as you like; there is ample vanilla cream to fill the middle and cover the outside of the cake, with enough left over to pipe on some additional decorations from a pastry bag fitted with a star tip. Candied fruit or violets also make an attractive, festive addition.

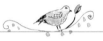

Whip the cream until it holds a peak but is still soft. Set aside.

Mix the instant pudding with the milk in a bowl according to the instructions on the box (using only half the milk called for on the box) until combined. As soon as it's combined, before it has a chance to start to set, fold in the whipped cream. Set the frosting aside. It will set and be ready to use within 15 minutes.

Cut the cake horizontally in half and place one of the halves on a serving plate. Spread the preserves over it and cover the preserves with a layer of the frosting. Place the second cake layer on top and cover the top and sides with frosting. If desired, spoon any remaining frosting into a pastry bag fitted with a star tip and add decorative touches to the cake.

Cut the cake into wedges and serve.

Instead of preparing a custard cream from scratch and combining it with gelatin to make a traditional Bavarian cream, I use vanilla ice cream and instant vanilla pudding to make this delicious dessert in only 30 minutes.

The dessert is particularly attractive when served in glass bowls or martini glasses. It is garnished with thinly sliced oranges sprinkled with orange liqueur. Serve with pound cake, sponge cake, or plain cookies, if you like.

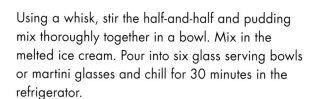

Using a whisk, stir the half-and-half and pudding mix thoroughly together in a bowl. Mix in the melted ice cream. Pour into six glass serving bowls or martini glasses and chill for 30 minutes in the refrigerator.

Meanwhile, peel the orange with a sharp knife, completely removing the peel and all the cottony white pith underneath. Then cut between the membranes to remove the orange wedges. Cut into 1-inch pieces.

Just before serving, arrange the orange pieces on top of the Bavarian cream. Sprinkle with the liqueur and serve immediately.

> **This rich, festive dessert is ready in just 30 minutes.**

ORANGE BAVARIAN CREAM

○ SERVES 6

1 cup half-and-half

One 3½-ounce package instant vanilla pudding

1 pint best-quality vanilla ice cream, melted

1 large seedless orange

2 tablespoons Cointreau, Grand Marnier, or mandarin orange liqueur

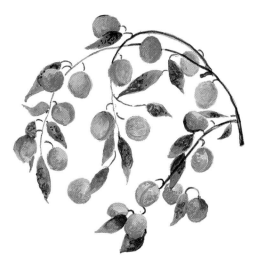

ORANGE CAKE WITH GRAND MARNIER SAUCE

◦ SERVES 6

1 round sponge cake (8 ounces), about 7 inches in diameter and 1½ inches thick

Suzette Butter

4 tablespoons (½ stick) unsalted butter, softened

1½ teaspoons grated orange rind

2 tablespoons orange juice

1 tablespoon confectioners' sugar

3 tablespoons orange juice

Sauce

1 cup sour cream

1 tablespoon Grand Marnier

1 tablespoon confectioners' sugar

Garnish

1 large seedless orange

I use a prepared sponge cake from the supermarket for this recipe, but you can bake your own. The Suzette butter, which I also use in the Gratin of Crepes Suzette (page 346), makes an easy and flavorful buttercream. The cake is served with a Grand Marnier sauce and garnished with thin slices of orange. I don't use much sugar in the Suzette butter or in the sauce, because commercial cakes are quite sweet.

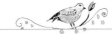

Split the cake horizontally into 2 layers. Place one layer on a serving plate.

Prepare the Suzette butter: Place the butter in a food processor and add the orange rind, orange juice, and confectioners' sugar. Process until combined. (At first the mixture may not blend; keep processing until the butter absorbs the juice.)

Spread the Suzette butter over the top of the first cake layer and place the other cake layer on top. Sprinkle it with the 3 tablespoons orange juice. (At this point, the cake can be wrapped in plastic wrap and stored in the refrigerator for up to 24 hours.)

Prepare the sauce: Mix the sour cream, Grand Marnier, and confectioners' sugar in a small bowl. Set aside.

Completely remove the skin from the orange, including the cottony white pith underneath, and cut the orange into slices.

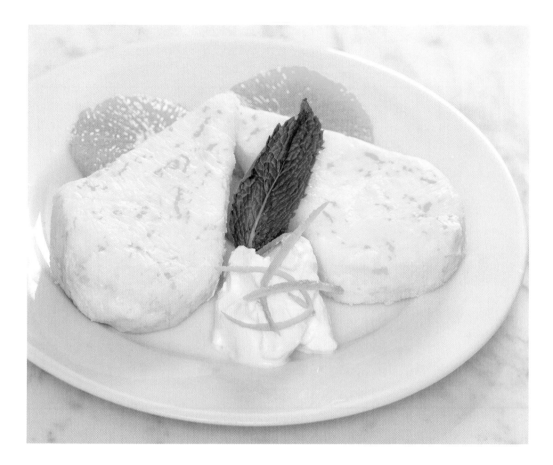

At serving time, cut the cake into 12 thin wedges. Place a spoonful of sauce on each dessert plate, arrange 2 small wedges of cake on the sauce, and top with an orange slice. Serve immediately.

> **You can prepare the cake ahead of time and then make the sauce in just a few minutes before serving.**

GRAPEFRUIT AND STRAWBERRIES WITH DRIED FRUIT

◦ SERVES 6 TO 8

2½ cups mixed dried fruits (pears, apricots, cherries, peaches, prunes, raisins, and/or currants)

1 large lemon

1 large lime

⅓ cup honey

2 tablespoons dark rum

2 red grapefruits

¼ cup Grand Marnier

2 cups strawberries

Store-bought pound cake, for serving

The dried fruits for this refreshing dessert can be mixed several days ahead, and the oranges prepared up to a day ahead.

Prepare the dried fruit mixture (do this ahead of time so it can macerate): If any of the fruit is extremely dry, as dried pears and peaches sometimes are, cover with boiling water and set aside for 5 to 10 minutes to soften, then drain. Cut all the dried fruit into ¼-inch pieces and place in a plastic bag.

Using a Microplane, remove about 1½ tablespoons of the rind from the lemon and lime.

Juice the lemon and lime (you should have approximately ⅓ cup combined juices). Add the juice, the lemon and lime rinds, the honey, and rum to the bag with the dried fruit and mix thoroughly. Tightly seal the plastic bag and set it aside in a cool place for at least 2 hours or up to 2 weeks. (The close confinement of the fruit and liquid facilitates the maceration process.)

Trim the grapefruits slightly at the base and top and remove the skin and white pith. Cut the grapefruit into ½-inch-thick slices. If the centers of the slices are seedy or tough, remove them with a serrated knife and discard.

Place the grapefruit slices in a gratin dish and pour the Grand Marnier over them. Cover with plastic wrap and set aside for up to 1 day.

Shortly before serving, clean the strawberries, cut them into ¼- to ½-inch-thick wedges, and refrigerate until ready to serve.

At serving time, arrange a slice of grapefruit, with some of the liquid from the dish, on each dessert plate. Cover the grapefruit with the medley of dried fruit and sprinkle with the cut-up strawberries. Serve with slices of your favorite pound cake.

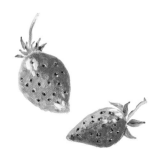

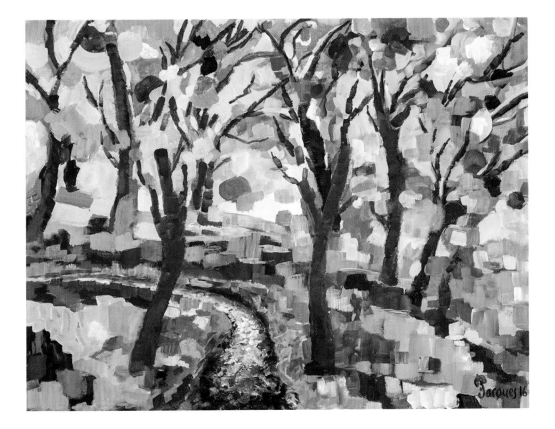

GRATIN OF CREPES SUZETTE

◦ SERVES 2

Crepes

½ cup all-purpose flour

1 large egg

1½ tablespoons unsalted butter, melted

¾ cup milk

½ teaspoon sugar

Pinch of salt

Filling

Suzette Butter (page 342)

½ cup orange marmalade

1 tablespoon sugar

1 or 2 tablespoons Cognac or other brandy

These crepes are large enough that two per person is a generous serving. They can be cooked and even filled ahead, ready to go into the oven for heating at the last moment. I fill them with orange marmalade and the Suzette butter I also use in the Orange Cake with Grand Marnier Sauce (page 342).

The crepe batter is easily made in a food processor. The recipe should yield about ten 8-inch crepes, if you use no more than 2½ tablespoons of batter per crepe. As soon as the batter touches the surface of the hot pan, it will begin to set, so how quickly you shake the pan to spread the batter will determine the thickness of the crepe. It's better to start with too little batter and then add some to the pan if necessary than to start with too much.

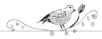

Prepare the crepes: Place all the batter ingredients in a food processor and process for a few seconds, just until the batter is smooth.

Heat a nonstick skillet with an 8-inch base until hot. Place about 2½ tablespoons of the batter in the hot pan and quickly tilt the pan one way and then the other to spread the batter thinly and evenly over the entire bottom of the pan. Cook for about 1 minute over medium to high heat. Then, using a fork, lift up one edge of the crepe, grab it with your other hand, set aside the fork, and turn the crepe over with both hands. Cook for about 30 seconds on the second side, then place on a plate, second side up. Repeat this procedure until all the batter is used, stacking the crepes on the plate as they are removed from the pan.

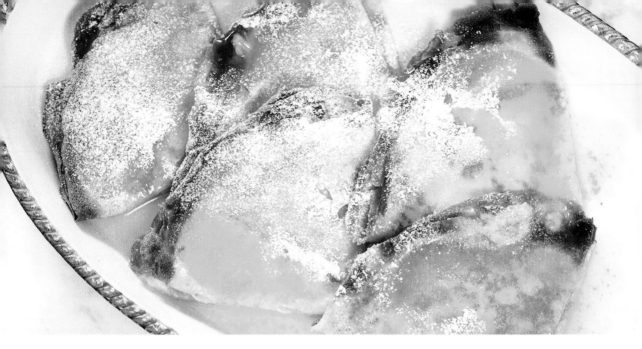

Prepare the filling: Mix the Suzette butter with the orange marmalade in a food processor, or mix by hand with a whisk. The mixture will separate initially but will eventually smooth out as you mix.

Arrange the crepes on a work surface, second (less browned) side up. Dividing it evenly, spread some of the filling on each crepe, then fold the crepes into fourths. Arrange them in a gratin dish, slightly overlapping, so that the folded point of each is visible. (At this point, the crepes can be refrigerated for up to 4 hours.)

At serving time, preheat the broiler. Sprinkle the crepes with the sugar. Place the dish under the broiler, 10 to 12 inches from the heat source, and broil for 7 to 8 minutes, until the crepes are heated through and nicely browned on top. Pour on the Cognac and carefully ignite it with a long match to flambé the crepes. Serve immediately, preferably with the crepes still flaming.

The crepes can be made and even filled ahead, so at serving time they need only to be heated under the broiler.

LEMON CAKE DELICE

○ 6 SERVINGS

1 fresh or frozen pound cake
(10 ounces), preferably all-butter

4 tablespoons (½ stick) unsalted
butter, softened

2 ounces cream cheese, softened

4 tablespoons lemon juice

⅓ cup confectioners' sugar

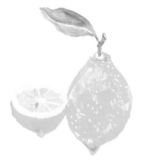

If you like lemon, you'll love this cake, which can be served on its own or in combination with ice cream or fruit. I use a good commercial pound cake and fill and frost it with a buttercream made in a food processor. Serve strong black coffee with the cake.

Trim the cake evenly to remove the brown exterior from the top, sides, and bottom. Slice the cake horizontally into 3 layers.

Combine the butter, cream cheese, 2 tablespoons of the lemon juice, and the confectioners' sugar in a food processor and process until smooth.

Sprinkle the cake layers with the remaining 2 tablespoons lemon juice and fill and frost the cake, coating each layer and the top and sides with the buttercream. Refrigerate for 10 to 15 minutes before slicing and serving.

> **A store-bought pound cake is transformed into company fare with a buttercream made in a food processor.**

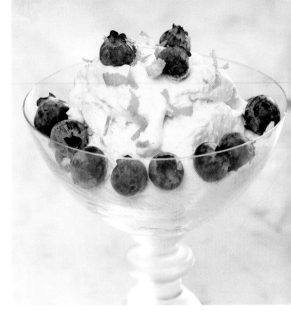

This recipe is amazingly easy to make. I do not remember where I got the idea of using condensed milk, but it may have been from my wife, who always uses condensed milk in her caramel custard, a favorite of our granddaughter, Shorey. (Remove the whole lid from the condensed milk can, rather than just puncturing it, so you can empty it completely using a rubber spatula.)

You can also make this dessert with orange, lemon, or other citrus fruits. The cream should not be beaten until stiff, only to a gentle peak. Overbeating the cream would make the dessert set too hard and give it a slight taste of butter rather than sweet cream.

Using a Microplane, remove 1 rounded tablespoon of rind from the limes. Place in a bowl, then squeeze the limes to get ½ cup of juice. Mix with the rind and add the bourbon.

Whip the cream by hand or with a mixer to a soft peak.

Open the can of condensed milk and add the contents to the lime juice mixture. Mix well with a whisk. Using a rubber spatula, fold in the whipped cream until well combined.

Spoon the mousse into a glass serving bowl or into individual bowls. Let set in the refrigerator for least 1 hour, then serve sprinkled with blueberries.

LIME MOUSSE WITH BLUEBERRIES

∘ SERVES 8

2 to 3 limes (depending on size)

2 tablespoons bourbon

2 cups heavy cream

One 14-ounce can sweetened condensed milk

1 pint blueberries (or other berries), for garnish

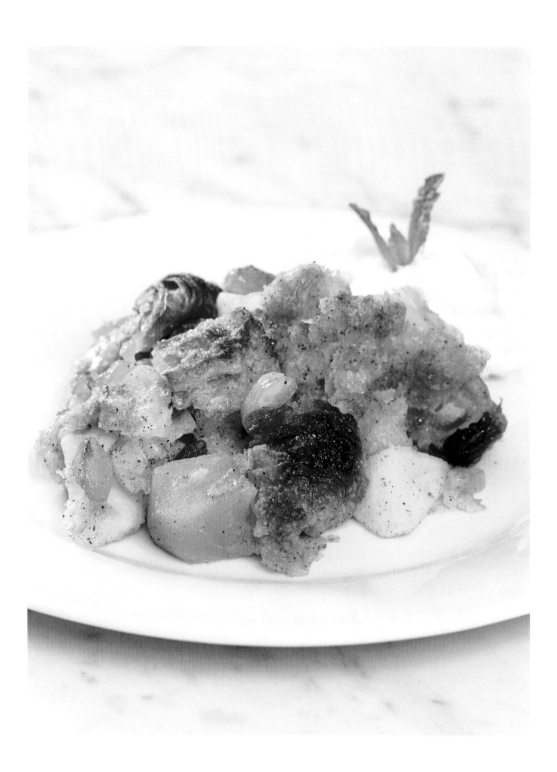

When I was working in restaurants, sometimes I would collect the leftover stale cakes, croissants, Danish pastries, muffins, pound cakes, pies, and cookies from the prior day to make—with great success—desserts like crumbles, brown Betty, bread pudding, and the like.

We always have fruit at our house, everything from bananas to apples, plums, peaches, and pears and after a few days, some of them get a bit overripe or wrinkled. Then it's time to use them in this recipe, which will vary greatly based on what fruit and baked goods you use, but the overall result is pretty consistent. I add preserves to the mix; sugar can be added or the preserves omitted from the recipe, depending on the sweetness lent by the other ingredients. This dessert is excellent with hard sauce, ice cream, whipped cream, or sour cream, as well as on its own.

Preheat the oven to 400 degrees. Mix the pear, apple, and remaining ingredients (except the garnishes) in a bowl until well combined. Spoon into a 6-cup gratin dish and place on a cookie sheet.

Bake for 45 to 60 minutes, until the fruits are very soft and the top is well browned. Serve warm, with crème fraîche and mint sprigs.

PEAR-APPLE GRATIN GLORIA

∘ SERVES 6

1 pear (about 10 ounces), peeled, halved, cored, and cut into 1-inch pieces (about 2 cups)

1 apple (about 10 ounces), peeled, cored, and cut into 1-inch pieces (about 2 cups)

About 8 ounces baked goods, such as a mix of croissants, Danish pastry, pound cake, muffins, pies, cookies, scones, and/or bread cut or broken into 1-inch pieces (about 3 cups)

4 tablespoons (½ stick) unsalted butter, melted

⅓ cup cherry or apricot preserves

⅓ cup golden raisins

¾ cup apple or orange juice

1 teaspoon ground cinnamon

Garnish

1 cup crème fraîche or sour cream

A few sprigs of mint, for garnish

BARTLETT PEARS IN PUFF PASTRY

◦ SERVES 6

6 tablespoons sugar

¾ teaspoon ground cinnamon

3 large ripe Bartlett pears
(about 8 ounces each)

3 tablespoons lemon juice

1 sheet frozen puff pastry
(about 8 ounces; ½ package),
partially defrosted

2 tablespoons unsalted butter,
softened

⅓ cup water

Crème fraîche or sour cream,
for serving (optional)

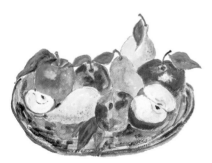

For this easy dessert, I cover pear halves with frozen puff pastry and serve them right in the gratin dish in which they are baked. You can use apples instead of pears, if you prefer.

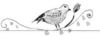

Preheat the oven to 375 degrees. Mix the sugar and cinnamon together and set aside.

Peel the pears and cut them lengthwise in half. Remove the core from each half and arrange the pear halves cut side down in one layer in a gratin dish. Sprinkle with the lemon juice and half the cinnamon-sugar mixture.

Unfold the sheet of puff pastry and cut it apart at the seams to get 3 pieces approximately 10 inches by 3 inches. Cut each of these crosswise in half to create 6 pieces. Lay a pastry piece on top of each pear half, and as the pastry starts to defrost a little more and relax slightly, press the pieces gently around the pears so they take on the shape of the pear halves. Spread the butter on the pastry and sprinkle the remaining cinnamon-sugar mixture on top.

Place the gratin dish on a cookie sheet and bake for about 30 minutes, until the pastry is browning nicely and the juices around the pears are bubbling and caramelized.

Pour the water around the pears and return them to the oven for 5 minutes. The water will melt the caramel and create a sauce. Serve the pears warm, with crème fraîche or sour cream, if desired.

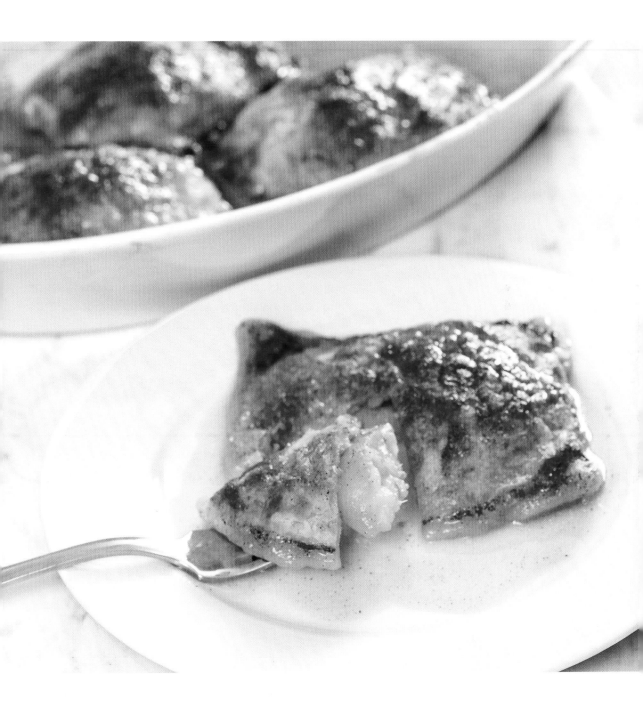

PEARS WITH CREAM CHEESE AND DRIED FRUIT

○ SERVES 6

4 ripe Anjou or Bartlett pears
(about 9 ounces each)

2 tablespoons lemon juice

Cream Cheese Balls

⅓ cup hazelnuts, crushed

One 8-ounce package cream
cheese, softened

1¼ cups mixed dried fruit
(apricots, cherries, raisins, and/or
pears), cut into ¼-inch dice

6 sprigs of mint, for garnish

This is an easy fall or winter dessert. The cheese balls can be made ahead. I mix different types of nuts and dried fruits into regular cream cheese and form it into balls. You might like to serve cookies alongside.

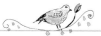

Preheat the oven to 400 degrees. Peel the pears, cut them in half, and remove the cores. Cut each half into 3 wedges. Roll them in the lemon juice and set aside.

Prepare the cream cheese balls: Spread the nuts out on a cookie sheet lined with nonstick aluminum foil and toast in the oven for 6 to 8 minutes. Let cool.

Mix the cream cheese, hazelnuts, and dried fruit in a bowl. Using a spoon or dampened hands, form the mixture into 6 balls.

At serving time, place one cream cheese ball in the center of each dessert plate and surround with 4 pear wedges. Place a sprig of mint in each ball and serve.

▷ **Make the cream cheese balls ahead for this cool-weather dessert.**

I make this dessert with frozen pineapple juice concentrate, which is a natural, pure reduction of juices, usually without added sweeteners. Soaking the ladyfingers in rum not only flavors them, but also prevents them from freezing in the dessert.

Break the ladyfingers into 1½- to 2-inch pieces into a glass serving bowl or soufflé mold. Mix the rum and water and sprinkle on the ladyfingers. Set aside.

Whip the cream until firm with an electric mixer or a whisk. When the pineapple concentrate is defrosted enough to be incorporated into the cream, place it in a bowl and add the whipped cream. Fold in gently with a rubber spatula until combined. Pour the mixture over the ladyfingers, mix lightly, cover, and place in the freezer for at least 3 hours.

Serve directly from the freezer, spooning the parfait into goblets or brandy snifters. Garnish with mint sprigs.

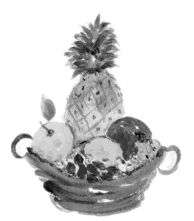

FROZEN PINEAPPLE PARFAIT

∘ SERVES 6

12 small packaged ladyfingers (about 1½ ounces each)

3 tablespoons dark rum

3 tablespoons water

1½ cups heavy cream

½ cup frozen pure pineapple juice concentrate, partially thawed

6 sprigs of mint, for garnish

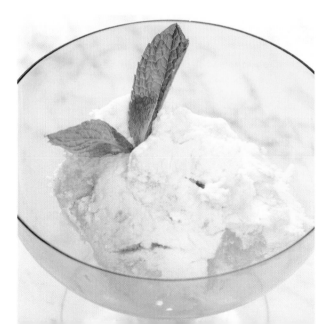

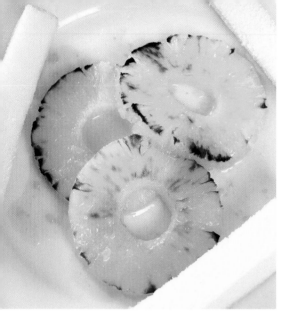

There is both a warm version and a cold version of this recipe here: In the warm version, sugared slices of pineapple are broiled and served warm with kirsch spooned over them and pound cake alongside. In the cold version, the pineapple is cut into chunks, marinated in a mixture of sugar and kirsch, and served chilled with a dollop of sour cream and a slice of pound cake.

A ripe fresh pineapple is the best choice for this recipe, but if that is unavailable, canned pineapple slices will do nicely. The kirsch, which is a cherry brandy, can be replaced with dark rum or Cognac for a different flavor.

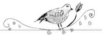

PINEAPPLE WITH KIRSCH

◦ SERVES 6

6 slices fresh pineapple (about ¾ inch thick each), core removed, or 6 slices canned pineapple, drained

3 tablespoons sugar

2 tablespoons kirsch

Sour cream or crème fraîche, for the cold version (optional)

Store-bought pound cake, for serving

For the warm pineapple: Preheat the broiler. Sprinkle the pineapple slices with the sugar and arrange them on a cookie sheet lined with nonstick aluminum foil. Place under the broiler, about 4 inches from the heat source, and broil for about 8 minutes, until the slices are sizzling on top. Arrange a slice on each dessert plate, sprinkle with the kirsch, and serve immediately, with slices of pound cake.

For the cold pineapple: Cut the pineapple slices into 1-inch chunks and mix them with the sugar and kirsch in a bowl. Refrigerate for a few hours to macerate and chill.

Serve the pineapple with sour cream, if desired, and slices of pound cake.

NOTE: If using fresh pineapple, remove the core from each slice with a sharp knife or a small round cookie cutter.

This tart is made with a store-bought frozen pie shell and IQF (Individually Quick Frozen) berries, but you can, of course, make your own pie shell and use fresh raspberries. This sweet-but-tart dessert is very good served with crème fraîche or Greek yogurt.

RASPBERRY TART

Preheat the oven to 400 degrees. Mix the berries, cornstarch, preserves, and sugar in a bowl. Pour into the frozen pie shell, place the shell on a cookie sheet and bake for 50 to 60 minutes, until the crust is nicely browned and the filling is bubbling. Set aside to cool for at least 1 hour before serving.

To serve, cut into wedges and top with the crème fraîche.

One 16-ounce bag frozen unsweetened raspberries

2 tablespoons cornstarch

One 12-ounce jar seedless raspberry preserves

2 tablespoons sugar

One 9-inch frozen pie shell

1 cup crème fraîche or Greek yogurt, for serving

NOTE: The filling will be a little runny, but I find it much more flavorful this way than if a greater amount of cornstarch were added to make it thicker.

▷ **The raspberry preserves help to sweeten and intensify the flavor of this filling.**

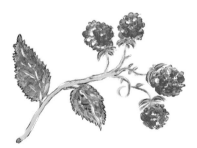

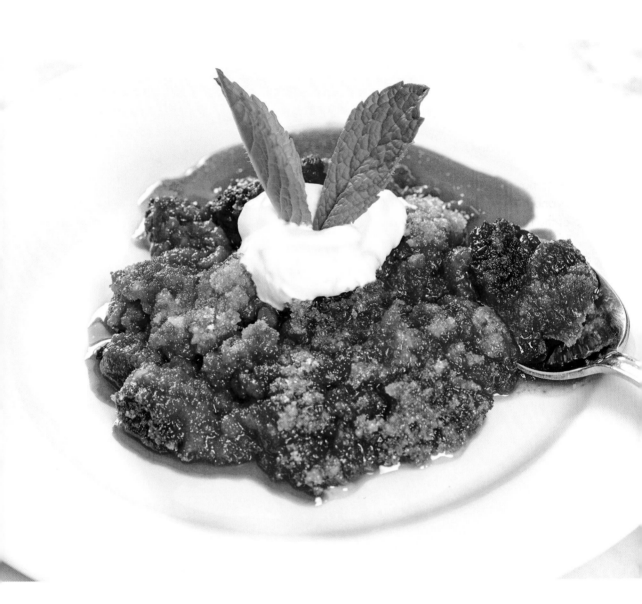

This tasty dessert can be made with fresh berries or IQF (Individually Quick Frozen) berries. I always have a few packages of frozen unsweetened berries in my freezer. Serve the gratin warm, with crème fraîche or sour cream.

RASPBERRY GRATIN

○ SERVES 6

Preheat the oven to 375 degrees. Place the berries in a 5-cup gratin dish.

Place the pastry pieces in a bowl. Add the melted butter and brown sugar and mix well. Sprinkle on top of the berries.

Bake for about 25 minutes, until the gratin is nicely browned on top. Serve warm, with crème fraîche.

> **Keep a supply of IQF (Individually Quick Frozen) berries in your freezer for use in fruit desserts.**

One 16-ounce bag frozen unsweetened raspberries, or 1 pint fresh raspberries

3 croissants or Danish pastries, or leftover cake, cut into ½-inch pieces (2 cups)

3 tablespoons unsalted butter, melted

½ cup packed light brown sugar

Crème fraîche or sour cream, for serving

STRAWBERRIES IN PEKOE TEA

∘ SERVES 4

1 orange pekoe tea bag
(or another tea to your liking,
from oolong to peppermint)

½ cup boiling water

½ cup apricot preserves

1 pint strawberries, cleaned
and hulled

Sour cream or whipped heavy
cream for garnish (optional)

4 sprigs mint or Thai basil,
for garnish (optional)

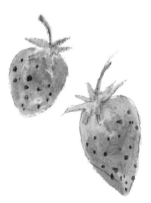

This unusual, refreshing dessert is best made in summer, when strawberries are at their peak. Flavored with tea and apricot preserves, the berries can be served at room temperature or cold, plain or garnished with a little sour cream or whipped cream.

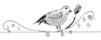

Put the tea bag in a medium bowl. Pour the boiling water over the tea bag and allow to steep, covered, for 5 minutes.

Remove the tea bag and stir the apricot preserves and strawberries into the tea. Set aside to macerate at room temperature for at least 1 hour or as long as overnight in the refrigerator.

Serve the strawberries in glasses as is or garnished with sour cream and topped with the mint sprigs.

> **Use only ripe, flavorful strawberries in this quick dessert.**

I especially like to make this dessert when tiny Black Mission figs appear at the market in midsummer. You can use larger figs too—but whatever variety you select, the figs must be ripe. However, if they are so ripe that their skin is splitting, reduce the cooking time as necessary to prevent them from falling apart.

Made in only a few minutes, this delightful dessert will keep and develop flavor in the refrigerator for at least a week. The juice of the figs turns it bright red, and the Campari gives it a slightly bitter, spicy taste. (If you are not fond of Campari, replace it with vermouth or eliminate it altogether.)

POACHED FRESH FIGS WITH CAMPARI

∘ SERVES 4

1 cup fruity white wine

⅓ cup sugar

¼ cup lime juice

1 pound small ripe Black Mission figs (about 20) or larger figs

2 teaspoons cornstarch, dissolved in 2 tablespoons water

2 tablespoons Campari

1 cup sour cream, for serving

Slices of pound cake or cookies, for serving (optional)

Combine the wine, sugar, and lime juice in a saucepan (preferably stainless steel) and bring to a boil. Add the figs, cover, and boil gently for 4 to 5 minutes, until the figs are tender when touched with a knife but not bursting open and falling apart. Using a slotted spoon, transfer the figs to a bowl.

There should be about 1 cup liquid in the saucepan; if there is more, boil it down to 1 cup. Add the dissolved cornstarch, stir, and bring to a boil. Pour the sauce over the figs and allow to cool to room temperature, then stir in the Campari.

Spoon 4 or 5 figs (or 2 or 3 larger figs) into individual deep dessert dishes. Spoon some sauce over the figs, place a dollop of sour cream in the center, and serve with a slice of pound cake (or a cookie), if desired.

CRUMBLED-COOKIE COFFEE ICE CREAM

◦ SERVES 4

4 ounces cookies

¼ cup golden raisins

2 tablespoons Cognac
or Armagnac

¼ cup orange juice

1 pint best-quality coffee
ice cream, for serving

Crumbled store-bought cookies form the base for this coffee ice cream dessert. I use all-butter cookies, but any of your favorite cookie will work. This dessert looks especially attractive served in small goblets or glass dessert bowls.

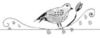

Coarsely crumble the cookies into a bowl. Add the raisins, Cognac, and orange juice, toss lightly to mix, and set aside.

At serving time, arrange a layer of the cookie mixture in the bottom of each of four goblets or glass dessert dishes and top each with a scoop of the ice cream.

▷ **You can create a special dessert with store-bought cookies and ice cream.**

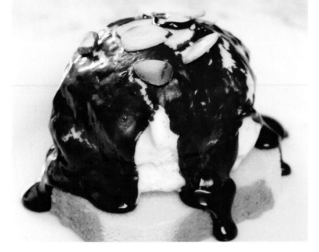

VANILLA ICE CREAM WITH CHOCOLATE SAUCE

◦ SERVES 4

This elegant dessert consists of vanilla ice cream served with a sauce made with melted chocolate and light cream. The vanilla ice cream is scooped directly out of its container and formed into small balls, then kept in the freezer.

¼ cup sliced almonds

1 pint best-quality vanilla ice cream

8 ounces bittersweet chocolate, broken into pieces

1 cup light cream

4 slices store-bought pound cake (½ inch thick)

Preheat the oven to 400 degrees. Spread the almonds on a cookie sheet lined with nonstick aluminum foil and toast in the oven until nicely browned. Set aside.

To make the ice cream balls, remove the ice cream from its container and cut it into 4 pieces. Place each one on a sheet of plastic wrap and wrap tightly, molding the ice cream into balls. Place in the freezer until serving time.

Place the cream in the microwave for 2 minutes, till very hot. Add the chocolate, stirring frequently, until the chocolate is melted; stir to combine.

At serving time, place a slice of pound cake on each dessert dish and set an ice cream ball on each piece of cake. Coat with the chocolate sauce and top with the toasted almonds. Serve immediately.

CHOCOLATE ROCHERS WITH NUTS IN VANILLA SAUCE

◦ SERVES 4

½ cup hazelnuts

½ pint best-quality chocolate ice cream

Sauce
___

½ cup crème fraîche

2 tablespoons milk

1 tablespoon sugar

½ teaspoon pure vanilla extract

Half a store-bought pound cake, for serving

Served with a creamy vanilla sauce and pieces of pound cake, this is a luxurious dessert.

Preheat the oven to 400 degrees. Spread the hazelnuts on a cookie sheet and toast them in the oven for 10 to 12 minutes, until lightly browned. Set the nuts aside until they are cool enough to handle. Rub the nuts in a paper towel to remove most of the skin, then crush them by hand or with a mortar and pestle until coarsely chopped.

Divide the ice cream into 4 equal pieces, place each one on a piece of plastic wrap, and wrap tightly, molding the ice cream into balls. Working quickly so the ice cream doesn't melt, roll the balls in the chopped nuts and return the balls to the freezer.

Prepare the sauce: Mix together the crème fraîche, milk, sugar, and vanilla in a bowl. Set aside.

Trim the pound cake and cut it into ½-inch-thick slices. Stack the slices and cut them into sticks, or "fingers," approximately 4 inches long and 1 inch wide.

At serving time, divide the vanilla sauce among four plates and position an ice cream ball in the center of each. Serve with the pound cake fingers.

> **Cut the ice cream with a sharp knife to divide it equally for shaping into balls.**

This is a variation on the famous drink Velvet Hammer often made with cream, rum, and Kahlúa. In my recipe I use ice cream, dark rum, and coffee liqueur. It works well with vanilla ice cream to produce a smooth, rich, rewarding taste.

VELVET HAMMER

∘ SERVES 4

Spoon the ice cream into a food processor and add the Kahlúa and rum. Process until well blended (the ice cream will become quite soft). Transfer the mixture to the original ice cream container or to a bowl, cover, and place in the freezer for 3 to 4 hours, until firm. (The liqueur and rum will prevent the ice cream from becoming too hard.)

To serve, spoon the ice cream into brandy snifters or dessert dishes and garnish with the coffee beans.

▷ **Assemble this quickly in a food processor and firm it up in the freezer.**

1 pint best-quality vanilla ice cream

2 tablespoons Kahlúa or other coffee-flavored liqueur

2 tablespoons dark rum

1 tablespoon whole coffee beans or chocolate-covered coffee beans, for garnish

INSTANT CHOCOLATE MOUSSE

° SERVES 4

1 cup heavy cream

¾ cup half-and-half

8 ounces bittersweet chocolate, broken or cut into ½-inch pieces

1 tablespoon Grand Marnier or other orange liqueur

A 1-ounce piece bittersweet or semisweet chocolate, for shaving

½ cup fresh raspberries, for garnish

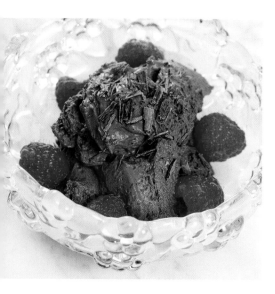

This is the fastest-possible way to make chocolate mousse. It is simply a mixture of melted chocolate and whipped cream flavored with a little Grand Marnier, which complements the flavor of the chocolate well.

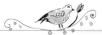

Whip the cream with an electric mixer or with a whisk until it holds a peak but is not too firm. Refrigerate.

Heat the half-and-half in a small saucepan until hot. Remove the pan from the heat, add the chocolate pieces, and stir gently with a whisk until the chocolate has melted and the mixture is smooth. Add the Grand Marnier and mix well. Cool to room temperature, testing by dipping your finger into the mixture periodically. Transfer it to a bowl.

Add all the whipped cream to the melted chocolate in one stroke and fold together with a large rubber spatula to incorporate it well. Cover and refrigerate for about 2 hours to set before serving.

To serve, spoon the mousse into glass dessert bowls or goblets. For the garnish, run the blade of a vegetable peeler along the edge of the 1-ounce piece of chocolate, letting the shavings drop directly onto the mousse. Garnish with the raspberries and serve.

> **To create this smooth, rich mousse, you just fold whipped cream into a chocolate sauce.**

These cinnamon sticks, like the savory Cheese Sticks on page 102, are made with packaged puff pastry. Each package contains two 10-inch-square sheets, each weighing about 8 ounces. The sheets are usually folded on themselves; allow the pastry to defrost just enough so that it can be unfolded. It is easier to handle, to cut, and to arrange on the cookie sheet while it is still slightly frozen, before it softens and becomes sticky.

Serve these on their own or with your favorite fruit or ice cream dessert. Store any leftovers in an airtight container in the freezer.

CINNAMON-SUGAR STICKS

○ MAKES ABOUT 20 STICKS

1 sheet frozen puff pastry
(8 ounces; ½ package)

2 tablespoons unsalted butter, softened

⅓ cup sugar

2 teaspoons ground cinnamon

Preheat the oven to 375 degrees. Place the frozen dough on a cookie sheet. After 15 to 20 minutes, while it's still partially frozen, unfold the dough (it will tend to crack at the seam) and rub the surface with half the butter. Mix the sugar and cinnamon together and spread half on the surface of the pastry, pushing it into the butter. Turn the dough over and repeat the procedure with the remaining butter and cinnamon-sugar mixture. Cut the square into 20 strips, each approximately ½ inch wide and 10 inches long.

Arrange the strips about 1 inch apart on a cookie sheet lined with nonstick aluminum foil. Bake for about 15 minutes, until the pastry is dark brown. Because the sugar on the underside of the pastry will have melted and caramelized, you need to transfer the sticks to a wire rack while they are still hot; if they are allowed to cool, the sugar will stick and the pastry will be difficult to remove from the cookie sheet. Let cool.

> **Work with puff pastry dough while it is still partially frozen. As it thaws, it becomes sticky, making it harder to handle.**

Index

Note: Page references in *italics* indicate photographs.

While the world is familiar with Jacques as a world-renowned chef, television personality, and culinary instructor, there are two additional facets to his life that are equally as impressive and important.

Founded in 2016 by Claudine Pépin and her husband, Rollie Wesen, The Jacques Pépin Foundation supports community kitchens that offer free life skills and culinary training to adults with high barriers to employment, including previous incarceration, homelessness, substance abuse issues, low skill and education attainment, and lack of work history. As Jacques has said, "We are all equal in the eyes of the stove." Through the important work done by the Foundation that bears his name, his belief is put into practice, changing lives through culinary education. For more information, please visit **jp.foundation**.

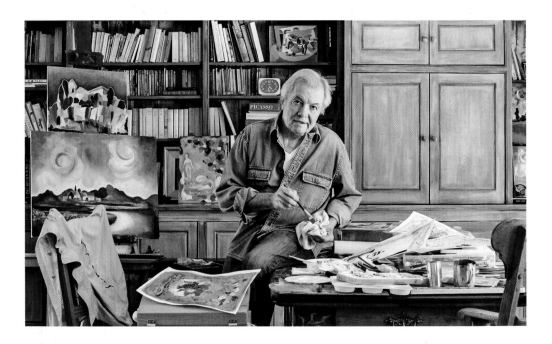

THE
ARTISTRY OF
JACQUES PEPIN

Jacques' passion and creativity are not limited to the kitchen. He has been painting for much of his life, and his works are lively, varied, and inspiring. While cooking is his "métier," his life's work, painting is something he does just for fun. That enjoyment comes across in all of his pieces. To learn more, please visit **jacquespepinart.com**.

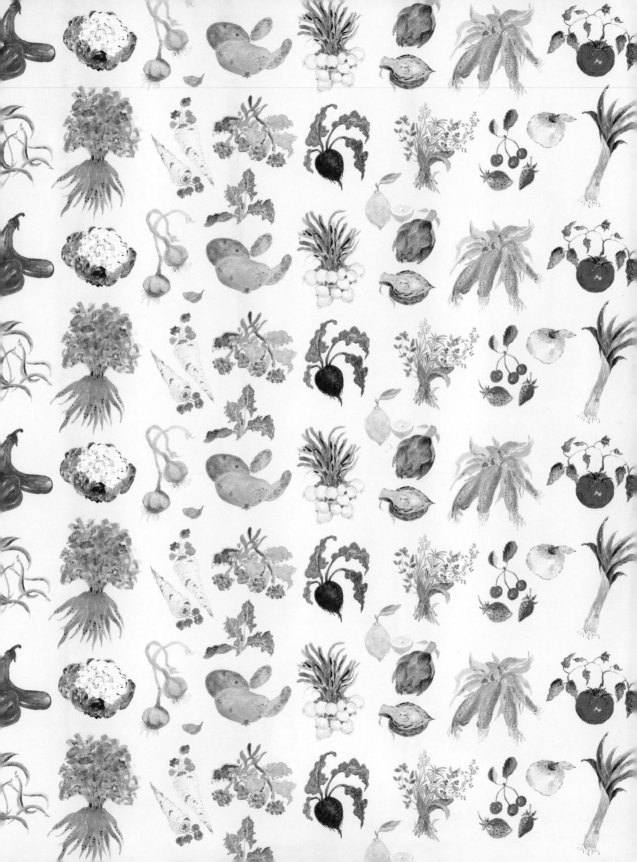

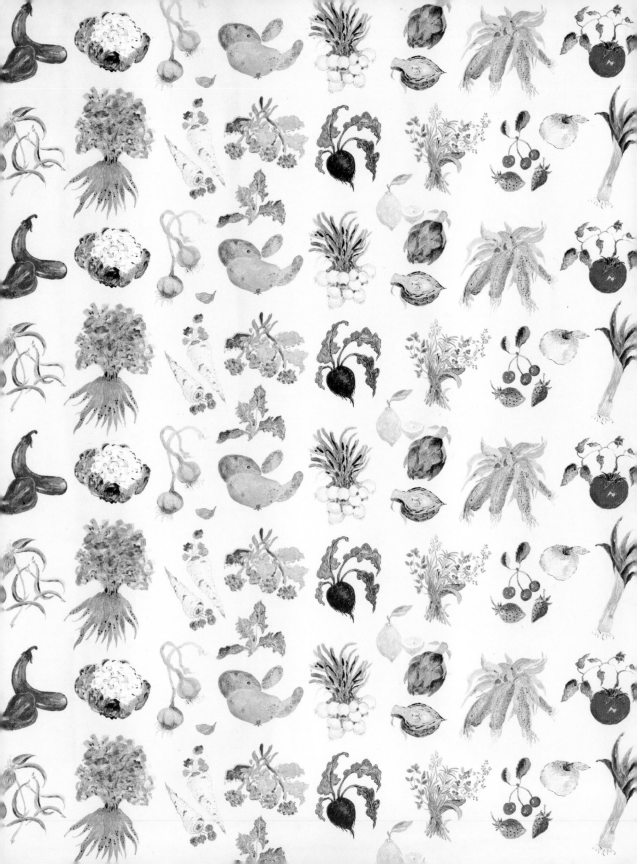